"Recent, global events highlight the vitality of mental healthcare to individual and collective well-being. The impact of these events on education, training, and delivery models of care has been tectonic. It has created gaps in healthcare delivery and exposed significant gaps in provider training. 'Necessity is the mother of invention'. It is the impetus for significant workforce development trends in family therapy training. Seminal texts (first order) that focus on systems theory and family therapy models often sacrifice application for overview. This critique has birthed additional family therapy clinical texts (second order) over time, that focus more on application, but none have managed to integrate systems theory and family therapy models in a comprehensive, applied way. *Foundational Concepts and Models of Family Therapy: An Introduction for Online Learning* achieves the Goldilocks Principle; it's just right. It's comprehensive, integrated, and applied. The editors and authors are to be commended, as this is a difficult feat, particularly when the application is for the online learning environment. Online healthcare education, training, and delivery is the future, and the demand is predicted to grow. The text represents the third order change the field of family therapy needs as educators and training programs continue to ramp up to outcome-based, data-driven healthcare education that is vital in the 21st century."

Christian Jordal, PhD, *Chair, Counseling and Family Therapy Department, Drexel University, Former Editor,* Journal of Family Psychotherapy.

"This book offers an amazing collection of helpful chapters which were written by seasoned MFT educators, teaching in an online environment. Readers are exposed to a strong introduction to systemic ways of thinking and practice and to a number of key MFT models of therapy. The book is written in a way that readers can engage with the ideas in an interactive way and it has a strong application component. This book is uniquely helpful for those learning MFT in an online environment."

Dale E. Bertram, PhD, *Professor of MFT, Campbellsville University Louisville.*

"Systems thinking and practice in family therapy has proven to advance the understanding and connection of relationships. Exploring the theories identified in this book has pulled together the most important ways to utilize and practice MFT. Therapists from a variety of underpinnings can involve themselves in broadening the scope of application to our larger population. Thank you for such a thorough comprehensive computation for the MFT field."

Tommie V. Boyd, PhD, LMFT.

Foundational Concepts and Models of Family Therapy

This textbook aims to introduce students to the foundational concepts of the marriage and family therapy field, providing a comprehensive overview of a range of models and their practical application.

Designed specifically for distance-learning, Yulia Watters and Darren Adamson bring together a collection of experienced marriage and family therapists to teach the absolute essentials of marriage and family therapy without peripheral or incidental information. Iterative in its presentation, the book introduces important systems concepts, provides a compelling history of family therapy, presents detailed exploration of classical and post-modern approaches to therapy, and covers clinical application and treatment planning. It uniquely follows the course structure of the first institution to receive Commission on Accreditation for Marriage and Family Therapy Education (COAMFTE) accreditation for both master's and doctoral online programs, giving students the fundamental knowledge they need to help them prepare for their licensing examination and subsequent practice as MFTs.

Written for students seeking to be MFT practitioners, this important volume adds a fresh perspective to teaching and application of family therapy.

Dr. Watters is a licensed Marriage and Family Therapist in FL and DE and has been the Director of Curriculum Development and Professor at Northcentral and then National University since 2012. She holds a PhD in MFT from Nova Southeastern University and a master's degree in Instructional Design from Northcentral University.

Dr. Adamson is a licensed MFT and has been a practicing Marriage and Family Therapist since 1987 and a Professor since 1989. He has been with Northcentral and then National University since 2010, currently serving as the Associate Dean for the Division of Social and Behavioral Sciences. He holds a Master's and PhD degree in MFT from Brigham Young University and is licensed as an MFT in Utah.

Foundational Concepts and Models of Family Therapy

An Introduction for Online Learning

Edited by Yulia Watters
and Darren Adamson

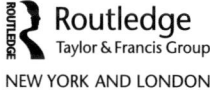

Routledge
Taylor & Francis Group

NEW YORK AND LONDON

Designed cover image: © Mary Peterson

First published 2024
by Routledge
605 Third Avenue, New York, NY 10158

and by Routledge
4 Park Square, Milton Park, Abingdon, Oxon, OX14 4RN

Routledge is an imprint of the Taylor & Francis Group, an informa business

ISBN: 978-1-032-46635-4 (hbk)
ISBN: 978-1-032-46634-7 (pbk)
ISBN: 978-1-003-38262-1 (ebk)

DOI: 10.4324/9781003382621

Typeset in Sabon
by Newgen Publishing UK

To the field of marriage and family therapy that we are devoted to and to all with whom we work as MFT scholar/practitioners – students, faculty, staff and clients. May this volume add to the preparation of the next generation of MFTs.

Contents

Contributors

Darren Adamson
Adamson is a Professor and Associate Dean of the Division of Social and Behavioural Sciences, a licensed MFT in Utah and an AAMFT Approved Supervisor.

Aurélia Bickler
Bickler is a Director of the Virtual Whole Person Center at National University, a licensed MFT in Florida and an AAMFT Approved Supervisor.

Valerie Q. Glass
Glass is a Professor at National University, a licensed MFT in Michigan and South Carolina, and an AAMFT Approved Supervisor.

Kristi Harrison
Harrison is a Part-Time Faculty at National University, a licensed MFT in Michigan and an AAMFT Approved Supervisor.

Michael Knerr
Knerr is an Associate Professor at National University, a licensed MFT and approved Supervisor in Ohio, and an AAMFT Approved Supervisor.

Vanieca Kraus
Kraus is an Associate Professor at National University, a licensed MFT in Oregon and an AAMFT Approved Supervisor.

Siva Perera
Perera is an Associate Professor and Associate Director of Faculty Support and Development at National University and a licensed MFT in Florida.

Patricia Postanowicz
Postanowicz is a Professor and MAMFT Program Director at National University.

Emily Schmittel
Schmittel is an Associate Professor and a Director of Doctoral MFT Clinical Training at National University, a licensed MFT in Illinois and Missouri, and an AAMFT Approved Supervisor.

Asha Sutton
Sutton is an Associate Professor at National University and the Department Chair for Marriage and Family Therapy at National University, a licensed MFT in Illinois and Michigan, and an AAMFT Approved Supervisor.

Amanda Veldorale-Griffin

Veldorale-Griffin is an Assistant Professor at National University, a licensed MFT in Florida and an AAMFT Approved Supervisor.

Yulia Watters

Watters is a Professor and Director of Curriculum Development at National University, a licensed MFT in Florida and Delaware, and an AAMFT Approved Supervisor

Foreword

I had the good fortune, and privilege, to join the Administrative Faculty at Northcentral University (NCU) in 2013 as the inaugural Director of Clinical Field Placement right after the master's program in marriage and family therapy (MAMFT) became the first distance-based MAMFT program accredited by the Commission on Accreditation for Marriage and Family Therapy Education (COAMFTE). This was a truly exciting time, not only for NCU, but for the field of marriage and family therapy (MFT). In retrospect the skepticism and challenges as to whether MFT education could be delivered online were substantial. After a decade, and a worldwide pandemic, many of those original concerns have been laid to rest and we now have an abundance of MFT programs offered online.

Prior to my joining the NCU faculty I remember being at the Association for Marital and Family Therapy Regulatory Boards (AMFTRB) annual meeting in Anchorage, Alaska and Branden Henline, the NCU MAMFT Program Director at the time, was asked to address the viability of MFT education virtually. I was, and still am, enamored with technology and was intrigued by the proposition that expanding the ability to train MFTs without having to give up two or more years of one's life to attend a brick-and-mortar institution was truly revolutionary. And, as it is with all things revolutionary, the critiques and doubts were significant. The technological limitations of the 2010s notwithstanding, the idea that someone could learn to be a family therapist without putting their lives on hold for two or more years was groundbreaking. At the time, marriage and family therapists (MFTs) were the smallest of all the behavioral health professions and had the most resource intensive training. Consequently, generating a significant number of competent MFTs outside of California was a serious challenge with the traditional brick-and-mortar COAMFTE accredited programs that were lucky to graduate 10–20 students per year.

The emergence of online MFT education also corresponded with the development and deployment of the MFT Core Competencies in the late aughts which provide an unprecedented opportunity for MFT programs to revise their training to be more focused on outcomes rather than inputs. It is the confluence of these factors from which sprung the innovation that is synonymous with the MAMFT program at NCU, now National University (NU).

Watters, Adamson and their MFT colleagues have embraced the innovative culture of NCU/NU to create a truly pioneering text. Sometimes being a trailblazer can distinguish and other times it can obfuscate. Fortunately, for MFT students and educators, the contribution of Watters and Adamson is the former. It is noteworthy the number of factors that seem to have contributed to the culmination of this text, including the experiences of students who might be considered "nontraditional" due to the significant age range, second careers and being first-generation graduate students. The NCU/NU MAMFT approach also did not use a cohort model, like the vast majority of MAMFT programs, including the nascent online programs emerging prior to the pandemic. The NCU/NU Mentor Model gave students a flexibility not yet available in the extant MAMFT programs. Combined with an open enrollment policy, the NCU/NU MAMFT program attracted a vast and diverse student population with unique needs and experiences, which makes this text possibly more valuable than most, at least in the online education world. Added to that list was the experience and commitment of the faculty contributors to the book. It is clear that the authors understand the developmental challenges that students can face when learning to become an MFT, particularly in an online, asynchronous environment, and the chapters reflect this in their organization, infographics, pullouts and case examples.

The goal of all MFT training programs is to provide the learning experiences necessary to become a competent, independent practitioner. Unfortunately, that process can take five years or more and the impact that any one text, course or learning experience has on the ultimate goal of becoming a licensed MFT, while minuscule, is also cumulative. The design of *Foundational Concepts and Models of Family Therapy* will serve well the neophyte trainee in understanding the field, role of family therapists and models of MFT, as well as preparing them for a future licensing exam.

The structure of the book provides readers with the scaffolding necessary to organize the material and the reiteration of concepts across chapters, highlighting different contexts, will also benefit trainees as they begin their MFT education. The first section of the book orients the reader to the foundation of the field and profession, including chapters on the use of theory, history of MFT, conceptualizing, postmodernism, treatment planning and clinical practices. The two sections on MFT models, classic and postmodern, provide an excellent primer for the models that inform extant MFT educational programs and practicing clinicians, from the pioneering work of Bowen, the MRI group and Philadelphia Child Guidance Clinic to the empirically supported models like Cognitive-Behavioral Therapy, Gottman and Emotionally Focused Therapy (EFT), and round things out with the postmodern approaches of Collaborative Language Systems, Narrative Therapy and Solution Focused. The chapters are robust enough to give entry level trainees a starting point to identify a model that might fit the family therapist to which she aspires. The references to primary sources will also assist students in identifying manuscripts that may further assist in the journey to becoming a competent family therapist prepared to assist families in addressing behavioral health challenges in broad and diverse contexts.

After the pandemic, and the concomitant shift to online learning for the vast majority of students to keep people safe, we have learned a lot about what can be done online and what cannot. Yet, NCU/NU has created an engaging and accessible MAMFT program that offers anyone who has the desire, time and commitment to learning the chance to become a family therapist. *Foundational Concepts and Models of Family Therapy* is a valued addition to the resources available to students and programs, not only who are doing online education, but in person, synchronous education as well. The content and organization of the book is accessible and robust. Watters and Adamson's vision of creating an engaging text firmly grounded in relational, systemic thinking was certainly realized and the incorporation of instructional design concepts is obvious. Whether it is the use of compelling infographics, case examples and text boxes, or drilling down to the nuts-and-bolts of starting a job, the complexity of the text does well to approximate the multifaceted and recursive aspects of learning how to think systemically.

William F. Northey, Jr., PhD, LMFT
CEO Q3 Analytics and Consulting and Clinical Director of the
Bellefonte Center for Children and Families Wilmington, DE

Acknowledgments

The editors, Drs. Watters and Adamson, express thanks to Dr. James Billings who encouraged and funded this project. His faith in us and the various faculty authors was instrumental in completing this volume. We also express appreciation to each of the chapter authors. Not only did they work to produce wonderful content, but they did it with diligence and grace. They are colleagues extraordinaire! We also express thanks to students, current and those who have graduated, for they were the inspiration for this project. They asked for a volume more focused on their unique situations (adult learners, career changers, first-generation graduate students). Finally, a heartfelt thanks to Heather Evans from Routledge who believed that this book would add to the body of knowledge for those seeking to learn about MFT. Her guidance in this process has been invaluable.

Introduction

1 Introduction

Systems Theory in the Context of Family Therapy

Yulia Watters and Darren Adamson

Several books have been written to explain the application of systems theory in the context of family therapy and to describe foundational family therapy models. What is different about this book?

This manuscript is a result of a collaborative effort of a group of Marriage and Family Therapy (MFT) faculty who have been teaching MFT in the context of the first-ever COAMFTE accredited online program (MAMFT). As with any teaching faculty, the professors involved in this project were trying to find different ways to engage students in considering the relational paradigm rather than continuing to see the world through a one-dimensional, linear lens of cause-and-effect interactions. The distance-based nature of the program added to the faculty's desire to make the material as interactive and engaging as possible. In addition, this book was inspired by their reflections regarding what concepts presented the most challenge to students, prompting them to provide more examples to effectively illustrate how these ideas relate to the MFT field. Finally, faculty found it important to introduce the founders of each model as well as the existing supporting research literature for each approach. More research is needed to support the important contribution of systems' trained practitioners to the mental health field. This book aims to contribute to this conversation.

The structure of this book is iterative by nature; readers are introduced to the systemic concepts multiple times throughout the book. Such organization is intentional as it allows students to read about the concepts in different contexts, examine their application and consider the foundational nature of systems theory in the creation of different therapeutic models. This structure was also found to be helpful in a distance-learning environment, where students are prompted to review materials multiple time as they progress through their coursework and engage in various conversations with their professors.

This book is divided into three parts. Part I presents the general introduction to systems theory concepts, history of family therapy, family conceptualization from an MFT perspective, an introduction to postmodernism and social constructionism, planning of the therapeutic process and guidelines for beginning therapists. Part II introduces family therapy models known as traditional or modern approaches in the field. It includes Milan Systemic Family Therapy, Structural Family Therapy, Strategic Family Therapy, Experiential Family Therapy, Bowen Family Systems Therapy, Emotionally-Focused Couple Therapy, Gottman Method Couple's Therapy and Contextual Therapy. Finally, Part III provides an illustration of how postmodern concepts were applied in family therapy and illustrates such postmodern approaches as Solution-Focused Brief Therapy, Narrative Therapy, Cognitive

DOI: 10.4324/9781003382621-2

Behavioral Family Therapy, Psychoanalytic Family Therapy and Collaborative Language Systems Therapy.

Part I – Foundational concepts of family therapy

Chapter 2 – Using Theory in the Practice of Marriage and Family Therapy – introduces the reader to the notion of theory and how it is used to answer fundamental questions pertinent to working as an MFT. Using a research practitioner approach and systemic lens, the author explores how the transition to becoming an MFT is supported by the life stance where the notions of multiple worldviews and ever-changing contexts serve as guiding principles, while a therapist builds a therapeutic relationship with a client or interacts within a larger environment.

Several situations are presented, challenging the reader to consider questions that they might ask to understand the worldview of another person – a client. Assumptions and how they can be effectively used in the therapeutic process helps the reader to explore their biases to ensure that they do not negatively affect their work in therapy.

This chapter explores the place of theory and systemic foundation in the framework of therapy models, core components of the process of therapy and the role of research in therapeutic practice.

Chapter 3 – History of Family Therapy – presents an overview of the MFT field from its early development in the 1960s to the present. It emphasizes the leading figures in the field, differentiates MFTs from other mental health professionals and addresses the current trends in the field. Readers are also introduced to therapeutic models, given an opportunity to explore the differences between traditional and postmodern models.

Chapter 4 – Building Blocks to Conceptualizing Family: A Family System's Perspective – introduces the understanding of the relational aspects involved in the formation and resolution of a problem within a family context. The role of a family, as a systemic unit, is emphasized as the foundation of the new epistemology that one is invited to embrace while becoming an MFT. Readers are also introduced to the foundational concepts of systems theory such as open vs. closed system, subsystems, complementary and reciprocal systems, first- and second-order change, causality (circular vs. linear), nonsummativity, equifinality and positive vs. negative feedback, while examining how these constructs are helpful in the understanding of relational patterns of interaction and promotion of a change process.

Chapter 5 – Postmodernism and Social Constructionism: Foundational Concepts – introduces the notions of postmodernism and social constructionism. Both constructs are of primary importance, as they introduced important paradigm change in the practice of MFT. Social constructionism emphasizes the idea that each individual's reality is constructed through the language interactions and cultural and historical background of the person. This construct is part of a larger philosophical paradigm of postmodernism, which postulates that all humans have a variety of lenses that they use to connect with the world, lenses that are the social constructs described above.

Chapter 6 – The Core Process of Therapy: Planning Therapy Guided by Theory – expands on the concepts introduced in Chapter 2, with an added focus on treatment planning and the use of theory to guide that effort. Terminology related to the primary aspects of treatment planning is delineated and described to enhance the understanding of the reader. Aspects of the therapeutic relationship that are important to accurate assessment and treatment planning are explored. Examples of types of treatment plans are shared and the experience of applying concepts to case scenarios is provided.

Chapter 7 – Clinical Practice: Preparing for Day 1 – introduces employment consider-ations for marriage and family therapists. What is the workplace going to be like? What expectations will there be for the MFT from employers, supervisors and colleagues? Ethics and legal considerations related to employment are also briefly discussed. The process of doing the work of an MFT is explored, including workflow and tasks that must be accomplished to support effective therapy. The final section of this chapter explores docu-mentation tools that support the work of therapy. Examples of these tools are presented, and full copies of various tools are provided in the chapter appendices.

Part II – Modern or classic models of family therapy

Chapter 8 – Milan Systemic Family Therapy – introduces one of the foundational trad-itional approaches in MFT. This chapter illustrates the systemic nature of this model and provides the overview of its cybernetics roots, its evolution and its significant influence in the current MFT field.

Chapter 9 – Structural Family Therapy – presents another traditional family therapy model. This chapter illustrates the systemic nature of the model by introducing the main concepts of this therapeutic approach, such as systems, subsystems, boundaries, roles and rules. As one of the original MFT models, Structural Family Therapy articulated funda-mental concepts related to the practice of MFT.

Chapter 10 – Strategic Family Therapy – introduces one of the foundational traditional models of family therapy; one of the first MFT models to be directly informed by systemic concepts. This chapter addresses the systemic foundation of the model, main representatives of this approach as well as the controversial interventions that were examined from an ethical perspective in the context of contemporary family therapy practice. Many of the concepts from this model have informed those that have come after it.

Chapter 11 – Experiential Family Therapy – introduces several models under the umbrella of the experiential approach: the Satir Growth model, Symbolic-Experiential Therapy, Emotionally-Focused Couples Therapy and Internal Family Systems. The common component of all these models being a warm and empathetic connection that establishes a joining process between the client and a therapist. This connection is the primary promoter of change in the client system.

Chapter 12 – Bowen Family Systems Theory – introduces one of the major theoret-ical approaches of MFT. This theory was developed by Murray Bowen and incorporates the understanding of evolutionary process and biological systems. Readers will be able to review such foundational concepts as differentiation, emotional systems, multigenerational transmission, emotional triangles, nuclear family, family projection process, sibling position and societal regression. Readers will also examine how these and other concepts apply to the family context.

Chapter 13 – Emotionally-Focused Family Therapy – is one of the most empirically- validated of the MFT models. It is firmly built on principles of systems theory and concepts from attachment theory. The goal of Emotionally-Focused Family Therapy (EFT) is second-order change, created through the use of experiential methods that, in the moment, identify problematic patterns of interaction. Intervention focuses on helping the couple to practice new, more secure connection and interactional patterns. The highly structured nature of the model, with stages and steps, allows for replicative studies that demonstrate its effectiveness. Information about how to gain a deeper understanding of the model is also provided.

Chapter 14 – Gottman Method Couple's Therapy – introduces the theory developed by John and Julie Gottman. This model focuses on assisting clients to build a strong foundation of friendship and positive sentiment in relationships. It is a directive model that is founded upon the divorce prediction and prevention research conducted for many years by John Gottman. There is a strong focus on assessment, psychoeducation and skills training. Clients engage in experiential learning and focus on the practice of new skills related to healthier patterns of interaction.

Chapter 15 – Contextual Therapy – introduces the theory developed primarily by Ivan Boszormenyi-Nagy. This model explores peoples' experiences from the past in relation to their present-day functioning within a system. It encourages family members to explore their experience of balance and fairness within the family unit across generations. This exploration allows family members to revisit their experiences and reconstruct a balanced level of "give and take" within their family unit. The goal is to allow fairness, trust and accountability to be established or reestablished within the family system.

Chapter 16 – Cognitive Behavioral Family Therapy – has its foundations in Cognitive Behavioral Therapy (CBT), which is very widely practiced across a range of mental health professions. Cognitive Behavioral Family Therapy (CBFT) takes that CBT foundation and incorporates a systems orientation. The primary focus is exploring how those with whom they are in a relationship reinforce people's behaviors and cognitions. One of the primary assumptions CBFT is that cognitions, behavior and emotions are mutually influential. Cognitive distortions affect interactional patterns in couples and families. Cognitions, behaviors and emotions are also the primary focus to create change.

Chapter 17 – Psychoanalytic Family Therapy – Historically, psychoanalysts (the most famous of which was Sigmund Freud) founded their work on the intrapsychic processes occurring within individual clients. Over time, some of these mental health practitioners began to consider the interaction between individuals and their families and how these relationships influenced relationships in later life. This convergence of individual and relational focus ultimately led to the development of the psychoanalytic family therapy approach. Psychoanalytic family therapy bridges the gap between the traditional intrapsychic focus and the relational nature of family systems and interactions. Object relations family therapy and family of origin therapy are all approaches to therapy that have developed from psychoanalytic family therapy.

Part III – Postmodern models of family therapy

Chapter 18 – Postmodernism and Social Constructionism in Family Therapy – returns the reader to the concepts of postmodernism and social constructionism to examine them in the context of family dynamics. This chapter introduces foundational concepts for the understanding and practice of postmodern family therapy approaches: Solution-Focused Brief Therapy, Collaborative Language Systems Therapy, and Narrative Family Therapy.

Chapter 19 – Solution-Focused Brief Therapy – introduces one of the postmodern approaches to family therapy. It includes the outline of the systemic foundation of the model and an introduction of the founders, Steve de Shazer and Insoo Kim Berg. The primary concept of shifting from a problem-saturated to a solution-focused view of the world and the clients' situation is also presented. Additionally, a description of the main interventions, such as: Miracle Questions, Scaling Questions, Exceptions Questions, Coping Questions and Relational Questions are delineated and described.

Chapter 20– Narrative Family Therapy – introduces the premises of the postmodern approach that was developed in Australia and New Zealand by Michael White and David Epston. Readers will become familiar with the foundational concepts of this approach, common interventions, as well as cultural competencies associated with this model.

Chapter 21– Collaborative Language Systems Therapy – refers to a postmodern approach to therapy that emphasizes the role of language and communication in the creation and maintenance of a problem. Social constructionism and hermeneutics are also introduced as the foundational concepts of the model, as well as the nonhierarchical position of a therapist that helps to create an opportunity for change in a dialogue between a client and a therapist.

Part I

Foundational Concepts
of Family Therapy

2 Using Theory in the Practice of Marriage and Family Therapy

Kristi Harrison

Preparing to learn about theory

Reflecting on personal assumptions about therapy

If you're reading this, chances are that you want to be a marriage and family therapist (MFT). You may already be a part of the mental health field or you might aspire to become a mental health professional. As you consider what it means to use theory to guide the practice of therapy, it's really important to consider your own views of the therapy process. How do you currently view therapy? What do you think is the purpose of therapy? From your perspective, how does therapy help people? Why do you personally want to be an MFT (or, if you're already in the field, why did you join the profession)? And how do your personal life experiences and your social context influence answers to these questions?

Take a moment to think about your view of therapy and why you want to be an MFT. As you consider what it means to use theory to guide you in the therapy process, it is especially important to consider this question: **how does therapy help people?**

Different therapeutic theories answer this question in different ways. A little later in this chapter, we'll look more closely at what a theory is, why theories are important in therapy and how you will go about learning to use theory in your work as an MFT. Here it is important to note that your learning process will involve critically evaluating the many therapy theories out there. Being a professional therapist involves figuring out which existing theory or theories may suit you while also challenging these theories regarding their biases and shortcomings. Your personal answer to this question – how does therapy help people? – will have a lot to do with which theories end up making the most sense to you, even with their potential limitations. By studying theories of therapy, you will expand your understanding of the multiple ways of seeing how therapy helps people, and hopefully your personal answer to this question – how does therapy help people? – will evolve and become more sophisticated as you learn.

At the same time, some of your core beliefs about therapy are likely to remain. It is essential for you to be aware of these beliefs so that you can examine and incorporate theory thoughtfully.

As you work on developing awareness of your own beliefs, the concept of reflexivity is important to understand. The term reflexivity involves critical examination of social context for beliefs (Givropoulou & Tseliou, 2021).

Ultimately, to be a competent therapist, you must be able to answer the question – how does therapy help people? – in a clear, direct way about your own work with clients. Your answer to this question will be unique to you; no two therapists answer this question the

DOI: 10.4324/9781003382621-4

same way. This question is one that you should think about again and again throughout your training process. And even people who are seasoned therapists ought to revisit their answer to this question periodically.

The decisions you make in therapy, including how you think about your work, what you do with your clients and how you document what you do – all need to be intentional. That is, you need to have reasons behind why you're approaching your work the way that you are. This is where professional knowledge comes into play (and it is why states require people to go to school before they can get a license to provide therapy!). You'll use various types of professional knowledge, including theory, research, ethical principles and self-awareness, to guide you in making decisions about your work as an MFT. As an MFT, this work will be based in a systemic perspective that views (and treats) problems within social and cultural contexts and employs familial and other relationships as key agents of change (Stratton, 2016). This approach has been shown to be effective across a wide array of client concerns and has been found to be more effective than individual approaches in treating many mental health issues (including mood disorders, eating disorders and substance use disorders). Systemic approaches also have a lower attrition rate than other types of therapy (Stratton, 2016).

Intentionality in therapy: becoming aware of the choices we make during the helping process

Imagine that a friend comes to you for help because they are having conflict with their spouse. This friend explains that they think their spouse drinks too much. They have tried everything to get the spouse to stop and nothing seems to work.

How would you go about helping this person? Take a few minutes to really think through this scenario and how you might handle it. Consider all aspects of the situation. How you would interact with your friend, what you might be thinking about, what you might say, how you might be feeling, etc. You'll get the most out of this exercise if you actually write out answers to these questions.

Now that you've taken some time to consider this scenario, let's take a step back.

It's time to reflect on your approach to this situation.

- What sorts of questions are you asking or conclusions were you drawing about the people involved?
- What assumptions were you making about the situation?
- What, if anything, did you identify as the 'problem' in this scenario? Did you see anything as a problem at all? If you did, did you start to develop a guess about the cause of the problem?
- Did you have ideas about what your friend might want or what this friend's end goal might be?
- How did you imagine interacting with this friend? How would your friend's expectations of you factor into your approach?
- What would you actually **do**? Would you ask questions? Would you try to figure out what was causing the problem? Would you offer advice? Would you just provide a listening ear? Would you offer reassurance or comfort? Would you think about what you might do if you were in the same situation?
- What sorts of things did you think might be helpful to this person? What process would you use to try to help them?
- What are the things you would need to do, both outwardly and in your own head, in order to be most helpful?

These questions are intended to help you identify all of the "ingredients" involved in being helpful to someone who is dealing with a concern like this.

Although this scenario could happen in a therapy context, it is not at all unique to therapy. As people in day-to-day life, we help others with problems all the time. Those who are interested in being therapists often find themselves in this helping role well before they enter professional training to be a therapist.

You may not have answers to all the questions mentioned so far, but chances are you have answers to at least some of them. Your answers to these questions reflect your assumptions, or the ideas that you take for granted in order to guide your action in a particular situation.

In day-to-day life, the term *assumption* is often viewed negatively (as in when we make "assumptions" about people and then turn out to be wrong about them). When studying theory, though, the term "assumption" is not bad; it simply refers to a belief or idea that is accepted as true or valid and that becomes the basis for some type of action.

For example, let's say you go to the refrigerator to get something to drink. When you pull the item out, you find that it's warm rather than being chilled as it should be. You've identified a problem that you want to solve. To take action, you must make one or more reasonable assumptions. You make the assumption that the fridge is not getting electricity the way that it's supposed to. On the basis of this assumption, you identify some steps you can take to try to solve the problem (make sure the fridge is plugged in, check the circuit breaker to see if a breaker has been tripped, check the power elsewhere in the house to see if it's out all over the house). This assumption that the fridge has lost electricity could end up being correct or incorrect (for example, maybe the item that you pulled out had just been placed in the fridge). Regardless, to solve the problem, you need to make some assumptions. Let's say that, based on the assumption that the fridge has lost power, you check everything you can think of that might have caused this and you haven't been able to fix the problem. What you would probably do at this point is return to your original assumption – that the power to the fridge was out – and see if this assumption might be flawed in some way. You return to the fridge and discover that the light inside is working and that the other items inside are still cold. This makes you wonder whether the original item you had pulled out had been put in recently; in other words, you've made a different assumption. You decide to reach for another drink from the back of the fridge. Lo and behold, it's cold.

This example might seem silly, and you may be wondering, "What does this have to do with being a therapist?" The logical reasoning process involved in this example is similar, in some ways, to what we do when we use theory in therapy. We notice something about a situation, we make assumptions, we take action, and we revise our assumptions until we've been successful in addressing the issue (Goodell, Sudderth & Allan, 2011).

One important thing that **does** make therapy different is that we must become conscious of our process of making assumptions. In day-to-day life, this problem-solving process is largely subconscious. Even when we're solving very important problems, many people are not conscious of their assumptions and of the process of revising their assumptions. The big difference involved in being a professional therapist is that we learn to be conscious of our assumptions, and we are transparent about the reasoning we are using to help people with the things that bring them to therapy (Goodell et al., 2011). This type of awareness of assumptions is why theory is so important.

Helping people with the situations that bring them to therapy requires assumptions or foundational beliefs about people, about how problems develop and about how to effectively help someone. There are many different assumptions we can make about people, problems and how to help people. For example, have you heard the saying, "You can bring a horse to water but you can't make them drink"? This is a common saying that refers to

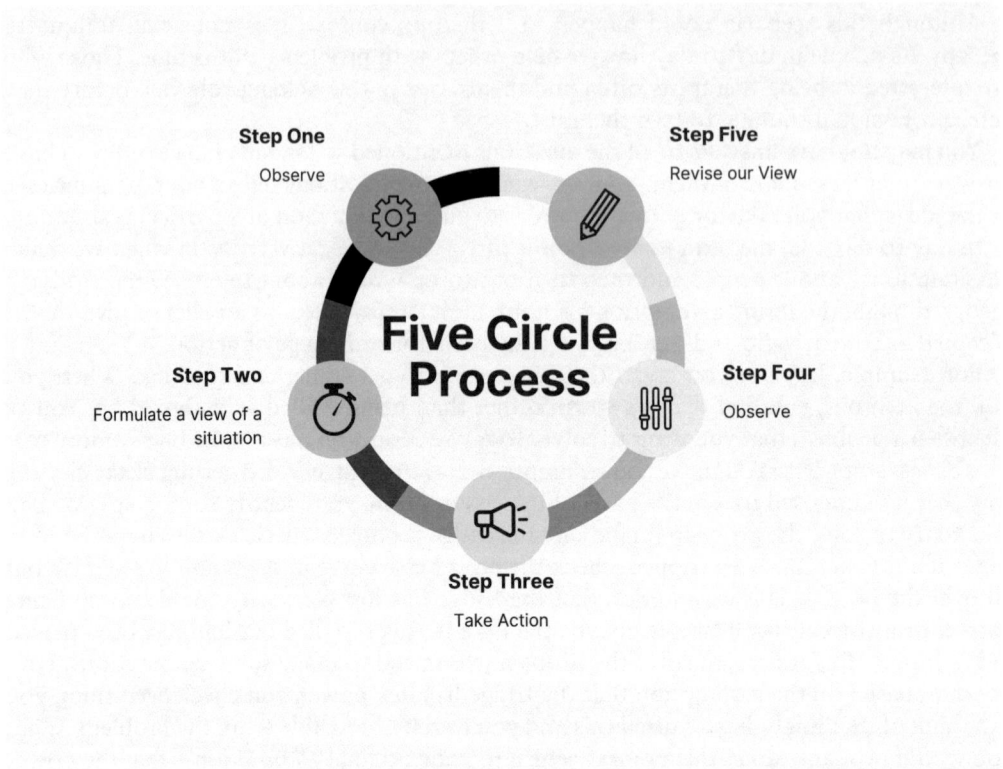

Figure 2.1 Infographic1: Interactive Process Five Steps.

the idea that you can't help someone who is not willing to help themselves. This is a popular assumption about the process of helping people. Have you ever found yourself saying this before? Have you ever questioned this assumption or thought about how it might close off possibilities for helping some people?

Thoughtfully analyzing this popular assumption is a great illustration of how training to be a professional therapist, and specifically becoming aware of assumptions, prepares us to be more effective helpers. Professional knowledge from the marriage and family therapy field partially questions the validity of this assumption, "you can't help someone who's not ready to be helped". In reality, people's openness to help often varies, depending on the situation. In one setting, a person may appear unwilling to change, while, in another situation, they seem more receptive to doing things differently. In a variety of ways, professional therapy theories help therapists work with people's motivation to help them change. If you're interested in learning more about this particular theory, you might check out Motivational Interviewing (see Levounis, Arnaout & Marienfeld, 2017), Solution-Focused Therapy (see de Shazer, et al., 2012) or research on the importance of building a strong therapeutic relationship (see Friedlander, Escudero, Welmers-van de Poll & Heatherington, 2018). The common factors literature (see Davis, Lebow & Sprenkle, 2012; Fife, Whiting, Bradford & Davis, 2014) also sheds

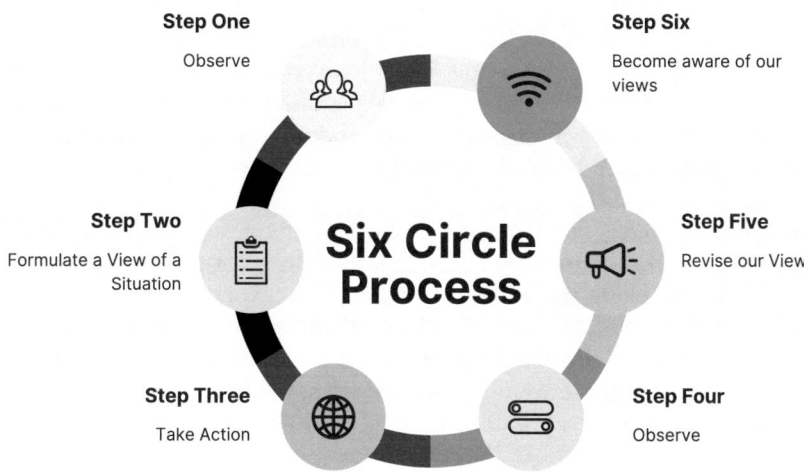

Figure 2.2 Infographic 2: Interactive Process Six Steps.

light on this idea of client motivation and therapist skill. Compared to the popular assumption – "you can't help people who aren't ready to help themselves" – therapeutic theory and research provides us with a more careful and nuanced view of people and of the helping process. To benefit from these theories, therapists and therapists-in-training need to learn to recognize their existing assumptions so that they can use theory to deepen their thinking.

One of the most essential things that separates professional therapists from people without professional training is that they learn to be explicit (clear and direct) about the assumptions they are making, and they help people using assumptions that have been evaluated in professional research and practice, rather than just using personal assumptions. This is where theory comes into play.

What is a theory and what is a therapy model?

Generally speaking (not just in the therapy world), **a theory** is defined as a set of ideas that explains some phenomenon. While people in day-to-day life may have their own "theories" or assumptions, in the social sciences, theories are carefully explained so that other professionals can consider the merits of the theory. Although theories may start out as one person's opinion about a situation, professional theories have been exposed to scrutiny in a variety of ways. Other professionals challenge them and contribute to revisions of the theory. Research is conducted to test different aspects of a theory and perhaps help with changing the theory.

The social sciences include all sorts of theories about human beings. There are theories about individual development, family life, relationships and all sorts of social phenomena. A **therapy model** is a special type of theory that guides therapists through the process of helping people in therapy. A therapy model is a theory that offers explanations in three domains. Psychotherapy theories include: (a) an explanation of human development and functioning across biological, psychological and social domains, (b) an explanation of how and why problems happen, and (c) an explanation of how therapy, as a process, helps people (Sharf, 2016).

To help someone effectively, we must make assumptions in all of these areas. To help someone as a professional therapist, we must make carefully thought-out assumptions in these three areas. This is where theory is important in our work as therapists and this is where a model of therapy (i.e., this special type of theory) is invaluable. As we'll discuss later, there are other types of theories (besides therapy models) that also supply us with important assumptions that guide what we do as MFTs, the process of helping people in therapy. A therapy model is a theory that offers explanations in three domains.

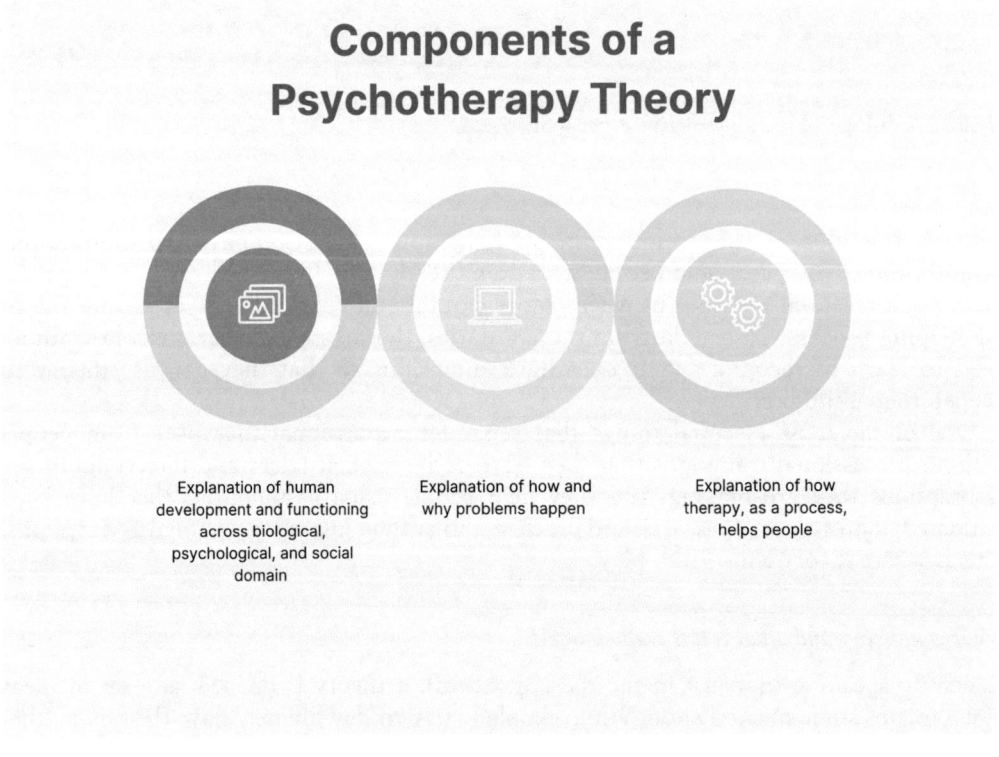

Figure 2.3 Infographic 3: Components of a Psychotherapy Theory.

A final note about how research and theory relate

The term evidence-based practice is commonplace in today's practice of therapy. What does **evidence-based practice** mean and how does using research evidence tie in with using theory?

As we're learning about the role of therapy in our work, it's important to look at how research relates to theory. **Research** is an organized process of collecting information about a particular thing. The scientific method involves gathering research in a way that is transparent and trustworthy.

Scientific or empirical research involves systematically collecting information about a particular phenomenon. The scientific method lays out a process of collecting information in a systematic (orderly) way (Goodson Beasley, 2011). When information is gathered in an orderly, transparent way, it increases our confidence in the results.

Imagine a friend tells you that chocolate is an effective treatment for depression. One of your first questions should be, "What is the basis for making this claim?" You would probably view this claim differently if your friend said, "Oh, I always feel happier after I eat a chocolate bar, so chocolate must help with depression, too." Or maybe your friend tells you that they saw a TV commercial for Hershey's kisses, suggesting that chocolate makes people happy. You would hopefully view this claim with skepticism. What if, instead, you read an article in a reputable professional journal discussing a study that compared chocolate to a commonly prescribed antidepressant. You might start to trust this information more than your friend's first-hand experience.

In the therapy world, it is possible to conduct scientific research about virtually every aspect of the therapy process, including the theories we use to guide therapy. Just because it is possible to conduct research about a certain aspect of therapy, doesn't mean that that research has actually taken place yet. In the professional practice of therapy, information gained from carefully conducted research is an essential part of making decisions about what you do in therapy (Goodson Beasley, 2011). This being said, scientific evidence should not be accepted without question, and scientific evidence is a supplement to theory, rather than a replacement for it.

Like the practice of therapy, conducting research always involves making assumptions and, in this regard, theory precedes research. Theories are made up of "systematically related propositions" (White & Klein, 2008, p. 10). That is, they are constructed of multiple related **hypotheses**, which we test through research. While the results of research can help us develop or revise theories, research alone is never going to be sufficient for providing a rationale for action the way that theory does. We always take the results of empirical research and interpret them; we insert them into our broader way of thinking about a particular issue. Empirical research is a necessary part of making decisions about the professional practice of therapy, but theory will always be necessary and more fundamental (Goodson Beasley, 2011).

Later in this chapter, we'll look more closely at what theory is and how it guides therapy. First, though, it is helpful to consider what therapy actually entails.

What is (psycho)therapy?

An overview of the therapy process to help prepare you for learning about theory and its role in treatment planning. Up to this point, we've referenced the therapy process repeatedly and asked you to consider your own existing beliefs about therapy. This involved the assumption that you have some existing knowledge of what therapy involves. While virtually everyone reading this will have at least some knowledge of what therapy involves, there are likely big differences in your understanding of the therapeutic process. To learn how to use theory in therapy, it is helpful to have some basic knowledge of what therapy involves, what therapists do and how theory plays a role in what therapists do.

What is therapy?

In popular culture, the term **"therapy"** is commonly used to refer to "talk therapy". You will sometimes also see the term "counseling" used, too. Although some people draw a distinction between these two things (therapy versus counseling), the terms are often used interchangeably. The distinction between these terms generally comes from the way that state licensing regulations have been written to define various types of mental health work (e.g., Marriage and Family Therapists, Licensed Professional Counselors, Psychologists, Clinical Social Workers). In the Marriage and Family Therapy field, the terms "therapy" and "therapist" tend to be used. In more general medical settings, the term "therapy" can refer to a wide range of health treatments, including treatments for the body (physical therapy, occupational therapy, etc.). The dictionary definition of the word "therapy" defines it as something designed to "cure" or "heal". In many mental health professions, there has been the tendency to view psychotherapy, or "talk therapy", as being similar to treatments for physical health problems. This is an assumption that is worth questioning. If you happen to have first-hand experience with (talk) therapy, think for a moment about how a therapist's work is different from that of a doctor. Why might members of the mental health profession want to classify what they do as "therapy" (i.e., as similar to what physicians do)? What might be some of the problems associated with this?

Viewing mental health through the same lens as we view physical health has some important implications. Comparing talk therapy to traditional physical medicine involves some powerful assumptions and we need to be aware of these assumptions and to think critically about them. This is an important point to keep in mind as you study theory.

What does it mean when we talk about "change"?

Change is a word you'll see mentioned a lot in discussions of therapy. You'll see questions like, "How does therapy help people to change?" or "What is the 'theory of change' in such-and-such model?" In many regards, therapy is all about helping people to make changes. The type of change will vary, both based on why people are seeking therapy and based on the therapist's approach. Some therapy involves healing psychological wounds. Some therapy involves personal growth and self-actualization. Therapy often involves changes in how we think and feel. And it almost always involves changes in what people do (behavioral change).

An important aspect of a therapist's professional development is formulating a clear theory of change. A therapist's theory of change is their unique explanation of how the therapy process works. A theory of change covers assumptions about a variety of different things, including basic ideas about human beings and what makes them tick, how people come to develop problems such that they might benefit from talk therapy and how the therapy process can help people to change. Keep in mind what was mentioned earlier about the different ways that therapy can involve change.

Where does therapy happen?

Traditionally, therapy has taken place in an office setting. More recently, therapists are taking therapy out of the office and into other spaces where people live and work. Examples include in-home therapy, walking therapy, workplace therapy (e.g., EAP), outdoor therapy, animal-assisted therapy and therapy offered as part of a hospital treatment (either residential or outpatient).

Reflection questions: How does the treatment setting relate to a therapist's theory of change? For example, what assumptions might a therapist hold such that doing therapy while walking outdoors makes more sense? What ethical considerations might come up as a result of where therapy is conducted?

What do we call the people providing the therapy?

A variety of terms are used to refer to the people involved in therapy. The terms counselor and therapist may both be used to refer to the professional delivering the therapy. This often varies by practice location and setting. More specific terms that are legally defined through licensing laws are also used (e.g., psychiatrist, psychologist, social worker, licensed professional counselor, licensed marriage and family therapist).

Take time to reflect: How does the terminology that we use to describe the therapy process help define or construct the way that the people involved view the process? How does the terminology specifically influence the way that **you** think about therapy? How does the language that you use to describe therapy relate to your assumptions about the therapy process?

In therapy offered in a healthcare setting, the medical term "patient" is sometimes used to describe the person seeking therapy. Some object to this term because of how it portrays the person seeking therapy. For some, the term "patient" invokes an image of someone passively receiving treatment, kind of like a person getting a shot at the doctor's office. In the specialty mental health sector, as well as in the marriage and family therapy field, the term "client" is generally preferred. "Client" tends to bring to mind a person who is actively seeking out a service. In some settings, the term "consumer" is used for the same reason (to emphasize the personal agency or free choice of the person seeking out therapy, see Onken, Craig, Ridgway, Ralph & Cook, 2007).

In therapy with more than one person (i.e., a couple or members of a family), the term "client" may also refer to the couple or family as a whole.

Besides talking, what do people do in therapy? What actually happens in therapy?

The process of therapy can take anywhere from a few minutes to many years. Some therapists can be really effective in a brief 15-minute session. Some traditional forms of individual therapy (e.g., psychoanalysis) tend to be carried out over the course of years. Regardless of the length of the therapy, there are some basic processes that all therapists carry out. These processes are important to be aware of. As you learn how to use theory to guide your work, you will want to think specifically about how theory informs these core therapeutic processes. One of your main learning objectives in this lesson is to develop an understanding of some of these core therapeutic processes.

Forming a relationship, sometimes called joining or developing rapport

Helping someone change requires having some type of relationship with them. We are not going to be receptive to a person or to an experience if we don't feel positively about the person and if we don't feel accepted (Sprenkle, Lebow & Davis, 2009). Even therapists who provide very brief therapy must form a relationship with the person they're working with. Arguably, therapists doing brief therapy need to be even more skilled at relationship-building, given that they have a very short window of time to make a difference (Taibbi, 2014). Developing a connection with your clients is important throughout therapy, but it is especially important early on. Joining happens in our very first contacts with our clients, which is often before we have our initial session. This process continues during our beginning meetings with clients and throughout the course of therapy.

Gathering and organizing information, sometimes called assessment, conceptualization or diagnosis

All therapy involves some type of information gathering and information organizing. Depending on a therapist's assumptions and the particular theory they use, this information gathering process will look different. The questions a therapist asks (or does not ask), how they go about gathering information and how they view the process of organizing this information into a cohesive "story" are all going to be influenced by a therapist's theory (Metcalf, 2011). Being aware of assumptions and biases (or viewpoints one has about a particular subject) is absolutely crucial for effectively gathering information and organizing it (Goodell et al., 2011). Typically, the active assessment process takes from one to three sessions. In general, it is expected that the main assessment process will be finished by the third session. That being said, therapists should continue gathering information throughout the therapy process.

Defining the change that is going to happen/Determining the goals of therapy

Therapy always has a point. As long as the client keeps showing up, there is a reason for them being there. These reasons can vary widely. Clients may be there because of a problem or need that they perceive, because someone else thinks they need to be there or because therapy fulfills some type of need. Understanding the client's reasons for being in therapy is a primary objective in the assessment process. In the goal-setting process, the focus is on defining what is going to be different as a result of therapy.

Change from what [defined in assessment] to what [defined in goals]

Agreeing on the goal of therapy is probably one of the most critical parts of the therapy process.

Change (sometimes called "intervening" or "intervention")

This is the process through which the therapy process helps clients to change. While the most active change process tends to come after several sessions, change can start before the client even comes to therapy. For example, research suggests that clients may experience some improvements in symptoms simply by being placed on a waitlist for therapy, though it should be noted that extended time on a waitlist can have a negative influence on later therapeutic encounters (Borkovec & Sibrava, 2005; Wampold, Minami, Tierney, Baskin & Bhati, 2005). Anything that a therapist does to promote positive change can be called an "intervention". In popular culture, the term "intervention" often brings to mind a meeting where family and friends confront an individual about a problematic behavior. In professional therapy, this type of "intervention" is very rare and is usually not what we mean when we refer to an "intervention". An intervention could involve having a family roleplay how to handle a particular scenario that tends to lead to conflict at home. It could involve a conversation where two members of a couple take turns listening to each other.

An intervention could be something as simple as helping the members of a family agree on a shared goal for therapy. All of these activities can help people start to make changes in how they think, feel, act and interact, thus they can all be called "interventions".

Documentation and evaluation

At various points in your training – including in your classes on ethics, assessment and research – you'll learn more about documenting therapy and evaluating your own effectiveness as a therapist. In the context of this lesson about the use of theory, documentation and evaluation are discussed so that you can understand how your use of theory (something you do conceptually) lines up with your written records of the therapy process and with your efforts to evaluate how therapy is going.

This overview of therapy highlighted five main processes: (a) joining, (b) assessment, (c) goal setting, (d) intervention, and (e) documentation and evaluation. These processes do not happen in a linear, step-by-step fashion but rather overlap and influence each other. These processes are, nonetheless, distinct and important in helping therapists plan their way of working with a client in therapy. These five processes are apparent in the therapy models you'll be studying as you prepare for your MFT work. Therapy models are tools for helping us move through these steps and, as you learn about each therapy model, you can be thinking about how the model facilitates each of these steps.

Anatomy of a therapy model – a guide for learning and applying theories of therapy

Throughout this chapter, we've repeatedly referenced the importance of being aware of assumptions. We've also talked about how the use of theory is a crucial way that we can be more aware of and explicit about our assumptions. Let's look more closely at how theory, include therapy models and other types of theory, comes together with other types of professional knowledge in order to guide us in therapy.

As noted earlier, a theory is a coordinated set of ideas that attempts to explain some phenomenon or situation. A therapy model is a specific type of theory that is designed to guide the therapy process. Models include basic assumptions about human beings, assumptions about how problems form and assumptions about how therapy can help people. In addition to a therapy model, other theories usually supplement our understanding of human beings. For example, there are theories of human development, sexuality, aging, grief and many other aspects of human experience that could supplement your use of a particular model. Usually, additional theories will supplement how you think about human functioning. Where you will rely most heavily on a particular therapy model is when it comes to your theory of change; that is, your theory of how therapy helps people change.

Let's look at the basic anatomy of a therapy model in order to better understand how you'll use a therapy model to guide your work as a therapist. Notice how the anatomy of a therapy model parallels the five processes involved in carrying out therapy.

Terminology note

Assumptions versus concepts: Concepts are a single idea that can typically be expressed in a word or phrase. Assumptions are complete thoughts that can only be articulated in a full sentence. ***Multidirected partiality*** is a concept in contextual therapy, whereas an example of an assumption would be something like, "People heal through feeling understood, thus contextual therapists help promote healing by validating each person's unique experience."

Core assumptions: How would you sum up this model in two or three sentences? What does the model say about people? Does it include a definition of individual or relational health? In what ways does the model reflect systems theory and social constructionism?

Joining and the role of the therapist's personality: All of the MFT models include some guidance about how therapists form productive relationships with clients. You'll see some commonalities among the models, as well as some notable differences. The question that you want to be able to answer about a therapy model is, "how does the model approach building a connection with clients?"

Problem formation: How does the model explain the formation of problems that bring people to therapy?

Assessment concepts: What concepts does the model use in order to view people and the problems that bring people to therapy?

Goals of therapy: What are the goals in this type of therapy? Are there universal goals that this model includes, in addition to goals that are specific to a client's situation? For example, in experiential therapy, self-actualization is typically a goal, over and above resolving the presenting concern.

Interventions: How does this model approach the change process? Each therapy model includes a strategy and set activities for helping clients to resolve their presenting concerns. How are clients expected to change? Does the model target changes in interaction (interpersonal behavior), thinking and meanings, feelings? What does a therapist using this model actually do in order to facilitate change? Do they have conversations with clients? Do they give clients new experiences? Do they promote insight? Do they coach clients on practicing new skills?

Research support: As mentioned earlier, another factor we consider when making decisions about how to conduct therapy is the results of scientific research. Research and theory go hand-in-hand. Theories can be tested in scientific studies and changed on the basis of research. While research can help refine a theory, research cannot exist without theory, that research cannot be carried without a set of guiding assumptions (Goodson Beasley, 2011). When you study theory, it is important to ask whether the theory has been evaluated in research. Being aware of whether a given therapy model has been evaluated in research helps you make decisions about how to work with particular clients and particular concerns.

Think about the five core therapy processes reviewed earlier: joining, assessment, goal setting, intervention and documentation/evaluation. Therapy models are tools for guiding therapists through these five processes. Notice how the anatomy of a therapy model overlaps with these five processes. Models include assumptions about how therapists form relationships (joining), about how problems are conceptualized (assessment), about the goals of therapy (goal setting) and about how change happens (intervention). The structure of a model helps you document, in writing, your therapeutic process (documentation) and the research base for your model is an important factor in evaluating your methods (evaluation). As you study theory and consider various therapy models, think about how each model supports therapists and clients in moving through the therapeutic journey.

The overarching focus in this lesson on theory and treatment planning is on how to use theory to guide you through the processes involved in competent therapy. Specific therapy models are an essential part of this; however, a therapy model is not going to supply all of the theory you'll need in order to be successful. As MFTs, other important theories support

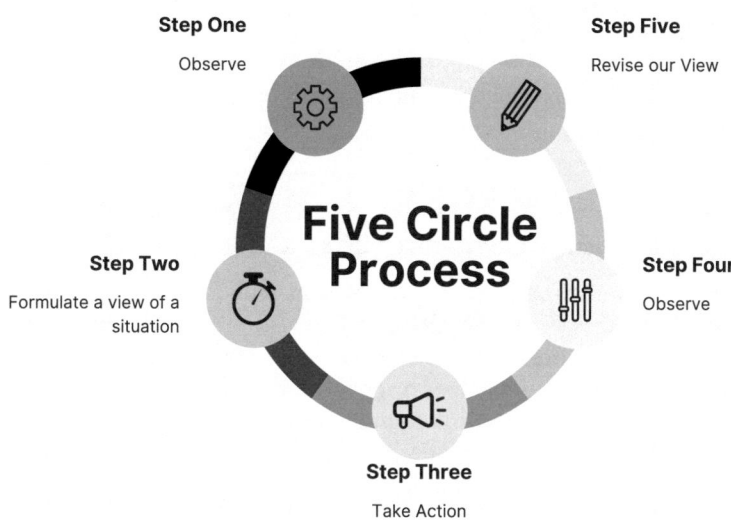

Figure 2.4 Infographic 1: Interactive Process Five Steps.

and complement our use of specific models. The next section will review some important theories that guide MFTs in the core therapy process. It briefly reviews systems theory and social constructionism in order to prepare you for considering how theory guides you in moving through the process of therapy.

Assumptions that are the foundation of how MFTs work with clients (key theories that cut across models)

Throughout this chapter, we've repeatedly referenced the idea that using theory in therapy is a matter of being explicit about the assumptions that are guiding you as you work with clients. A specific therapy model makes up part of your theory foundation, but there are other important theories that will also guide your work as an MFT. Two theories – systems theory and social constructionism – are so important that you study these theories separately before learning about the various therapy models that emerged from these theories. Systems theory and social constructionism were influential in the development of our field's main models, and they are important enough that we continue to study them separately from the therapy models. Understanding the defining assumptions of systems theory and social constructionism is essential for preparing you to work as a marriage and family therapist. The assumptions of systems theory and social constructionism are some of the most consequential for how you will actually work with people as a therapist. Even if you end up carefully studying one of the particular MFT models you'll learn about during your graduate study, if you don't internalize the assumptions of systems theory and social constructionism, you won't be fully prepared to succeed as an MFT.

This chapter is not intended to be a comprehensive overview of systems theory and social constructionism. A brief review of the defining assumptions is included here in order to help you understand how these assumptions form the foundation for therapy processes, regardless of which particular model you're using.

Systems theory as a set of assumptions that form the basis for MFT practice and that are essential to the therapy models that MFTs use

Earlier in this chapter we presented a simple scenario in which a friend approached you for relationship help. The purpose of this thought exercise was to introduce the idea of examining assumptions. The process of helping someone can go many different ways, depending on the assumptions that the helper brings to the process. In the MFT field, there is a particular set of assumptions that are the foundation for the way that MFTs work with clients. This set of assumptions – known collectively as "systems theory" – is what unites professionals from many different backgrounds under the common identity "Marriage and Family Therapist".

We will briefly review the core assumptions of systems theory. It is important because the assumptions of systems theory have implications for how **all** MFTs conduct therapy, regardless of what particular model or models of therapy they use. In your training as an MFT, being able to carry out therapy in a way that is consistent with systems theory is essential to your professional identity. This is what makes you an MFT. At many points along your professional journey, you will need to demonstrate your ability to use systems theory to carry out therapy. This is a requirement to graduate from NCU's master's and doctoral programs in MFT. This is also a primary focus during the post-degree supervision process for therapists who want to be licensed as MFTs. And, perhaps most significantly, being grounded in systems theory assumptions is a primary focus in the MFT licensing examination.

Watzlawick, Beavin Bavelas and Jackson (1967) outline several key assumptions of human communication that form the basis for systems theory. These include:

Circular causality is necessary to understand the vast majority of human issues. In most situations, things happen simultaneously, and they mutually influence each other.

The idea of a system focuses on any group of parts that is capable of exchanging information and adjusting behavior on the basis that that information is going to develop **patterns of interaction**.

All behavior makes sense when viewed in the appropriate context. All behavior is communication; that is all behavior is **interpersonal/contextual**.

Social constructionism as the foundation to MFT practice and MFT models

Social constructionism is a theory with its roots in Enlightenment era philosophy that was brought into the social sciences in the late 20th century (Mercadal, 2019). It explains how people develop stories or narratives to make sense of their experiences. This storytelling process is fundamentally social in that our stories always have an audience and individuals inherit many stories from their social circles, including their immediate families, communities and broader cultural contexts. Individual personal narratives are frequently a tapestry that weaves together societal stories. Social constructionism has important implications for how MFTs approach assessment, regardless of what model or models of therapy a therapist might use.

Key social constructionist assumptions

Human beings are meaning-making creatures. We are always in the process of making sense of things. We put experiences into stories.

How we make sense of things is personal but also socially influenced. This means that there are always multiple perspectives on a situation and that how we make sense of experiences is influenced by our contexts (Mercadal, 2019).

Meanings are fluid (evolving) and this evolution happens in the context of relationships. *The power dynamics of social relationships affect the meaning-making process.* Therapists usually have power. The therapy process is not just a discovery process; it is a meaning-making process. How you ask about a situation will shape the way that the situation is understood (Gergen, 1985).

Summary

The material you just reviewed focused on two theories that are foundational to the way that MFTs think and work: systems theory and social constructionism. The assumptions that make up these two theories are woven throughout the specific therapy models you'll study in your MFT training. Moreover, the assumptions of systems theory and social constructionism provide essential theoretical guidance for therapists moving through the core processes of therapy. At this point, we will look specifically at how therapists move through and plan out the therapeutic journey. Throughout this chapter, we will consider how theory (including systems theory, social constructionism and specific therapy models) acts as a map or guide for the therapeutic journey with our clients.

References

Borkovec, T. D. & Sibrava, N. J. (2005). Problems with the use of placebo conditions in psychotherapy research, suggested alternatives, and some strategies for the pursuit of the placebo phenomenon. *Journal of Clinical Psychology, 61*, 805–818.

Davis, S. D., Lebow, J. & Sprenkle, D. H. (2012). Common factors of change in couple therapy. *Behavior Therapy, 43*(1), 36–48.

de Shazer, S. & Dolan, Y., Korman, H., Trepper, T., McCollum, E. & Berg, I. K. (2012). *More than miracles: the state of solution-focused brief therapy*. New York, NY: Taylor & Francis.

Fife, S. T., Whiting, J. B., Bradford, K. & Davis, S. (2014). The therapeutic pyramid: a common factors synthesis of techniques, alliance, and way of being. *Journal of Marital and Family Therapy, 40*(1), 20–33.

Friedlander, M. L., Escudero, V., Welmers-van de Poll, M. J. & Heatherington, L. (2018). Meta-analysis of the alliance-outcome relation in couple and family therapy. *Psychotherapy, 55*(4), 356–371.

Gergen, K. J. (1985). The social constructionist movement in modern psychology. *American Psychologist, 40*(3), 266–275.

Givropoulou, D. & Tseliou, E. (2021). Developing reflexivity through group processes in psychotherapy training: an interpretative phenomenological analysis of Systemic Family Therapy trainees' experience. *Family Process, 60*(2), 346–360.

Goodell, K. A., Sudderth, B. G. & Allan, C. D. (2011). The self of the therapist. *Marriage and Family Therapy: A Practice-Oriented Approach*, 21–38.

Goodson Beasley, E. M. (2011). Research in marriage and family therapy. In L. Metcalf (Ed.), *Marriage and family therapy: a practice-oriented approach* (pp. 443–474). New York, NY: Springer.

Levounis, P., Arnaout, B. & Marienfeld, C. (2017). *Motivational interviewing for clinical practice*. Arlington, VA: American Psychiatric Association Publishing.

Mercadal, T. (2019). *Social constructionism*. Salem Press Encyclopedia. New Jersey, NJ: Grey House Publishing, Inc.

Metcalf, L. (2011). *Marriage and family therapy: a practice-oriented approach*. New York, NY: Springer Publishing Company.

Onken, S. J., Craig, C. M., Ridgway, P., Ralph, R. O. & Cook, J. A. (2007). An analysis of the definitions and elements of recovery: a review of the literature. *Psychiatric Rehabilitation Journal*, 31(1), 9.

Sharf, R. S. (2016). *Theories of psychotherapy and counseling: concepts and cases* (6th ed.). Boston, MA: Cengage Learning.

Sprenkle, D. H., Lebow, J. & Davis, S. D. (2009). *Common factors in couple and family therapy: the overlooked foundation for effective practice*. New York, NY: The Guilford Press.

Stratton, P. (2016). *The evidence base of family therapy and systemic practice*. London, UK: Association for Family Therapy.

Taibbi, R. (2014). *Boot camp therapy: brief, action-oriented clinical approaches to anxiety, anger, & depression*. New York, NY: W. W. Norton.

Wampold, B. E., Minami, T., Tierney, S. C., Baskin, T. W. & Bhati, K. S. (2005). The placebo is powerful: estimating placebo effects in medicine and psychotherapy from randomized clinical trials. *Journal of Clinical Psychology, 61*, 835–854.

Watzlawick, P., Beavin Baveles, J. & Jackson, D. D. (1967). *Pragmatics of human communication: a study of interactional patterns, pathologies, and paradoxes*. New York, NY: Norton.

White, J. M. & Klein, D. M. (2008). *Family Theories* (3rd ed.). Thousand Oaks, CA: SAGE Publications.

3 History of Family Therapy

Patricia Postanowicz

Introduction

Marriage and family therapy (MFT) has existed as a field for approximately 60 years. But the groundwork for this career was laid decades prior (Bond, 2009). This chapter will focus on the history and development of this field. The goal is to provide a high-level view of the journey it took for MFT to become a separate entity from other helping professions such as psychiatry, psychology, social work and counseling. It will also cover the direction the field is moving in currently and the exciting things happening now that will impact the future of the field.

MFTs will often say when asked that being an MFT is more than just a job, it is a way of life, a life perspective, and the principles of relational thinking and ideals infuse not only in our professional lives, but also in our personal lives. MFTs are taught to see the wide-angle lens, considering the influence of multiple factors on individual and relational problems. However, it can be argued that many people considering a career as an MFT already have this perspective. It is almost hard-wired into their vision, and that this way of seeing problems is less about learning a new skill and more about sharpening a tool that already exists in a student's tool belt. But, for some students, this is a new way of thinking and it can take some time to move from a more traditional way of seeing interpersonal issues to one that takes into account the influence of others on the identified client or patient.

To say that therapy is a mix of art and science is an understatement. Therapy done well is a symphony of give and take between therapists and clients, and there is great care and planning that goes into this exchange. However, there is also an underlying compassion and empathy that therapists must have in order for clients to feel safe enough to explore difficult and often very confusing situations (Moyers & Miller, 2013). These qualities provide the basis for creating a strong therapeutic alliance, which has been shown to lead to better outcomes for clients (Horvath, del Re, Flückiger & Symonds., 2011).

Our journey begins as one that was very much connected with many fields, including psychology, social work, psychiatry, biology and engineering (Bond, 2009), but it diverged over time to become a field all of its own. But it is important to acknowledge that our field is one of many that provides counseling and services for mental health concerns. We offer a unique perspective in the larger mental health arena, but we often overlap with psychology, social work and case management as part of our daily work.

Before we move into what makes marriage and family therapy different to other disciplines, it is important to acknowledge that our history is one that is difficult to tell. Not because there is not a good record of our developments, but because of one of the key

DOI: 10.4324/9781003382621-5

perspectives of systemic thinking – that multiple perspectives exist. In essence, the telling of our history reflects the perspective of the person writing the narrative. What is included, or ignored, emphasized or downplayed, all show the bias of the narrator. To which we only have one answer and that is to own that perspective. It would be impossible to trace every person's story who was a part of the foundation of our field and, as you will soon see, there are so many overlaps in both people, theory and perspective that the family tree of MFT is a large, winding, often confusing ball of roots and branches. Untangling all of that to show how this field developed is challenging, but it is an important venture, so it is with the knowledge that there is no one definite version of the information that we forge ahead. The field of MFT began with a series of questions: do families operate in a way that is predictable and changeable, can we implement change within a family at the individual level and see that change throughout the family? And what causes a family to resist change, at the emotional and psychological cost of its members?

The roots of family therapy are shared with other **helping professions** (e.g., in the use of talk therapy). Jung, Freud, Adler, Skinner and Rogers all were heavily influential in our work and while these therapists may not have directly worked with families, their belief in creating an environment for change through the process of counseling is essential to our development as a field (Bond, 2009). There is also another important movement to acknowledge and that is the **child guidance movement**. The 1920s saw a shift in emphasis away from institutionalization of those with mental health issues to a focus on prevention and addressing early childhood causes for later mental health concerns (Weinstein, 2013). It also shifted the view of what caused problems from issues of class or heredity to "bad parenting" (Weinstein, 2013, p. 20). While the movement away from institutionalization and to a more context-based and preventive approach was positive and important, the movement was criticized for allowing doctors and therapists to blame parents (usually the mothers) for the children's behavior. Eventually, child guidance workers saw that the work with families was even more effective than the work with children alone, and they moved away from placing blame on parents to "situating pathology within relationship interaction" (Bond, 2009, p. 130).

The understanding that a child's behavior may be a symptom of a larger family issue was not a new thought but it was revolutionary to shift the focus of assessment and treatment from the child to the family. The fact that these pioneers were considering children at all was also a relatively new phenomenon. For the greater part of human history, children were not seen as a particularly protected class. The concept of a "childhood" is one that is only a few hundred years old and was only present in Western industrialized cultures (Aries, 1965; Lowe, 2009; Thane, 1981). To even consider that children needed to be protected and nurtured was a step in a radical direction and to involve family in this discussion was an even more radical step. This shift in the way that children are perceived in the social and family contexts, paired with the growth of the child guidance movement, sowed the seeds for the creation of a counseling field, dedicated to understanding the complex interactions and behaviors of a family; family therapy was about to be born.

The early days

Marriage and family therapists regularly use the term "systemic". It is important to know what this means. A **system** can be defined as "an organized whole" whose parts are "necessarily interdependent" (Minuchin, 1985, p. 289). In other words, a system is a group where the members of the group are affected by and affect each other. As such, no one family member can take all the blame or responsibility for any other family member or the family as a whole (Bateson, 1972).

The very idea that families could be considered systems is a relatively new concept. Systemic thinking reflects an understanding that members influence one another in a group and that behavior isn't as simple as A causes B, but rather A is impacted by B and B is impacted by A. For instance, in traditional linear psychotherapeutic thinking, a client might present with the complaint that "my wife is ignoring me so I drink and stay out with my friends". The client is using linear causality; his drinking is caused by his wife's attitude. However, using a systemic perspective, the problem becomes more complicated, wife ignores husband, husband is hurt, he drinks and stays out with friends as avoidance and punishment, wife is hurt and withdraws from husband, and so on and so on, the pattern is circular. This understanding is what makes the work of MFT different from the other helping professions and it came from the work of many early founding therapists.

In the1940s, Joseph Macy brought together a number of scholars and researchers in order to discuss how groups of things operate and influence each other and from this **General Systems Theory** was born (Bateson, 1972). From this conference, many exciting things happened and one of them was that Gregory Bateson, along with several others, formed the Bateson research group in 1953 to begin to consider how to best approach the idea that families could be considered systems (Bateson, 1972). From the work of the Bateson group, another important set of ideas emerged: cybernetics.

Cybernetics is a field of study focused on the ways in which systems self-regulate through the use of feedback. Through the lens of cybernetics, actions are viewed as having a circular (rather than linear) causality and the context is viewed as paramount in understanding any event (Bateson, 1972). Cybernetics looks at the behavior of all sorts of things that are capable of adjusting their behavior based on information from the environment. Just as the captain of a ship makes adjustments in response to waves and wind and other factors, family members are continually adjusting their behavior in response to what they are seeing from those around them.

Cybernetics began a conversation that continues to this day, which includes questions such as: How do families develop the characteristic patterns that make them unique? What leads families to stay the same over time, and how do families change? And what role can a therapist have in this change? Bateson and several others (Jay Haley, Don Jackson, John Weakland, to name a few) formed the Bateson group, which considered the question of communication within families. The Bateson group contributed heavily to our field but the most well-known contribution to come out of this group was the concept of the double bind. Bateson and his colleagues worked primarily with patients who had been diagnosed with schizophrenia and from this work they conceptualized that the symptoms of schizophrenia were a result of unusual communication patterns created out of family interactions characterized by double binds (Bateson, 1972; Duncan, 2001). In this way, we began to understand that individual behavior is connected to the behaviors of others and is a product of those interactions and not just an issue that exists within the psyche of the patient (Bateson, 1972).

This, of course, is not to say that issues of mental health are caused by families. In the years since the Bateson group and others worked in the field of schizophrenia, it is clear that science supports a primarily genetic component to this and many other severe mental illnesses. Researchers have found that schizophrenia has "high heritability" with estimates of 64%–81% (Bergen et al., 2019, p. 29; Sullivan, Kendler & Neal, 2003). However, the primary point is still valid. What we know is that an individual's experience is shaped by those around them and that our behaviors are products of the interactions we have with those in our family and other systems influential to us. This reflects the concept that "the whole is greater than the sum of its' parts", which means that an individual cannot be understood unless the individual's system is considered and analyzed (Watzlawicz, Beavelas & Jackson, 1967). Something as complex as a family cannot be broken down into small parts and examined to explain the larger family problem. We need more information, not less, and, when it comes to families, what we need is to see the entire family in action to truly understand the nuanced way a family operates.

The Bateson group did some wonderful work and spurred another group that would be foundational to the movement of family therapy, **the Mental Research Institute (MRI)**. Founded in Palo Alto, CA in 1962 by Don Jackson and Virginia Satir, among others, it focused on developing a more relationally and communication focused approach that brought family therapy to the forefront (Bond, 2009). Soon Jay Haley, Richard Fisch, Paul Watzalwick and John Weakland joined the group (notice the overlap between Bateson's group and MRI). MRI's lasting impact on family therapy would be in the form of two very important contributions: one is the creation of strategic therapy and the other is the formation of the field's first academic journal, *Family Process* (originally edited by Don Jackson and Nathan Ackerman), which exists to this day.

The 1960s saw a flurry of activity in the development of this field and it is worth noting that, while much of that activity was happening on the west coast of the U.S., Salvador Minuchin was doing his part to bring the conversations about systemic thinking to the east coast. In 1965, he founded **the Philadelphia Child Guidance Clinic** and began work on creating one of the foundational theories of family therapy: structural family therapy (Gehart, 2014). This modality operated on the fundamental principle that families had an "underlying organization" (Bond, 2009). While the Palo Alto group worked mainly with families where mental illness was the presenting complaint, Minuchin worked with families whose socioeconomic status put them at high risk for a variety of family problems. In 1967, Jay Haley came across the country to join Minuchin and the Philadelphia Child Guidance Clinic is still in operation to this day, working with families and training therapists in the use of structural family therapy (Gehart, 2014).

In addition to the work of Bateson and Minuchin, the 1960s and 1970s were a significant growth period for work in couple and family therapy. Therapists all over the U.S. and the world were collaborating and innovating in various areas of therapeutic theory and intervention. Some of the most important strides in the history of MFT came in a relatively short period of time. From Bowen's work in **natural systems theory** to develop **intergenerational family therapy**, to Nagy's work in **contextual family therapy** and Whitaker's work with **symbolic experiential therapy**, there was a tremendous excitement in this period and it led to an explosion of new ideas and theories. Some were based in traditional **psychodynamic and behavioral approaches**, augmented to accommodate a systemic perspective and others were rooted firmly in **humanistic work** based on Rogers and Erickson (Bond, 2009).

This time period was also one of great social unrest, particularly in the U.S. The 1960s and 1970s brought about significant social change in terms of civil rights and the rise of feminism. Many people were challenging the notions of separate but equal, and racism and sexism, along with classism and the rise of the gay rights movement, were creating an environment of pushing back against the status quo. Lives were lost, people were arrested and jailed, riots broke out across the country, all in the name of fighting for rights previously denied for many American citizens. The notion that "all men were created equal"

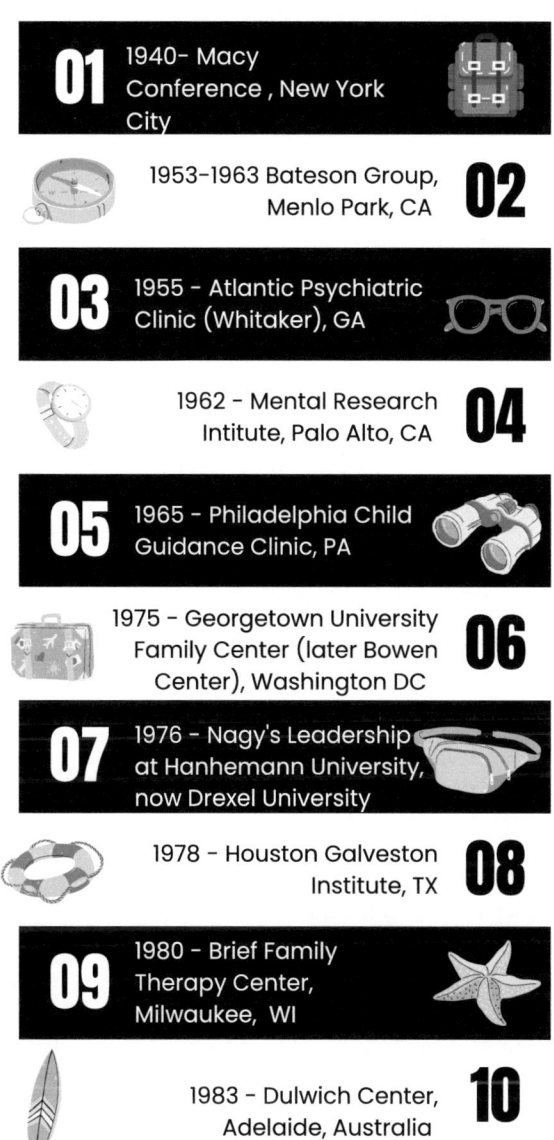

Significant Moments in
MFT

01 1940– Macy Conference , New York City

1953–1963 Bateson Group, Menlo Park, CA **02**

03 1955 - Atlantic Psychiatric Clinic (Whitaker), GA

1962 - Mental Research Intitute, Palo Alto, CA **04**

05 1965 - Philadelphia Child Guidance Clinic, PA

1975 - Georgetown University Family Center (later Bowen Center), Washington DC **06**

07 1976 - Nagy's Leadership at Hanhemann University, now Drexel University

1978 - Houston Galveston Institute, TX **08**

09 1980 - Brief Family Therapy Center, Milwaukee, WI

1983 - Dulwich Center, Adelaide, Australia **10**

Figure 3.1 Infographic 4: Significant Moments in MFT Infographic.

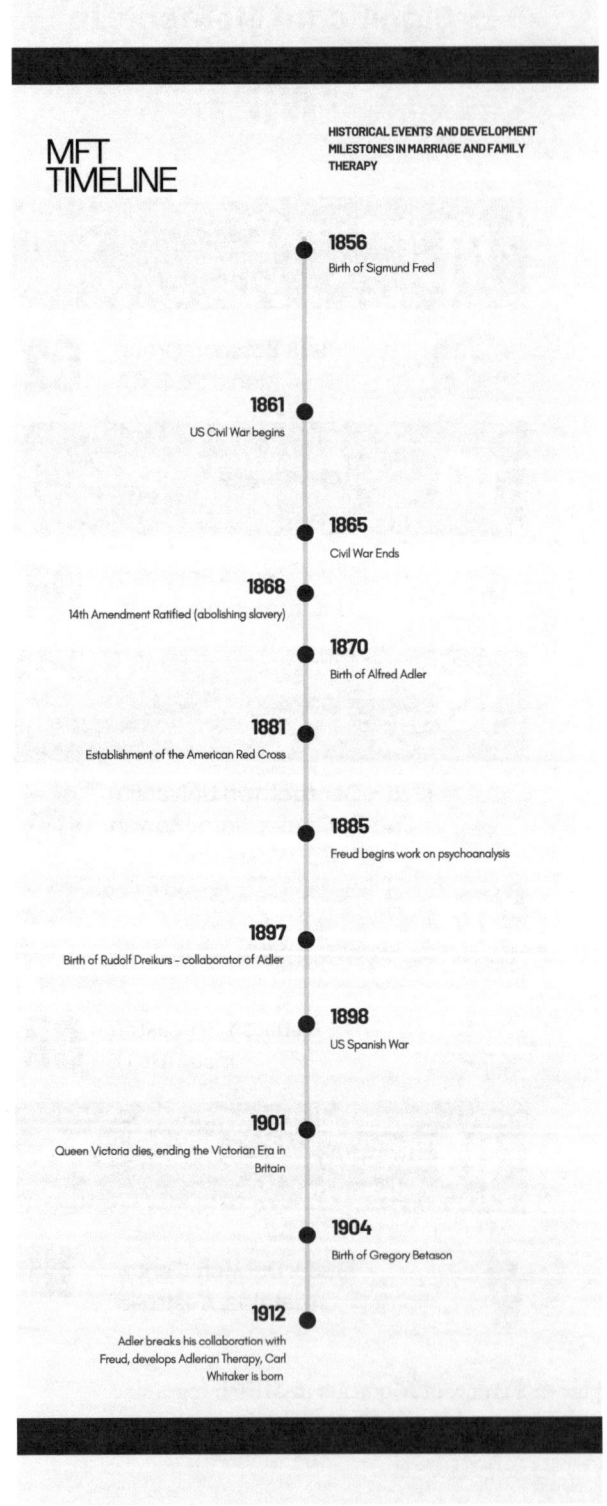

Figure 3.2 Infographic 5: MFT Timeline Development and History Infographic.

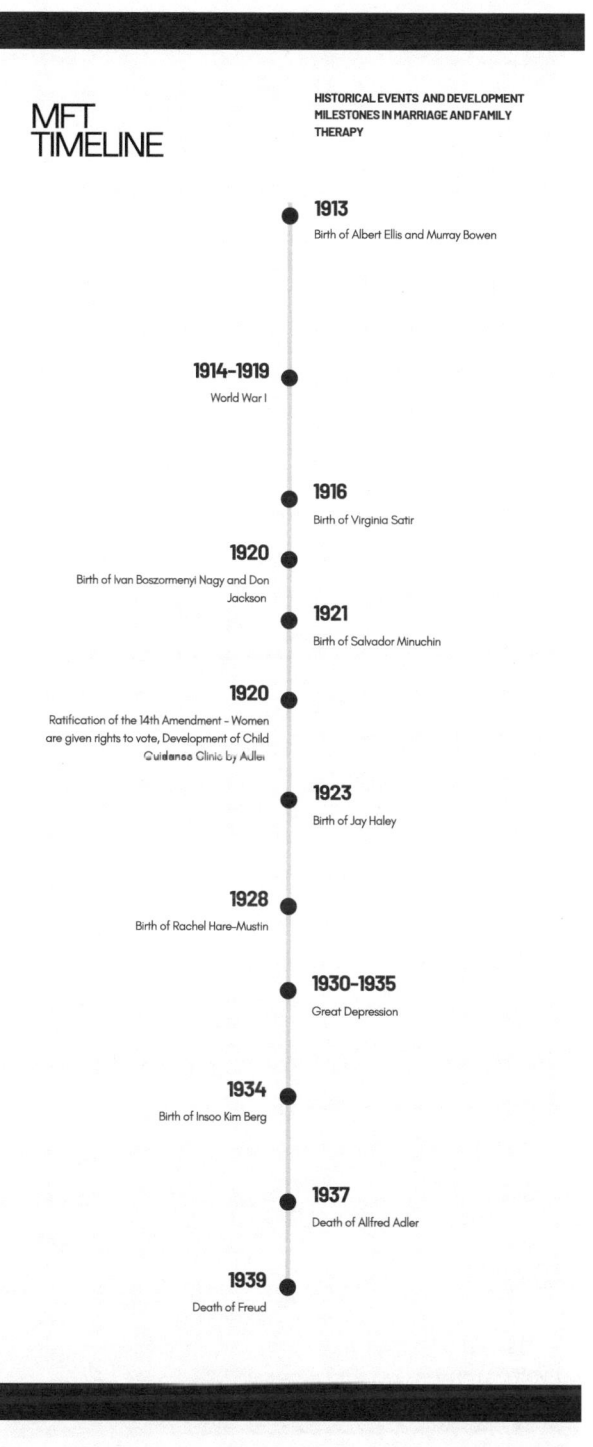

Figure 3.2 (Continued)

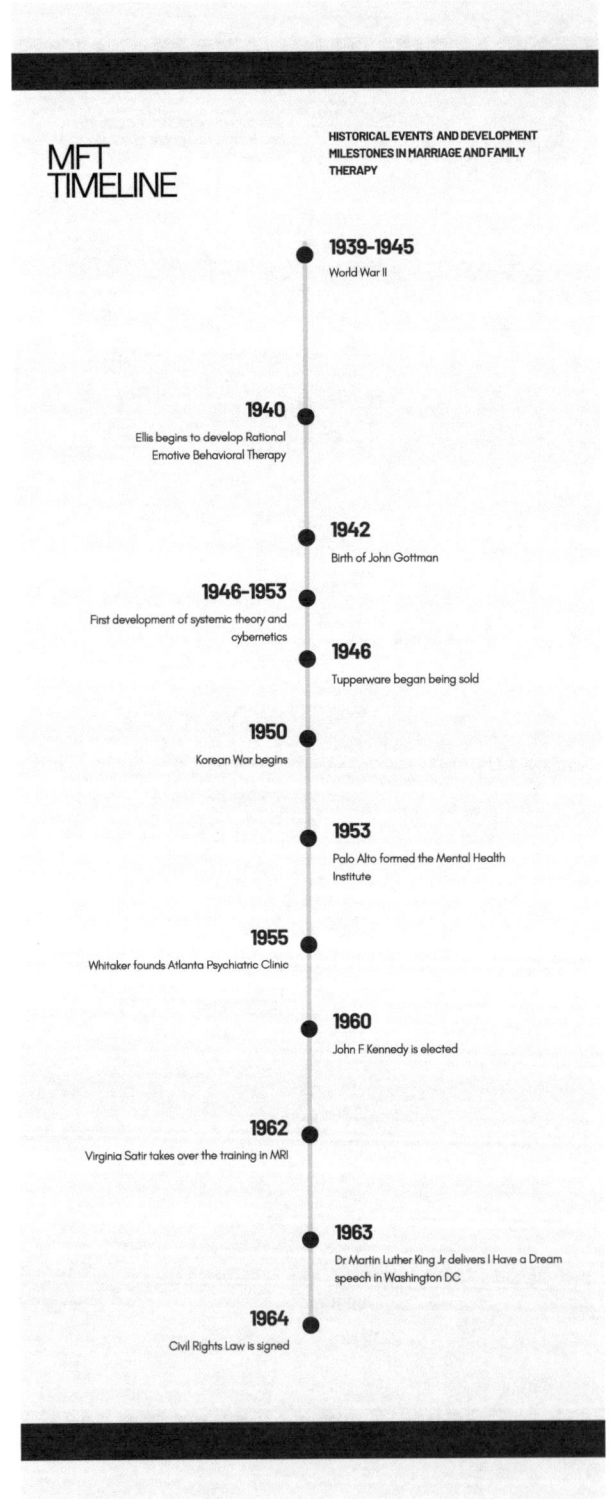

Figure 3.2 (Continued)

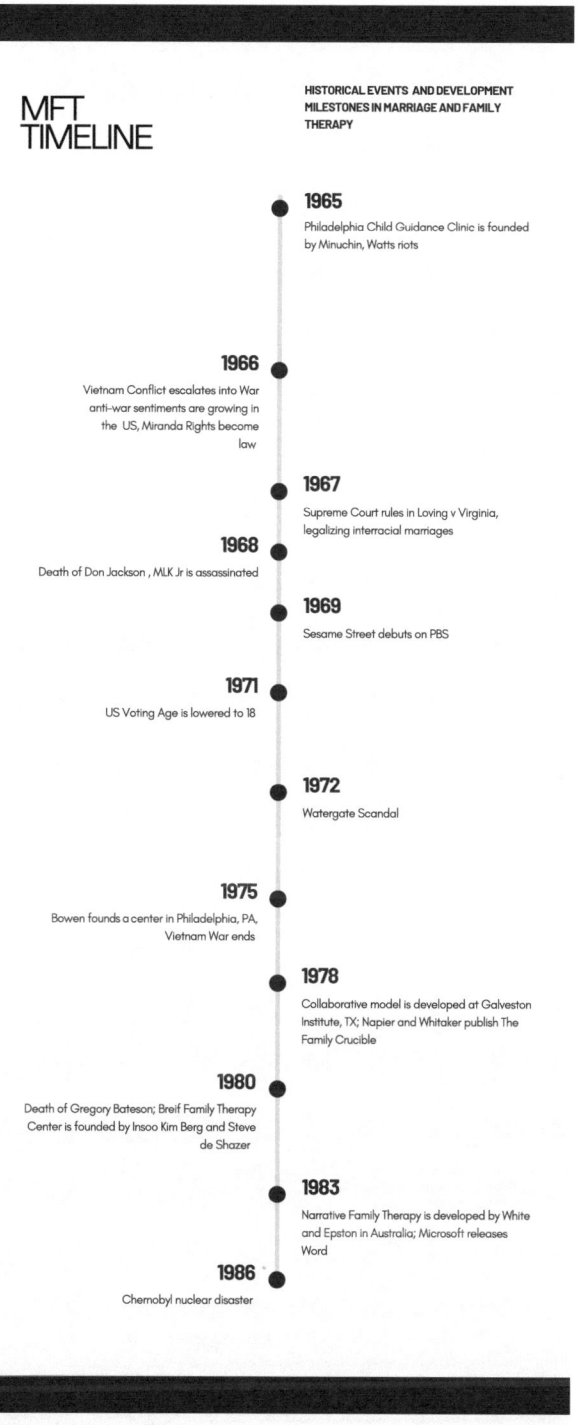

Figure 3.2 (Continued)

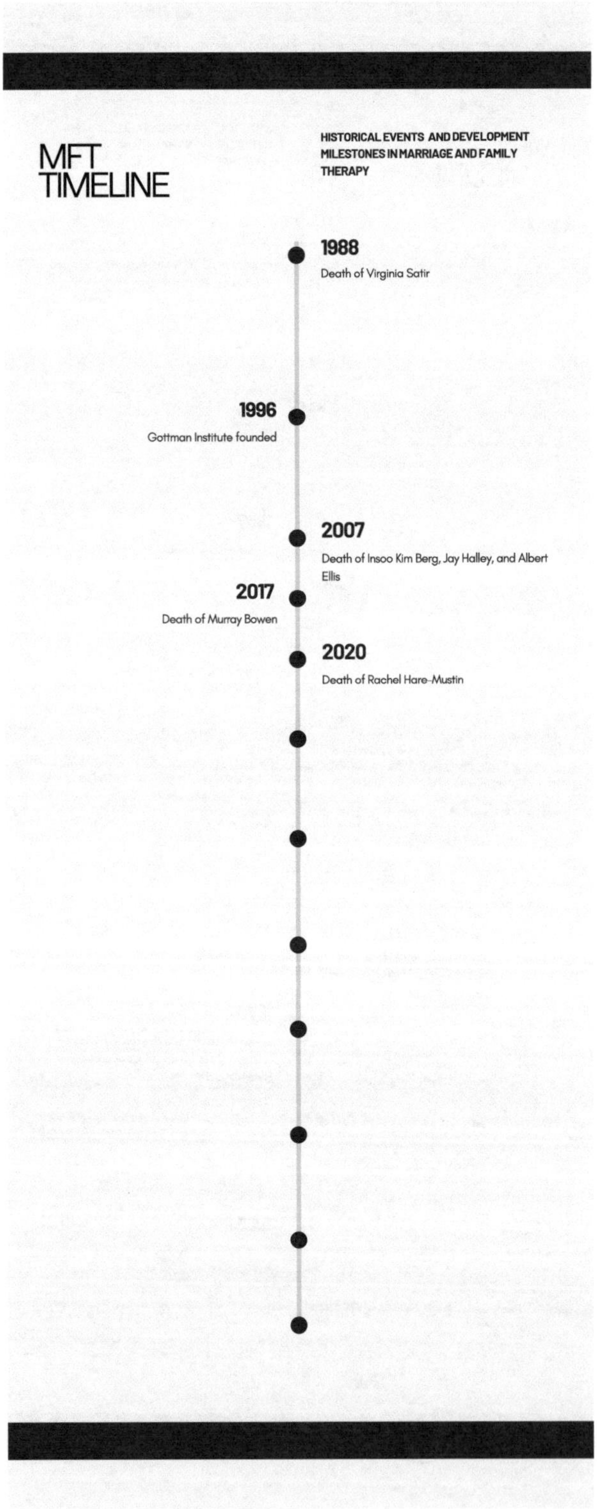

MFT TIMELINE

HISTORICAL EVENTS AND DEVELOPMENT
MILESTONES IN MARRIAGE AND FAMILY
THERAPY

1988
Death of Virginia Satir

1996
Gottman Institute founded

2007
Death of Insoo Kim Berg, Jay Halley, and Albert Ellis

2017
Death of Murray Bowen

2020
Death of Rachel Hare-Mustin

Figure 3.2 (Continued)

was given significant lip service, but, in reality, many people in our country were victims of hate, intimidation and violence all because they weren't White, male, heterosexual or middle class.

MFT as a field did not exist in a vacuum and was certainly influenced by the changes that were happening in the larger society. Even though the work of the founding mothers and fathers of our field was based in real life experience with clients, there was also a shift happening in the very paradigm of therapy. Students of the therapists mentioned above were beginning to question the very nature of their relationships with clients, the bedrocks of the therapeutic endeavor, and new voices began to emerge at the dawn of the 1970s, which moved family therapy into a direction of focusing more on **social justice** and the **postmodern perspective**. The late 1980s also brought feminist critiques of the modernist models. These critiques focused on the failures of the models to address power dynamics and gender roles in how families and family issues were conceptualized (Bond, 2009).

Transition from modern models to postmodern models

There has been discussion within our field for years as to the differences between modern models (known in some readings as the traditional or classic models) and the postmodern models. Some focus on the difference in the metaphors each uses; the modern models use a systems metaphor to look at families, while the postmodern models use a social constructionist lens. Others look at the differences in the role of the therapist in the therapeutic relationship, and still others look at the role the therapist plays in advocacy for issues of social justice, power dynamics and empowering the lived experience in underserved and underrepresented communities.

However, it is important to consider that, while all of the above is likely accurate to some extent, the important thing to understand is that there is a difference and that both sets of approaches are useful and relevant in our work today. It is also important to understand the sociocultural environment that led to the shift in our field. It is believed that the social unrest of the late 1960s and early 1970s had a dramatic impact on how leaders in our field saw their roles in working with clients. The rise of civil rights concerns, the increase in discussion about the role of **feminism** in our work and the shift in the role of the therapist as "expert" were all contributing to a rise in new approaches to therapy that would carry us into the 21st century. These new, postmodern models sought to shift the therapist into a **non-pathologizing** stance where they are able to honor multiple perspectives and "refrain from privileging their knowing over the client's knowing" (D'Arrigo-Patrick, Hoff, Knudson-Martin & Tuttle, 2017, p. 576).

At this point, it is likely to be helpful to provide some definitions of concepts like postmodernism and social constructionism. These concepts will be covered more in detail when specific therapies fitting the postmodern lens are discussed, but in terms of an introduction:

Postmodernism a philosophy that rejects the existence of an objective reality or "truth" and questions the necessity for a search for one truth, but rather encourages the embracing of multiple perspectives. There are several postmodern assumptions; the most important of which is that reality is constructed by our experiences and the interactions in which we engage. This philosophy eschews the idea of Objective Truth, in favor of the view that all knowledge is filtered through our perception and is, thus, inherently subjective (Maturana & Varela, 1987).

Social constructionism a specific theory of knowledge that was an important part of the postmodern movement. Social constructionism, as a theory, suggests that what we consider to be true and real is largely shaped by the complex interactions of social groups. At its most basic level, social constructionism states that our understanding of our world and everything in it is based on the collective, subjective truths of our society (Gergen, 1985). Why does green mean "go" and red mean "stop"? Why do we consider a 17-year-old a child and an 18-year-old an adult? What makes driving on the right-hand side of the road the correct way? For that matter, why do we call it "left and right"? These are the sorts of questions asked by social constructionists.

Perhaps the most important part of social constructionism is the understanding that **language** is not a representation of reality but rather shapes how we see the world.

When we attach words to the world around us, we are actively attributing meaning to the world. It is through social processes, particularly our use of language, that things take on meaning. Social constructionists are essentially saying that human beings are storytellers. We construct meaning around experiences by putting experiences into language (Gergen, 1985). This process of attaching language to experience is determined by our social setting. There is not one correct "story" to attach to each experience. The same experiences and facts can be "storied" in many different ways.

In terms of work with clients, it is important to understand that the words they use may mean different things to them than they do to us and we can never assume we know what they mean; we need to ask.

Postmodern models

There are several MFT models that fall under the umbrella of postmodern. However, there are three models that stand out for their influence and contribution to moving the field of MFT forward in both their ability to be effective with a diverse clientele and their brevity, which has become more and more the desired type of model used by therapists in the field. All of these models will be covered more in depth later in subsequent chapters, but an introduction to the therapists responsible for these theories follow here.

The first of these models is **Solution-Focused Therapy** and it was created by Insoo Kim Berg and Steve de Shazer at the Milwaukee Brief Family Therapy Center in the early 1980s and evolved into several different types of solution-based therapies, including Solution-Oriented Therapy, developed by Bill O'Hanlon and Michelle Weiner-Davis (O'Hanlon & Weiner-Davis, 1989). Berg and de Shazer published extensively about the model and it has become one of the most researched models in family therapy (Berg, 1994, Berg & Jaya, 1993, Berg & Szabo, 2005, de Shazer, 1985; de Shazer, 1988;). In an interesting aside, Scott Miller, who was trained under Berg and de Shazer, has gone on to spearhead the common factors movement. That movement focuses on the study of multiple counseling theories to discover what they all have in common that helps clients achieve success in therapy (Miller, Seidel & Hubble, 2015).

The next model is **Narrative Therapy** and it was created by Michael White and David Epston in Australia and New Zealand in the early 1990s (Gehart, 2014). Narrative Therapy focuses on how people construct the stories of their lives, and how often people will become stuck because they are in a problem-saturated narrative; thus, they become convinced that change is impossible. But Narrative Therapy seeks to shift the focus from the narrative that contains the problem to a narrative that contains the solutions to the problem, thus breaking the cycle and telling a new story (White, 1995; White & Epston, 1990). Narrative Therapy is often connected to the third approach, Collaborative language systems therapy in that it shares many of the same assumptions and the therapist's role is very similar in how change is initiated.

Collaborative Language Systems Therapy was the product of Harlene Anderson and Harry Goolishian, who worked together in Houston, TX and established the Houston Galveston Institute, which was influenced by the work done decades earlier at the MRI. In addition to Anderson and Goolishian, Tom Andersen, Lynne Hoffman and Peggy Penn have all been influential in developing Collaborative Language Systems Therapy (Gehart, 2014). This therapy approach is perhaps the most postmodern in the approaches listed above in that it sets out to have the relationship between the therapist and clients as collaborators in the journey of therapy. The role of expert is shared between the therapist and the client, with both contributing to the journey of the therapy and the therapist posing questions to the client in an open and curious way. To the layperson, Collaborative Language Systems Therapy can sound like a conversation between friends over coffee, but, in fact, it is a complex set of carefully crafted give and take between therapist and client (Anderson, 1997; Anderson & Goolishan, 1992).

The exciting work of those listed above and many others continue to push the field of MFT into new and diverse directions. In a field that continues to grow both in terms of acceptance in the community and interest for those wanting to pursue a career in the helping professions, it is an exciting time to be an MFT. As exciting as this growth is, there are also hurdles to overcome and a changing landscape of health care to navigate.

New horizons

Currently all 50 states and the District of Columbia, as well as Puerto Rico, offer licensure in MFT (AAMFT, 2017). More and more countries all over the world are also recognizing this profession through licensure and with the creation of the International Family Therapy Association (IFTA), as well as the Canadian Association of MFT and several other country-specific associations; the field is growing larger than ever. However, this was not always the case. In fact, licensure for marriage and family therapists is a relatively new process. California was the first state to offer licensure and that was in 1967. And the relationship between licensure and insurance coverage is one that is important to understand. In the early days of our field, therapists were practicing without much oversight and were not regulated by the states they were working in. Often, they might have licensures in psychology or social work, but they were practicing MFT. But they were having trouble getting paid for their services because MFT was not a recognized profession due to lack of licensure. And, so, the necessity of licensure and oversight of our profession began.

This level of oversight is important for both the client and the therapist to be protected and it adds a level of importance to the work we do. But, as in many cases where good intentions lead to difficult consequences, the legitimization of our profession led to an increase in the influence of third-party payers.

In the beginning of the MFT relationship with insurance agencies, it was believed that the addition of MFT services would benefit clients who wanted therapy but were unable to pay out of pocket for sessions. However, currently there is a challenge that MFTs face; staying true to our philosophical roots of systemic treatment while attempting to work within a health care system that requires that diagnosis be given for payment of services. Several therapists have written about their experiences with managed care, for better or worse, and it continues to be an ever-evolving relationship that gets more complicated as health care reform gets debated and decided in the federal government (Ackley, 1998; Duncan, 2001; Freeny, 1994). It is important not to be discouraged though, it is important to be informed. The pace at which the field is changing and growing is quite rapid and the work we are doing now as advocates for our clients has been groundbreaking in terms of both change at the individual system and the community system levels.

Currently, there are more than **48,000 licensed** marriage and family therapists in the U.S. (AAMFT, 2017). In addition to private practice, MFTs work in agencies (both state and federally funded), hospitals, schools, prisons, churches, residential treatment centers, outpatient treatment centers, private and publicly-owned companies and corporations as consultants and members of employee assistant programs, and many, many other settings (Bureau of Labor Statistics, 2016). As our world becomes more and more connected, and as traditional definitions of a family and a marriage become more evolved and inclusive, we find ourselves working with clients from diverse religious, cultural, racial and ethnic backgrounds. We are tasked to grow in our understanding of sexual orientation and gender identity, polyamory and open relationships, and a variety of subcultures related to family relationships. While this can be overwhelming for new therapists, rest assured that you will get many opportunities for learning and exposure to groups and issues that may be foreign to you in your experiences thus far.

Another exciting development is how technology will impact our work. Ten years ago, there were no master's or doctoral programs in MFT that were both available online and accredited by Commission on Accreditation for Marriage and Family Therapy Education (COAMFTE). Now there are three universities that have accredited online master's programs and one with an accredited online doctoral program, with more on the way. More and more therapists are integrating technology into their practices in terms of electronic case notes and real time updates to treatment plans in session with clients. Perhaps the most exciting development in our field in recent years is the presence of **teletherapy**. The impact of the 2020 pandemic cannot be understated in the growth of the use of teletherapy. The massive shift of many services to an online format in the years of the pandemic forced many hold outs for the viability for online therapy to have to quickly switch to using this platform, with varied success. The frenzied way that therapists were left to accommodate a massive public health crisis served as a reminder that we need to stay flexible in our approaches to mental health care to best serve our clients. There are many exciting developments that have come as a result of this crisis: many states are accounting for the delivery of telehealth services in their licensing standards, COAMFTE has adjusted their stance on web-based therapy delivered by student therapists and insurance companies have continued to reimburse providers for telehealth at the same rates they are reimbursing for in-person therapy. This isn't to say that the use of telehealth services for therapy is a closed subject. There is still a lot of discussion and debate to be had about how to regulate this space and how to protect client privacy and confidentiality. Those that are interested in the subject may consult works by Derrig-Palumbo and Zeine (2005) and Luxton, Nelson and Maheu (2016) and the systematic review on telemental health done in 2021 by de Boer et al.

The future of MFT is bright and it is a very exciting time to be a part of this profession. The foundations of this field have been laid by the work of great women and men. Our work sits on the shoulders of these theorists and therapists and we can pave the path into our future knowing we are standing on solid ground. As more and more students are pursuing this degree path, our field will continue to evolve to meet the needs of our clients. What started out as debates on patterns of communication, cybernetics, boundaries and hierarchies, and developed into discussions of power and equality and social justice, continues to evolve to capture new ideas, perspectives and technologies. What wasn't possible even ten years ago is now not only possible but thriving and pushing the envelope of the way mental health care is conceptualized and delivered. What a wonderful time to be or become an MFT!

References

Ackley, D. (1998). When three's a crowd. *Family Therapy Networker, 22*(1), 1–7.

American Association for Marriage and Family Therapy (2017). *Find MFT Licensing Boards*. Retrieved from: www.aamft.org/iMIS15/AAMFT/Content/directories/MFT_licensing_boards.aspx on September 28, 2017.

Anderson, H. (1997). *Conversations, language, and possibilities: a postmodern approach to therapy*. New York, NY: Basic Books.

Anderson, H. & Goolishan, H. (1992). The client is the expert: a not-knowing approach to therapy. In S. McNamee & K. J. Gergen (Eds.), *Therapy as social construction* (pp. 25–29). Newbury Park, CA: Sage Publications.

Aries, P. (1965). *Centuries of childhood: a social history of family life*. New York, NY: Random House.

Bateson, G. (1972). *Steps to an ecology of mind: collected essays in anthropology, psychiatry, evolution, and epistemology*. Northvale, NJ: Jason Aronson, Inc.

Bateson, G., Jackson, D. D., Haley, J. & Weakland, J. (1956). Toward a theory of schizophrenia. *Behavioral Science*, 1, 251–264.

Bateson, G., Jackson, D. D., Haley, J. & Weakland, J. (1963). Toward a theory of schizophrenia. In N. J. Smelser & W. T. Smelser (Eds.), *Personality and social systems* (pp. 172–187). Hoboken, NJ: John Wiley & Sons Inc.

Berg, I. K. (1994). *Family based services: a solution-focused approach*. New York, NY: Norton.

Berg, I.K. & Jaya, A. (1993). Different and the same: family therapy with Asian-American families. *Journal of Marital Family Therapy*, 19, 31–38.

Berg, I.K. & Szabo, P. (2005). *Brief coaching for last solutions*. New York, NY: Norton.

Bergen, S. E., Ploner, A., Howrigan, D., O'Donovan, M. C., Smoller, J. W., Sullivan, P. F. (2019). Joint contributions of rare copy number variants and common SNPs to risk for schizophrenia. *J Psychiatry*, 176, 29–35. doi: 10.1176/appi.ajp.2018.17040467

Bond, S. (2009). Couple and family therapy: the evolution of the profession with social work at its core. *Intervention*, 131, 128–138.

Bureau of Labor Statistics (2016). Occupational Employment Statistics: Occupational Employment and Wages, May 2016. Retrieved from: www.bls.gov/oes/current/oes211013.htm

D'Arrigo-Patrick, J., Hoff, C., Knudson-Martin, C. & Tuttle, A. (2017). Navigating critical theory and postmodernism: social justice and therapist power in family therapy. *Family Process, 56*(3), 574–588.

Derrig-Palumbo, K. & Zeine, F. (2005). *Online therapy: a therapist's guide to expanding your practice*. New York, NY: Norton.

de Boer, K., Muir, S. D., Silva, S. S. M., Nedeljkovic, M., Seabrook, E., Thomas, N. & Meyer, D. (2021). Videoconferencing psychotherapy for couples and families: a systematic review. *J Marital Fam Ther*, 47, 259–288. https://doi.org/10.1111/jmft.12518

de Shazer, S. (1985). *Keys to solutions in brief therapy*. New York, NY: Norton.

de Shazer, S. (1988). *Clues: investigating solutions in brief therapy*. New York, NY: Norton.

Duncan, B. (2001). The future of psychotherapy. *Psychotherapy Networker, 25*(4), 1–11.

Freeny, M. (1994, Sep). Getting well in the fast lane. *Family Therapy Networker*, 18(5), 1–6.

Gehart, D. R. (2014). *Mastering competencies in family therapy*. Belmont, CA: Brooks-Cole, Cengage Learning.

Gergen, K. (1985). The social constructionist movement in modern psychology. *American Psychologist*, 40, 266–275.

Horvath, A. O., Del Re, A. C., Flückiger, C. & Symonds, D. (2011). Alliance in individual psycho-therapy. *Psychotherapy, 48*(1), 9–16.

Lowe, R. (2009). Childhood throughout the ages. In T. Maynard & N. Thomas (Eds.), *An Introduction to Early Childhood Studies* (pp. 21–32). California, CA: Sage Publications.

Luxton, D. D., Nelson, E. L. & Maheu, M. M. (2016). *A practitioner's guide to telemental health: how to conduct legal, ethical, and evidence-based telepractice*. Washington, DC: American Psychological Association.

Miller, S. D. Seidel, J. A. & Hubble, M. A. (2015). Common factors in therapy. In E. S. Neukrug (Ed.), *The Sage encyclopedia of theory in counseling and psychotherapy* (pp. 207–208).

Maturana, H. R. & Varela, F. J. (1987). *The tree of knowledge: the biological roots of human understanding*. Boston, MA: Shambhala Publications, Inc.

Minuchin, P. (1985). Families and individual development: provocations from the field of family therapy. *Child Development, 56*(2), 289–302.

Moyers, T. B. & Miller, W. R. (2013). Is low therapist empathy toxic? *Psychology of addictive behaviors, 27*(3), 878–884.

O'Hanlon, W.H. & Weiner-Davis, M. (1989). *In search of solutions: a new direction in psychotherapy*. New York: Norton.

Sullivan P. F., Kendler, K. S. & Neale M. C. (2003). Schizophrenia as a complex trait: evidence from a meta-analysis of twin studies. *Archives of General Psychiatry, 60*, 1187–1192.

Thane, P. (1981). Childhood in history. In M. King (Ed.), *Childhood, welfare and justice* (pp. 6–25). London, UK: Batsford.

Watzlawick, P., Baveles, J.B. & Jackson, D. D. (1967). *Pragmatics of human communication: a study of interactional patterns, pathologies, and paradoxes*. New York, NY: Norton.

Weinstein, D. (2013). *The pathological family: postwar America and the rise of family therapy*. Ithaca, NY: Cornell University Press.

White, M. (1995). *Re-authoring lives: interviews and essays*. Adelaide, Australia: Dulwich Centre Publications.

White, M. & Epston, D. (1990). *Narrative means to therapeutic ends*. New York, NY: Norton.

4 Building Blocks to Conceptualizing Family

A Family System's Perspective

Valerie Q. Glass

Background of systemic thinking

Systemic thinking, for some, means trying on a new and unique lens when considering "presenting problems" that arise in therapeutic settings. Most mental and emotional health backgrounds study individual cognitive and emotional processes, systemic thinking means a shift in looking at one person to looking at a whole system. Keeney (1983) calls this change in professional theory an **epistemological shift**.

Epistemology, most basically, is the way one understands what is in front of them, and the root with which decisions are made. Helping fields all develop from different epistemologies. Psychiatry views medicine and biology as their epistemological construct of how or why people act the way they do. Much of the epistemological focus of social work fields embraces the necessity or connecting to resources and social support as a catalyst for change. Psychology explores the make-up of the individual's mind and develops steps for change. Family systems, and the main focus of this chapter, dive into the epistemology of looking at families through the constructs with which we might look at various systems. You are at the beginning of a new epistemological journey. As part of that journey, new concepts will be presented that allow you to consider the role of systems in presenting problems and in change.

Mechanical and biological systemic terminology will be used to highlight how families work like systems to both maintain "presenting problems" as well as healing or changing these "presenting problems". This epistemological stance might fit with your natural understanding of the world and how problems arise or are maintained or these ideas may deviate slightly from your perspectives on problems. Marriage and family therapy (MFT), as a profession, holds a foundational epistemological view that family systems play a major role in how we view clients, presenting problems, the maintenance of problems, and the keys to change and growth (Jackson & Weakland in Ray, Stivers and Brasher, 2011).

Biological and mechanical systems

The major representation of the idea of family systems is in the construct of "**system**". If you think about anything where a bunch of separate parts work together to generate a working system, this idea of a system can be visualized. Consider a natural ecosystem where you have plants bringing in air and growing from nutrients in the soil and sun. Then you have animals eating the plants and bigger animals preying on the smaller animals. Finally, you have dead animals decaying to provide nutrients to the soil. This is

DOI: 10.4324/9781003382621-6

an example of an ecological system. If you view the one plant separate from the system, it does not make sense, you cannot break apart how the plant works and grows without including the other parts of the system. Additionally, if the plant does not survive, it does not do this alone; it is dependent on the system around it and their role in the plant's survival.

A second example of a system could be a mechanical system. Consider a car; it has a bunch of different systems working together to help it run properly. If you saw just a steering wheel by itself, that would not make sense and would not function without the rest of the mechanical system. Also, if one part of a car's system does not work – let's say the tire is low on air – the rest of the system compensates (the driver has to hold the steering wheel tighter in one direction, the engine works harder, the other tires wear because they are pushed in a different direction).

We could name many different systems (e.g., a human body, an air-conditioning system, a ship, a sports team, a traffic light, a computer), the list is endless. The commonality is that systems need all the parts to "function". The parts can "function" independently. Using this background of mechanical or biological systems, apply these ideas to family functioning. A family works to maintain their "normal" (or homeostasis, which we will talk about later). Each member in a family system has a job or a role in helping that family function in the way that is normal to them. To see a person independently, we cannot understand their role in that family system without seeing or learning about the family context. These systemic constructs help us view family dynamics from this systemic perspective. They lead us to consider how that system is working, what the system's "normal" is, and the identification of the strengths and weaknesses in the entire system. Family therapy helps the system find a new (healthier) way of working.

Historical backdrop of systemic theory

The process of looking at family through a systemic lens is known as "systems theory", "general systems theory" or "family systems theory." Minuchin (1985) describes a system as an "organized whole" (p. 289) or a group or parts that organize around one idea or function. Considering theory is important to your work as a family therapist, because your identity as an MFT, from this point forward, will take into account the very foundational idea that family is a whole system and functions much like mechanical and biological systems. There is not one major contributor to the idea of systemic thinking and the application to families; however, there seemed to be somewhat of a movement that began around 1950 and solidified as a specific theory within the next 20 or so years. We will only consider some of the names that were involved in developing the metaphor of systems as they are applied to thinking about family dynamics (Smith-Acuña, 2011).

Don Jackson. In the 1960s, Jackson developed what he coined an "Interactional Theory" where he explored the idea that families seem to want to maintain a normality, or their sense of normality (called homeostasis, which will be defined later) (see Jackson, 1968a; Jackson, 1968b, as found in Ray et al., 2011). In addition, Jackson identified that working with the family allowed clinicians to observe family systemic interactions and utilize them as part of treatment.

Harry Stack Sullivan. Sullivan influenced some of Jackson's ideas by stating that clinicians cannot look at the mental health of one individual independently from the family context. He argued that mental health is a result of both internal and external forces (Stack Sullivan, 1939).

Gregory Bateson. Bateson worked closely with two other familiar names in MFT history: John Weakland and Jay Haley (Ray & Brasher, 2010). Together, they solidified some of the foundational research in the field of systemic thinking by researching the role of homeostasis and communication patterns in families. Bateson opened the door to systemic thinking about how patterns were part of family systems (Keeney & Thomas, 1986). Bateson also worked with other founders of systemic thinking, such as Watzawick (see below); they theorized the connection of cybernetics in family patterns (Bateson, 1979).

Watzlawick, Fisch and Weakland. Weakland expanded on his work with Bateson and Haley to develop a theory of family therapy with Watzlawick and Fisch titled MRI Brief Therapy (Ray & Brasher, 2010). MRI Brief is often labeled as the foundational theory of family systems therapy. One of the major assumptions of the MRI group was that therapy should explore the interactional patterns between people. In addition, these therapists explored the roles of family members in maintaining problems (Watzlawick, Bavelas & Jackson, 1967).

Ludwig Von Bertalanffy. Von Bertalanffy was an Austrian biologist who eschewed the reductive view of systems that had previously existed and embraced the idea that scientific principles were bigger than the one object or idea. He stressed that context had to be considered to better understand the element (Bond, 2009). Von Bertalanffy's ideas about systemic thinking were applicable to all areas of the world: ecology, biology, politics or global systems, humankind or groupings of any kind. He argued that global solutions could not be addressed without considering the larger systemic context.

Alfred Adler. Adler predated family systems thinking; however, he did add to the construction of systemic thinking in the mental health and psychology fields (Carich & Willingham, 1987). Adler argued that there was an individual that was examined from a psychological context; however, the psychologist should still remember their social environment and the role this might play in who they are. In addition, Adler discussed the role of causation in mental health. He labeled causation as "circular processes" (similar to circular causality that will be discussed later). This is the idea that psychologists cannot just hone in on one specific cause for mental health issues, he stated that there was a more complex process involved that included the client's context and social interactions.

The convergence of ideas or a shift in epistemology, brought on by great thinkers from many fields, led to the constructs of systemic thinking. The over-arching ideas presented the foundation for many concepts that help family systems theorists discuss and define family dynamics. In the next section, many concepts that have emerged will be presented, defined and applied to families.

Systemic concepts

Summary

For systemic therapists, these foundational constructs become part of the understanding of how a presenting problem is maintained. Our role as systemic therapists is to help families find new equilibriums, to help families figure out what is reinforcing the unhealthy homeostasis, or to assist families in defining and developing second-order change (Chae, 2017; Keeney & Thomas, 1986). Since the origins of systemic thinking and the application to families in the mid-1900s, subsequent clinicians and theorists have added to these constructs to determine methodology and direction for making these homeostatic shifts. Some theorists

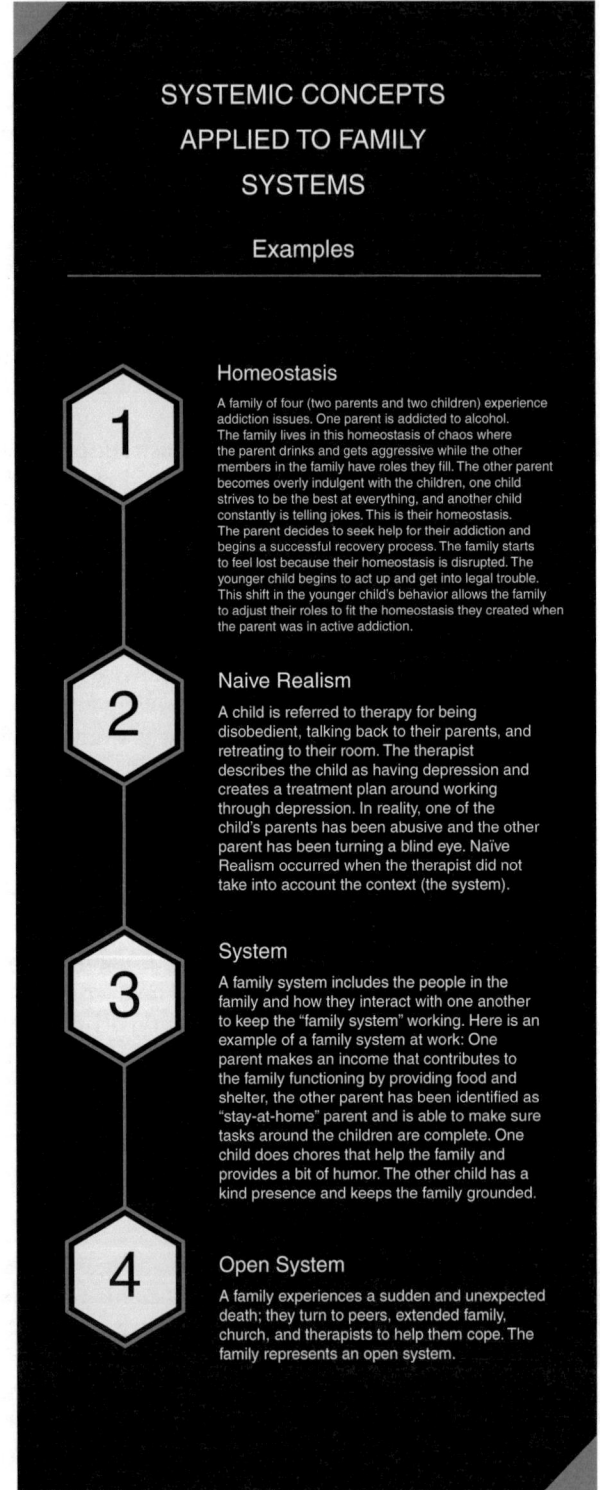

Figure 4.1 Infographic 6: Systemic Concepts Examples.

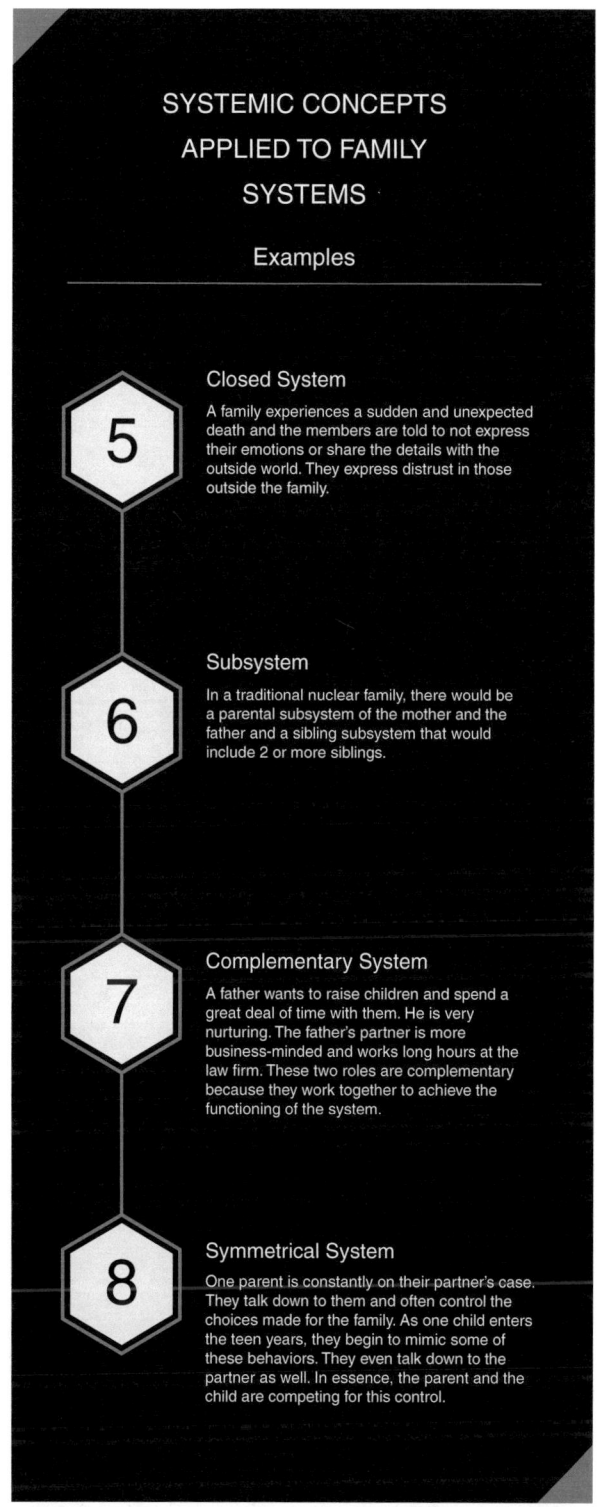

SYSTEMIC CONCEPTS APPLIED TO FAMILY SYSTEMS

Examples

5 Closed System

A family experiences a sudden and unexpected death and the members are told to not express their emotions or share the details with the outside world. They express distrust in those outside the family.

6 Subsystem

In a traditional nuclear family, there would be a parental subsystem of the mother and the father and a sibling subsystem that would include 2 or more siblings.

7 Complementary System

A father wants to raise children and spend a great deal of time with them. He is very nurturing. The father's partner is more business-minded and works long hours at the law firm. These two roles are complementary because they work together to achieve the functioning of the system.

8 Symmetrical System

One parent is constantly on their partner's case. They talk down to them and often control the choices made for the family. As one child enters the teen years, they begin to mimic some of these behaviors. They even talk down to the partner as well. In essence, the parent and the child are competing for this control.

Figure 4.1 (Continued)

SYSTEMIC CONCEPTS APPLIED TO FAMILY SYSTEMS

Examples

9

Reciprocal System

Both parents in a family work and they divide their time to care for the children and collaborate to make family choices.

10

First Order Change

A child is having a temper tantrum when the family is out to dinner because they want dessert. The family goes ahead and gives the child a dessert in order to shift the behavior in the moment. It does work; however, there is not lasting change (the child will have temper tantrums in the future).

11

Second Order Change

A child is having temper tantrums in restaurants. The parents work together and incorporate a plan at home to combat temper tantrums through dialog and positive reinforcement. Over time, the child's behavior shifts and creates lasting change.

12

Continuous Change

A couple comes to therapy and one partner feels like the other partner is constantly dismissing her feelings. The therapist works with the couple step-by-step, first by helping create a safe space for letting out feelings, then, by helping them articulate their feelings, and then by helping them learn to listen and take in what the other person says. In this step-by-step process, change occurs.

Figure 4.1 (Continued)

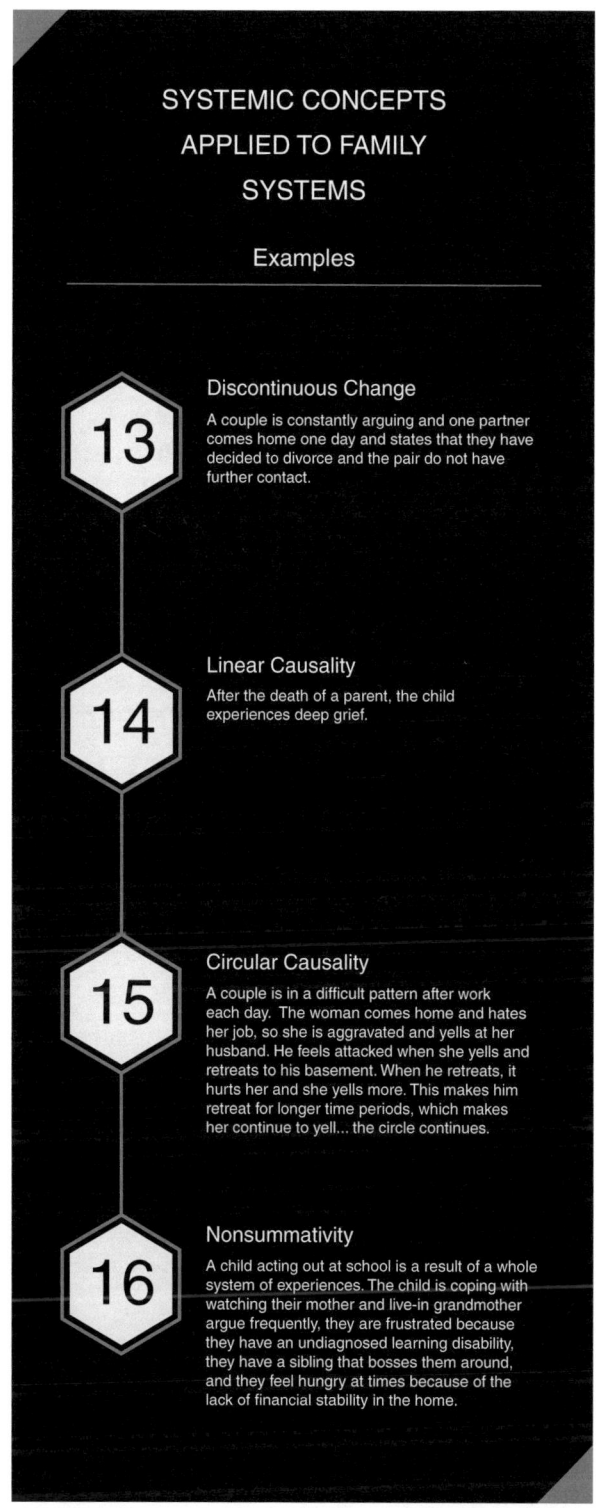

SYSTEMIC CONCEPTS APPLIED TO FAMILY SYSTEMS

Examples

13 Discontinuous Change
A couple is constantly arguing and one partner comes home one day and states that they have decided to divorce and the pair do not have further contact.

14 Linear Causality
After the death of a parent, the child experiences deep grief.

15 Circular Causality
A couple is in a difficult pattern after work each day. The woman comes home and hates her job, so she is aggravated and yells at her husband. He feels attacked when she yells and retreats to his basement. When he retreats, it hurts her and she yells more. This makes him retreat for longer time periods, which makes her continue to yell... the circle continues.

16 Nonsummativity
A child acting out at school is a result of a whole system of experiences. The child is coping with watching their mother and live-in grandmother argue frequently, they are frustrated because they have an undiagnosed learning disability, they have a sibling that bosses them around, and they feel hungry at times because of the lack of financial stability in the home.

Figure 4.1 (Continued)

SYSTEMIC CONCEPTS
APPLIED TO FAMILY
SYSTEMS

Examples

17

Equifinality

The child in the example for nonsummativity could be acting out because of any one of these experiences or any combination of these experiences (watching mom and grandma argue, a learning disability, sibling issues, or poverty).

18

Cybernetics

A couple has been married for 25 years and one partner is known for constantly putting down the other. The other partner is known for being passive and just taking the emotional abuse. They seek counseling and start to have moments where this pattern shifts and they think things are better, so they stop counseling and something will happen where the partner finds fault and the putting down pattern (their homeostasis) continues.

19

Double Bind

A partner shares with her partner that she really wants to spend more time together; however, every time the partner makes suggestions of things to do together, she states she is too tired to do those things or is uninterested in that activity.

20

Multifinality

A major event happens in a family (divorce) and there are multiple repercussions. One child withdraws, one child has behavioral issues, one parent is diagnosed with depression.

Figure 4.1 (Continued)

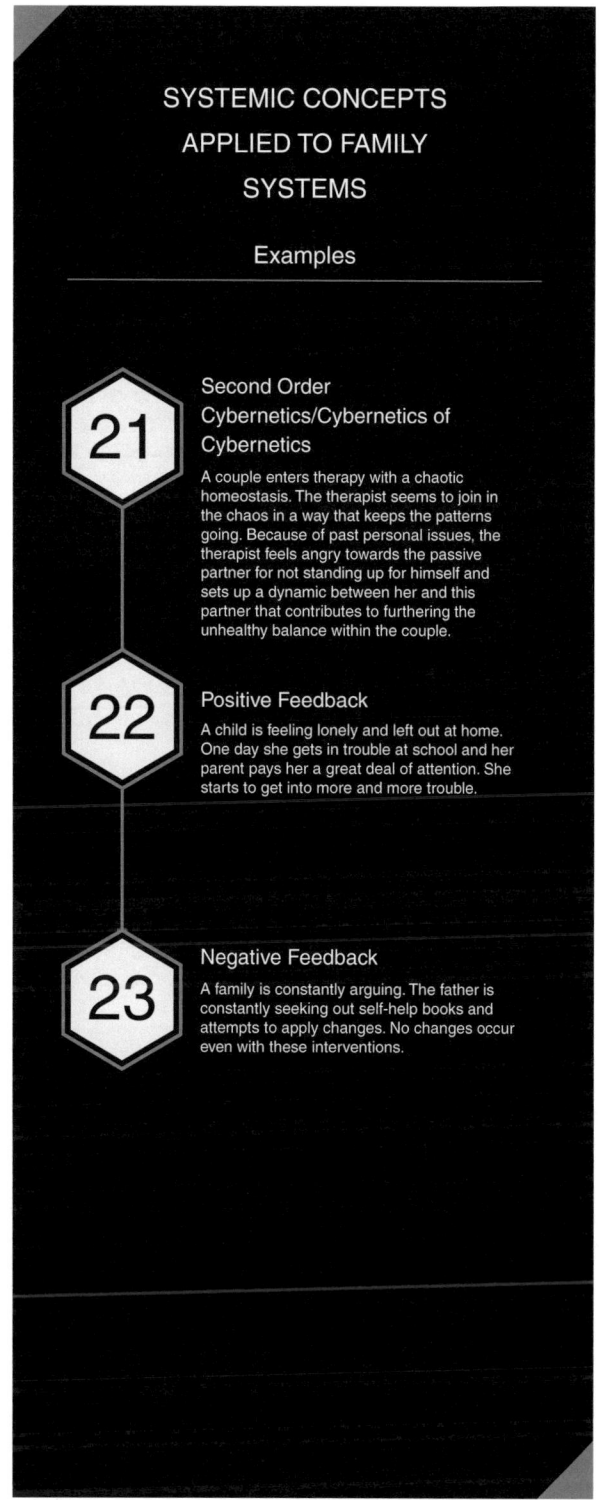

Figure 4.1 (Continued)

feel that more directive and specific interventions can lead to systemic change, other theorists focus on collaborative relationships and their functioning in change dynamics. In addition, there was limited research on these constructs initially and more recently researchers have begun to build in research related to these constructs to continue to define them as a discipline. Regardless, MFTs, as a whole, work from and visualize families through these foundational constructs.

References

Bateson, G. (1979). *Mind and nature: a necessary unity*. New York, NY: E. P. Dutton.

Bond, S. (2009). Couple and family therapy: the evolution of the profession with social work at its core. Retrieved from Intervention.org.

Carich, M. S. & Willingham, W. (1987). The roots of family systems theory in individual psychology. *Individual Psychology: The Journal of Adlerian Theory, Research & Practice, 43*(1), 71–78.

Chae, K. B. (2017). Second-order change. In J. Carlson & S. B. Dermer (Eds.), *The SAGE encyclopedia of Marriage, Family, and Couples Counseling* (pp. 1461–1462). Thousand Oaks, CA: SAGE Publications, Inc.

Keeney, B. P. (1983). *Aesthetics of change*. New York, NY: Guilford Press.

Keeney, B. P. & Thomas, F. N. (1986). Cybernetic foundations of family therapy. In F. P. Piercy & D. H. Sprenkle (Eds.), *Family therapy sourcebook*. New York, NY: The Guilford Press.

Minuchin, P. (1985). Families and individual development: provocations from the field of family therapy. *Child Development. 56*, 289–302.

Ray, W. A. & Brasher, C. (2010). Brief systemic therapy: creating our future while embracing our past. *Journal of Systemic Therapies, 29*(4), 17. doi:10.1521/jsyt.2010.29.4.17

Ray, W. A., Stivers, R. J. & Brasher, C. (2011). Through the eyes of Don D. Jackson M. D. *Journal of Systemic Therapies, 30*(1), 38–58. doi:10.1521/jsyt.2011.30.1.38

Smith-Acuña, S. (2011). *Systems theory in action: applications to individual, couples, and family therapy*. Hoboken, NJ: John Wiley & Sons, Inc.

Stack Sullivan, H. (1939). A note on formulating the relationship of the individual and the group. *American Journal of Sociology, 44*(6), 932–937.

Watzlawick, P., Bavelas, J. B. & Jackson, D. D. (1967). *Pragmatics of human communication: a study of interactional patterns*. New York, NY: W. W. Norton & Company, Inc.

5 Postmodernism and Social Constructionism
Foundational Concepts

Valerie Q. Glass

Introduction

The concepts of postmodernism and social construction can feel confusing at first because they are rooted in abstract philosophical ideas. In addition, the assumptions of these constructs can challenge our understanding of our own realities. This chapter will provide a foundation for understanding the history of these two concepts and a description of the major tenets of these models. In general, social construction describes the way we learn about the world around us and that this world is defined through language and conversation with others. Postmodernism describes our understanding that everyone we engage with has a different set of social constructions.

Social construction

How do you think you know that what you know is real? How do you know what you know? Social constructionism came out of the idea of epistemology (Berger & Luckmann, 1966). Epistemology is the philosophical concept that asks the question "How do we know what we know?" This construct takes into account all the information present in our knowledge banks that lead us to say "yes, I know that for sure". Throughout time, many philosophers have attempted to address this question. **Descartes'** famous statement, "I think therefore I am", has provided to many generations a question to ponder about what it really means to "be". Similarly, **John Locke** introduced the idea of a tabula rasa – this idea indicated that humans' minds were blank or empty and are "filled" as they interact with the world around them. Many great thinkers, theorists and philosophers have attempted to answer this idea of epistemology. Social construction is one of those theories that evolved from this question. Social constructionists' answer to epistemology is that people "construct knowledge" through the process of connecting to others socially through language (Burr, 1995).

Science is a reflection of this idea of epistemology. Most of us feel science is a proven answer to addressing reality and what is real. Consider that, at one point, scientists argued that the Earth was flat. More recently, scientists noted that there were only the eight planets and one solar system. These ideas have been "proven" wrong by scientific means. Because we believe in these scientific measures, we "know" that we "know" they are right. How do you know that you are breathing right at this moment?

At some time in your life, you learned that air coming in and out of your nose and mouth signaled you were alive and breathing. This is the crux of epistemology; how do we know what we know? Philosophers question this idea of epistemology and argue how do

DOI: 10.4324/9781003382621-7

we know that what we know is reality? If you meet two very different people from two very unique cultures and ask them about religion or morals, you will get two very different responses. How do you know which one is right? Philosophers in the late 1960s started to question that there is not one "right" way to view things.

Social construction takes this idea of epistemology a step further by indicating that what we know is based on our interactions with others (Berger & Luckmann, 1966). What we know of as a reality is formed by language behind that reality and how that language is used in connecting to others. Humans are born with the ability and yearning to connect socially. This social connection is how we understand the world around us. This ability to communicate and understand language and social symbols is part of our biological make up.

Social constructionist philosophers

In general, social constructionism was a movement of the ideas of many. There was not one major philosopher that "invented" social construction; rather, much like the concept suggests, it was a progressive discourse that led to the inception of this philosophy. As previously mentioned, early European philosophers asked questions that catapulted human questioning about how we know things (e.g., Descartes, Kant and Locke among others) (Berger & Luckmann, 1966). **Max Schelor** (a German philosopher) and **Lev Vygotsky** (a Russian developmental psychologist) argued in support of the idea that humans were born with a tabula rasa (blank slate) and that our understanding came from experience. Taking into account this idea of a tabula rasa, the emergence of social construction developed to further explain where knowledge and understanding come from.

Many attribute **Michel Foucault** to modern-day social constructionism, poststructuralism and postmodernist ideas (Burr, 1995). Foucault was a philosopher in the mid-to-late 1900s and presented ideas on political science, economics, social sciences, history and medicine. He profoundly believed in the idea that social discourse creates understanding. One element Foucault frequently discussed was the socially constructed elements of sex and sexuality. He argued that, historically, humans have taken on different sexual morals that have driven social expectations and definitions around sex and pleasure. In addition to sexual behavior, Foucault identified the role of power in social constructions overall. He implied that elements of human control and identity are shaped by the constructions of those in power – by negating or dehumanizing those that are not in power as a way to maintain one's privilege. Modern day postmodernist and social justice advocates are informed by Foucault's ideas and have further indicated the importance of deconstructing our own position or privilege as a way to establish a more equitable community.

Kenneth Gergen, a professor of social psychology, has contributed many texts on the topic of social constructionism (Aceros, 2012). His premise is that discourse creates knowledge and understanding and that dialogue between people is an active process of "constructing". Through his authored texts, Gergen (2001) has provided a base for the role of social construction in human sciences, more specifically, in therapy settings. There were many "voices" and continue to be many "voices" that expand on the understanding of social construction and the influence of social construction on our lives personally and professionally.

Assumptions of social construction

Social constructionism identifies three major assumptions: reality, knowledge and learning (Kukla, 2000). Reality is created through social interactions within one's environment.

Reality is an active process of engaging with others. Social interaction creates what we know of as reality. As we engage with others in our surroundings, we have experiences that we come to better understand through the dialogue that we have with those around us. Essentially, people are putting language and meaning to what we are doing and experiencing. We begin to internalize those messages and they become our reality.

Major concepts of social construction

Social construction is a "construction" and through time and conversation the idea of socially constructing gains depth. Many concepts help to describe the process of constructing reality. This section will focus on a few of the most notable constructs: reality, language, identity, discourse and positioning.

Reality. Berger and Luckmann (1966) introduced the idea of the "reality of everyday life" (p. 36). They indicated that each of us lives our life on a daily basis and just believe that this is our reality. Our reality is shaped by the world around us, more specifically, our social interactions. If language or communication does not invent it, it does not exist.

Within social constructionist philosophers, there is a slight division on the existence of reality. Some agree that there really is not a reality outside of language (e.g., Gergen), while others feel that there is a reality; however, our social constructions are more of a "lens" that, if we get to a place where we question this reality (e.g., Foucalt), we engage in conversation to better understand. These conversations contribute to a new reality that is socially constructed.

Language. Language is the mechanism through which we socially construct our surroundings. I remember hearing once that adults do not recall memories from when they were babies because they did not have words for what was experienced as a baby to imprint what was going on into memory banks. In essence, babies do not have any social constructions; they are at the start of that journey. Consider that language is not just about language we are experiencing in the moment, it is also about historical language - language from our families, language we see on street signs, in body language, in the media, in expression of emotion and so on (Berger & Luckmann, 1966). Words and discourse label events, emotions, identities, things, interactions, expectations and the list goes on.

Identity. Our identity is formed through our language (Berger & Luckmann, 1966). "Identity is a phenomenon that emerges from the dialect between individual and society" (Berger & Luckmann, 1966, p. 194). Consider all the elements of "self" that you might define (i.e., are you are parent, a child, what is your profession, are you shy or outgoing, are you active or reserved, are you intelligent, what is your religion, your race, your cultural background, and so on). These aspects of defining yourself have evolved as you have understood who you are, using language as a way to define "self". The evolution of identity occurred through language and discussing with others. Consider what this means when we attempt to understand the identity of others. Our understanding of what is "different" to us is completely based on the language we use around that difference. For example, if you hear someone share with you, "I am from southern Alabama and consider myself a true southern boy". What images arise in your own mind that are similar or different to your own identity? You are constructing what you feel this "true southern boy" identity means based on **your** experiences with language and social construction, which may not match their experiences. This idea that we see through our own social constructions and define the world through these constructions moves us into postmodernism, which I will dive more into detail about later in this chapter.

Discourse. Discourse is all of the understandings that surround a word, symbol or representation (Burr, 1995). Consider a picture of "thought bubbles" over someone's head; when a word is spoken, there are tons of "thought bubbles" that have developed from our own experiences, our social connections and our previous conversations around that word. These "thought bubbles" influence how we react with this word. How does it make us feel? What do we associate it with? Is it "good or bad"? When a person says, "that woman is stunning", for example, the discourse (the "thought bubbles") around both "woman" and "stunning" mean something different for each person. These different meanings are developed by our interaction with people in our past. If you asked a man native to the Yoruba Tribe of Nigeria and a man from central London, England to describe a "stunning woman", their descriptions would be based on their discourse – their social interchanges throughout their lives that have brought meaning ("thought bubbles") to the concepts of "woman" and "stunning". Symbols can evoke different discourses for people. Consider the American Flag and the "thought bubbles" that this symbol evokes for you. These "thought bubbles" vary by individuals within the U.S. and across the world based on the discourses that each person has developed through language and experience.

Positioning. In social construction, positioning is the awareness of our own "position" related to our personal constructions (Burr, 1995). Put simply, this is the understanding that people are going to have differences of opinion. These opinions are developed from

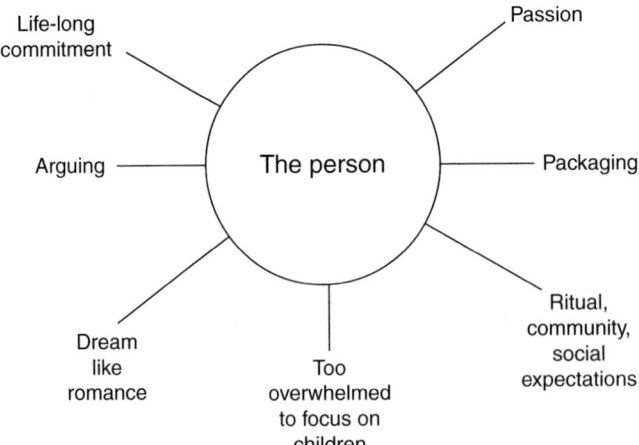

Figure 5.1 Infographic 6: The Process of Social Construction.

our social experiences. Another way to think of the concept of positioning is to consider an element of your identity (for example, how you identify your gender) and recognize that you experience and understand the world from that "position", that experience of being that gender. Being a cis-gendered woman, I would view the world from this perspective and do not see the world from a male perspective. This idea of positioning can lead to change and influences what postmodern therapist attempt to do. By positioning, one can de-construct or recognize that position that they are taking and how this might influence their reality. Consider someone who's identity is a woman and she has "positioned" herself in that identity and her understanding of that identity for a while. She starts to consider why people seem to take advantage of her. In de-constructing her own understanding of what a "woman" is, she realizes that she may have adopted her social construction of womanhood as passive and decides that being a woman can also mean being assertive. This realization (or new construction) changes her pattern.

Social construction is one of the foundational concepts of postmodernism. Postmodernism embraces the major tenets of social construction. One way I differentiate these ideas is that I consider social construction to be the "verb". On a daily basis, we are socially constructing a new reality through our dialogues.

Postmodernism in a larger sense is that we understand that all of our social constructions differ. It is the awareness of different constructs in people's "thought bubbles".

Modernism

Modernist ideas serve as the precursor of the emergence of postmodernist thinking (Burr, 1995). Modernism was a dominant epistemology and paradigm during the turn of the 1900s, during the time of the industrial period and the evolution of science.

Modernism highlights that science is an accurate and complete explanation for knowledge and understanding of why things are the way they are. Modernism is the idea that, if we look hard enough, there is one "answer". One example of modernism is when research is done and a result is calculated, this calculation is the "answer", the reality. Modernist research is about looking at the most accurate and "proven" methodology. A modernist therapist (e.g., psychoanalytic, cognitive-behavioral, structure, intergenerational, strategic) would explore the problem, identify or label the problem and highlight supported techniques that would assist in the problem.

Early philosophers did touch on some ideas that are found in postmodern thinking; however, the 1970s brought a more detailed and clearer theoretical frame to the concept of postmodernism (Anderson, 1997). Postmodernism was one way of thinking that emerged from the scientific growth of the early 20th century as well as much of the one-sided thinking within politics and religion at the time. Essentially, people were saying "there is not one way of viewing things".

Often you hear about the idea of postmodernism as represented in art, literature and architecture (as well as other artistic expressions). The concepts of modernism and postmodernism vary slightly when thinking about their application to artistic venues; however, the foundation of these concepts is still present. Modernist art has one meaning that it attempts to get across in the presentation, whereas postmodern art stresses the idea that the person viewing the art is the one that interprets the meaning. Many of us have seen art in galleries or in others' homes and people seem to be touched by the art, but we just can't locate that same feeling within us about the work. We all have a different perspective and bring something different to what we see.

Postmodernism

Postmodernism has evolved into an understanding of different perspectives and constructions. Many current theorists define postmodernism in a variety of ways, yet each definition highlights that all humans have a different set of lenses with which they view the world. Harlene Anderson (1997), the founder of one of the postmodern models of marriage and family therapy (collaborative), stated that "human systems are complex entities composed of individuals who think, interpret, and understand" (p. 37). She described the process of how we develop meaning, that meaning is derived from conversations humans have with one another. Postmodernism directly challenges the ideas of "one truth". Burr (1995) defines postmodernism as "the rejection of 'grand narratives' in theory and the replacement of a search for the truth with a celebration of the multiplicity of (equally valid) perspectives" (p. 204). As you can see from these definitions, postmodernism is both an awareness that reality is different for those you encounter, but that this reality is based on the context of language and how language helped to develop this sense of understanding. Postmodernists claim that the world can be viewed as a mixture of multiple ways of viewing the events around us.

Postmodern assumptions

The most thorough way to explore theory related to postmodernism is to specifically highlight each assumption. There are several assumptions of postmodernism that vary by the user, this paper will explore two noted lists of assumptions that have been generated by postmodern marriage and family theorists: 1) Freedman and Combs' Postmodern Narrative context and 2) Anderson's Collaborative approach.

Narrative therapists Jill Freedman and Gene Combs (1996) identified four major assumptions of postmodernism that provide the backdrop of the narrative model:

Reality is socially constructed. Naturally, humans interact using language (Freedman & Combs, 1996). It is this *languaging* process that leads us to an understanding of what is around us. Gender is an example of this type of message. The context and conversation around us define what "gender" means. One person's understanding of gender and expectations of gender may differ completely from a person who lives in a different context. The reality of what gender is can be seen as being in the eye of the person defining it.

Consider, for example, a person is born to a family that sees women as submissive, nurturing and family caretakers. A child is born to that family and biologically their world sees them as female. From the moment they are born, their society represents this perspective. This person sees women in their life taking on these roles, they are taught that messages in their religion hone in on the importance of women taking these roles, they see these roles in the media and words are constantly being used to reinforce these constructions. They might be rewarded if they are cooking or cleaning. They might hear words that describe them as "nurturing" or "obedient" that are not used for other genders. Overtime, they develop constructions around what is a "good woman" or a "bad woman" that becomes part of their understanding of the world. Social constructions can change. Assume this same person finds themselves in a different community where the constructions of gender look very different. They will "add to" their constructions and incorporate those as part of their understanding of the world.

There is an understanding that these realities are not only changing but existed before us. Social construction is a constantly changing phenomenon because communication is all around us – images, symbols, gestures, facial expressions and conversations constantly change our perspectives and views about the meaning and context of what is around us.

Realities are constructed through language. Much like social construction, we understand a situation based on the narrating around it (Freedman & Combs, 1996). Language is not just about talking and verbal communication, as in this previous example. Language can include a lot of different communication tools: conversations, debates, stories, body communication, facial expressions, non-verbal expressions, media, written language and so on. Another consideration about the role of language is to consider the context of who created the language around certain ideas. Typically, in social settings there is often a "dominant" voice that can almost dictate the meaning of certain contexts. Using gender in this example, many patriarchal societies have defined men as powerful and women as weaker. The language around "men" and "women" has followed these realities or expectations. Being a woman in a patriarchal society can eliminate the woman's voice or perspective because the "dominant discourse" around their identity as a woman is defined as weak or unvalued. This process of negating or dismissing certain groups of people can lead to many alternative realities that are misunderstood or unknown.

Realities are organized and maintained through narrative. There is a constant shifting of reality that occurs with the passage of time (Freedman & Combs, 1996). We understand our context only to be challenged by a shifting of ideas – new constructions. These constructions become part of our narrative of understanding.

Consider how a dominant story in your family of origin may create this dominant narrative (expectation or experience) based on that story. Consider, for example, if a family has a family member share that they have depression, maybe the family talk about this person in detail and frequently discuss this person's symptoms of "not getting out of bed" or "being lazy". In gatherings, the family will share with others "at home he just does nothing…" – this has become the reality that continues to be maintained by this frequent retelling of the story. The retelling of this story reiterates these negative cycles and, in some ways, keeps that person with depression in that mode, in that reality. Think about the systemic concept of homeostasis and consider how these stories work within this reality that we seek to maintain; this could be an example of how the families' "reality" is maintained through the story.

There are no essential truths. An essential truth is the idea that there is only one specific way of seeing things and that we, as humans, seek this one appropriate and correct answer (Freedman & Combs, 1996). To explain this idea of no essential truths a bit more, let us look at an example. Consider you know a person and they share with you that they really struggle with their mother being overbearing and strict. They mention this a lot and you have developed a perception of this mother in your mind. Then, you happen to meet a sibling who starts to talk about the mother fondly. Your previous "truth" has been rattled. Consider another example, from a clinical perspective. A client can be diagnosed with a mental health disorder, yet they do not fit all the criteria or maybe experience them differently on a continuum of seriousness.

When I think about this assumption that there are no essential truths, as a therapist, I think it is important to recognize that the person in front of you may not have the same understanding of reality that the therapist does. To make it even more complicated, all the people in the room (the family members) are likely to have different understandings of "truth" that they are bringing to therapy. That is where postmodern therapies are very useful. They tap into these multiple realities to better understand the complete story.

Harlene Anderson (1997) embraces **six assumptions of postmodernism** in her collaborative approach; these are as follows (p. 3):

1. Human systems are language- and meaning-generating systems
2. The construction of reality is in forms of social action rather than independent individual mental processes
3. An individual mind is a social composition and self, therefore, becomes a social, relational composition
4. The reality and meaning that we attribute to ourselves and others and to the experiences and events of our lives and interactional phenomena created and experienced by individuals in conversation and action (thought language) with one another and with themselves
5. Language in generative gives order and meaning to our lives and our world, and functions as a form of social participation
6. Knowledge is relational and is embodied and generated in language and our everyday practices

Anderson noted that postmodern therapeutic practice embraces these assumptions as the major force of change in therapeutic practice.

Postmodernist assumptions note that we each come from a different context and have a different reality or understanding of a situation. In addition, these assumptions imply that change and perception can adapt over time because of *languaging* and storying that occur within one's social context. Consider this example: imagine you were in a treatment team meeting talking about a heterosexual couple and shared a moment when the husband in this scenario cried in session. Then, another therapist asked, "How did the wife feel about this outburst?" You may remember the wife looking at the husband and, based on your own social constructions of empathy, share you feel she was empathetic. You could make a guess, based on your own social constructions of emotion; however, her feelings were probably different to your perception, likely her feelings differed from her husband's perceptions of her reactions.

This is the idea of postmodernism; we see and feel things differently even though we are all in the same moment.

Limitations and arguments

When learning about the constructs of social constructionism and postmodernism for the first time, people can have a variety of reactions: some may stop to pause and consider these ideas a bit more, others might feel these constructs fit their reality and understanding, other times people have an adverse reaction and feel these constructs threaten their understanding of reality. Frequently, I have heard marriage and family therapy students share that their religious convictions are reality; therefore, they cannot accept the premise of these concepts. Social construction and postmodernism are not without philosophical arguments. In this section, I hope to present the external voices of some philosophical arguments toward these philosophies and address some personal challenges that individuals might experience when it comes to these concepts.

One common argument toward social construction and postmodernism is that the major premise of "no absolute truth" is made null and void by even stating that assumption (North, 2016). By stating that there is no absolute truth, would postmodernism as an idea even exist? How could you practice under a "postmodern philosophy" if there was not a "truth" to the term postmodernism? Similarly, postmodernism was a reaction to the modernist approaches, to state that there is no "reality" is counter to arguing that the "modernist" approach is not the appropriate reality (North, 2016).

Another argument toward these philosophies is geared toward the larger social understandings of what is right and wrong (North, 2016). As therapists, there are certain narratives that clients bring to the table that we must argue are "wrong" (e.g., general harm toward self or others). Considering the client's reality, it can become difficult to identify direction or what "change" should look like.

Embrace and challenge

As a growing scholar and therapist, it is essential to both embrace and challenge those "facts" that are presented to you throughout your learning (North, 2016). Having discussions with your peers and mentors about these concepts (and any others that challenge your thinking) can only strengthen your understanding of your professional self. I have witnessed the most resistant students embrace social construction and postmodernism and, on the flip side, I have seen students who found solace in these concepts argue their influence on their own clinical work.

When I consider the major kickback that I see from students who feel these concepts threaten what they believe whole-heartedly is real (for example, I commonly hear arguments that postmodernism and religions are incompatible), I think these concepts help us understand religion and the context of religion in our own lives. In addition, it allows us to both embrace our own spiritual identity while allowing the spiritual identities of those around us to also flourish.

It is undeniable that the constructs of postmodernism and social constructionism have opened up the dialogue to issues of power, privilege and difference (Giroux, 1990). These philosophies embrace that we need to understand ourselves and our own context in order to help others understand theirs. These concepts allow us to argue against what we feel does not fit into our greater understanding and allow us to look outside ourselves and our own experiences. These constructs have opened up a way of understanding our role as therapists in the change process.

References

Aceros, J. C. (2012). Social construction and relationalism: a conversation with Kenneth Gergen. *Universitas Psychologica, 11*(3), 1001–1011.

Anderson, H. (1997). *Conversation, language, and possibilities: a postmodern approach to therapy.* New York, NY: Basic Books.

Berger, P. L. & Luckmann, T. (1966). *The social construction of reality: a treatise in the sociology of knowledge.* New York, NY: Penguin Books.

Burr, V. (1995). *Social constructionism.* New York, NY: Routledge.

Freedman, J. & Combs, G. (1996). *Narrative therapy: the social construction of preferred realities.* New York, NY: W. W. Norton.

Gergen, K. J. (2001). Psychological science in a postmodern context. *American Psychologist, 56*(10), 803–813. doi:10.1037/0003-066X.56.10.803

Giroux, H. A. (1990). Rethinking the boundaries of educational discourse: modernism, postmodernism, and feminism. *College Literature, 17*(2/3), 1.

Kukla, A. (2000). *Social constructivism and the philosophy of science.* New York, NY: Routledge.

North, A. (2016). A millennial mistake: three arguments against radical social constructivism. *Journal of Counseling & Development, 94*(1), 114–122. doi:10.1002/jcad.12067

6 The Core Process of Therapy

Planning Therapy Guided by Theory

Kristi Harrison

Planning how you will carry out therapy with a client is no small undertaking. This topic encompasses the majority of the knowledge, skills and attitudes associated with being an effective therapist. Planning the therapy process requires knowledge of how therapy is executed (joining, assessing, formulating goals, intervening and documentation). It also requires an integrated understanding of theory that the therapist uses to identify the overall aim of therapy.

The term **treatment planning** itself is a bit ambiguous. In one respect, it refers to the therapist's process of planning out therapy. Treatment planning also refers to the preparation of a formal, written document that identifies the reason for therapy (presenting problem(s)), the goals and objectives of therapy, and the interventions or plan for accomplishing those goals. A comprehensive plan for therapy (literally a plan for treatment) will involve a plan for carrying out the five major processes we've considered throughout this chapter: joining, assessment, goal setting, intervention and documentation. The written documentation (the formal "treatment plan") may not explicitly address all five of these processes, even though competent therapy will still need to involve all these things.

Formal treatment plans (written treatment plans) will vary in terms of their format and contents. Generally, they are created in order to document the organizing focus (problem and goals) and methods used in therapy (Patterson, Williams, Edwards, Chamow & Grauf-Grounds, 2018). A formal (written) treatment plan is created with several audiences in mind, including the client and potentially other third parties invested in therapy (e.g., insurance company, court system, child protective services, etc.).

A therapist's conceptual plan for treatment is much more thorough than what is included in a typical written treatment plan, but this conceptual plan for therapy covers lots of details that may not be helpful for clients and other stakeholders to see. Formal (written) treatment plans highlight therapeutic goals and interventions in a way that a client or an outsider could quickly determine what the focus of therapy is.

Additionally, the formal treatment plan accomplishes something essential: it establishes behavioral, measurable statements of both the problem and the goals that therapy is aiming to accomplish. As you move through your training, both forms of treatment planning (literally planning out the therapy process and writing formal treatment plans) will be important. As you study various models, think about treatment planning in these two different ways. How does a given model help you move through the therapy process with the client? How does a given model provide helpful guidance for writing a formal treatment plan?

The remainder of this section will consider the five core processes of therapy – joining, assessment, goal setting, intervention and evaluation/documentation – giving

DOI: 10.4324/9781003382621-8

specific consideration to how theory informs and coordinates these processes. As part of considering goal setting and intervention, we will look specifically at written treatment plans and how theory and therapy models are important in developing written treatment plans.

Core therapy process 1 – joining

Joining is the process by which therapists metaphorically walk beside their clients and demonstrate a deep understanding of their concerns (Panichelli, 2013). Compared to the sections that follow (assessment, goal setting and intervention), this section on joining will be relatively short. But don't let that fool you. Forming a relationship with clients is incredibly important. In many regards, success in therapy is **all** about joining!

More and more research evidence points to the therapeutic relationship as one of the biggest determinants of whether therapy will be successful (see Asay & Lambert, 1999; Blow & Sprenkle, 2001; Fife, Whiting, Bradford & Davis, 2014; Sprenkle & Blow, 2004).

Simply put, establishing a relationship of mutual trust is the basis for everything that can come from therapy.

Much of the above comes out of the "Common Factors" research, which identifies factors that are common across different types of therapy that show positive outcomes. Allow this information to sink in for a moment… the quality of the therapeutic relationship matters a lot, and the client's perception of the relationships is especially important in predicting therapy outcomes. In light of this, Shaw and Murray (2014) advocate for monitoring how our clients perceive their alliance with us. Consider this information in light of your study of theory and of the various marriage and family therapy (MFT) models. All of the MFT models give specific considerations to how therapists form relationships with clients. In strategic therapy, there is the concept of "client position". In structural family therapy, therapists "join and accommodate" the client system. In experiential therapy, therapists attend to the "battles for structure and initiative". Narrative therapists meet the client separately from the problem. These are just a few examples of how concepts from specific models can be related back to Common Factors research on the importance of forming a strong therapeutic alliance.

As we are talking about joining and the formation of a therapeutic alliance, it is important to note that the therapeutic alliance is more than just the bond between therapist and client. The therapeutic alliance is usually thought of in terms of three dimensions first identified by Bordin (1979), who defined alliance as involving client-therapist agreement on (a) therapeutic goals, (b) the tasks or methods to be used in therapy and (c) the relational bond. What this means is that joining with our clients is intertwined with all aspects of planning therapy, particularly the formation of goals and the selection of therapeutic interventions. Developing a written treatment plan that identifies the goals and interventions in therapy (which relates to the documentation process) is intertwined with joining and how we form relationships with clients. Moreover, Shaw and Murray's (2014) point about monitoring the quality of the alliance also reminds us that joining is relevant in evaluating therapy. Consistently measuring clients' perceptions of the therapeutic alliance can be a helpful way to evaluate the services we're providing. Theory and research, including specific therapy model and research like the Common Factors research, provide essential guidance that allows us to be intentional in how we form bonds with clients, develop shared goals and develop a shared plan for therapy.

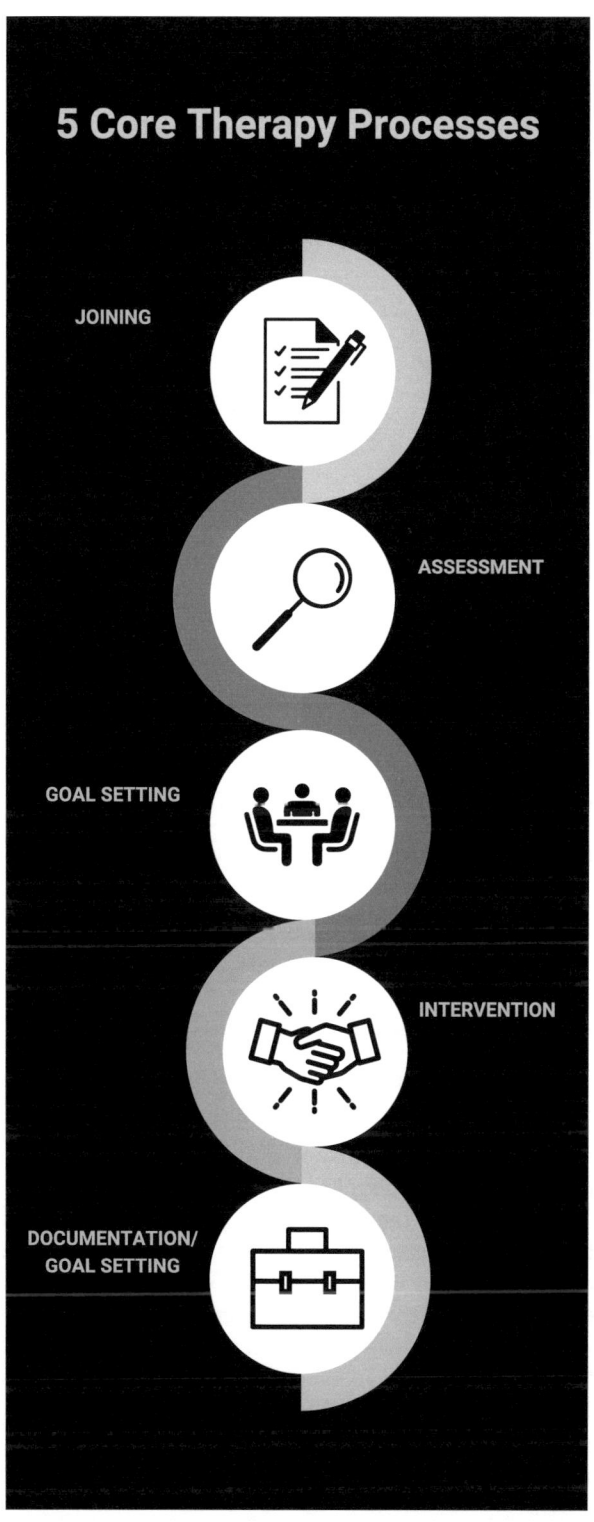

Figure 6.1 Infographic 7: Five Core Processes.

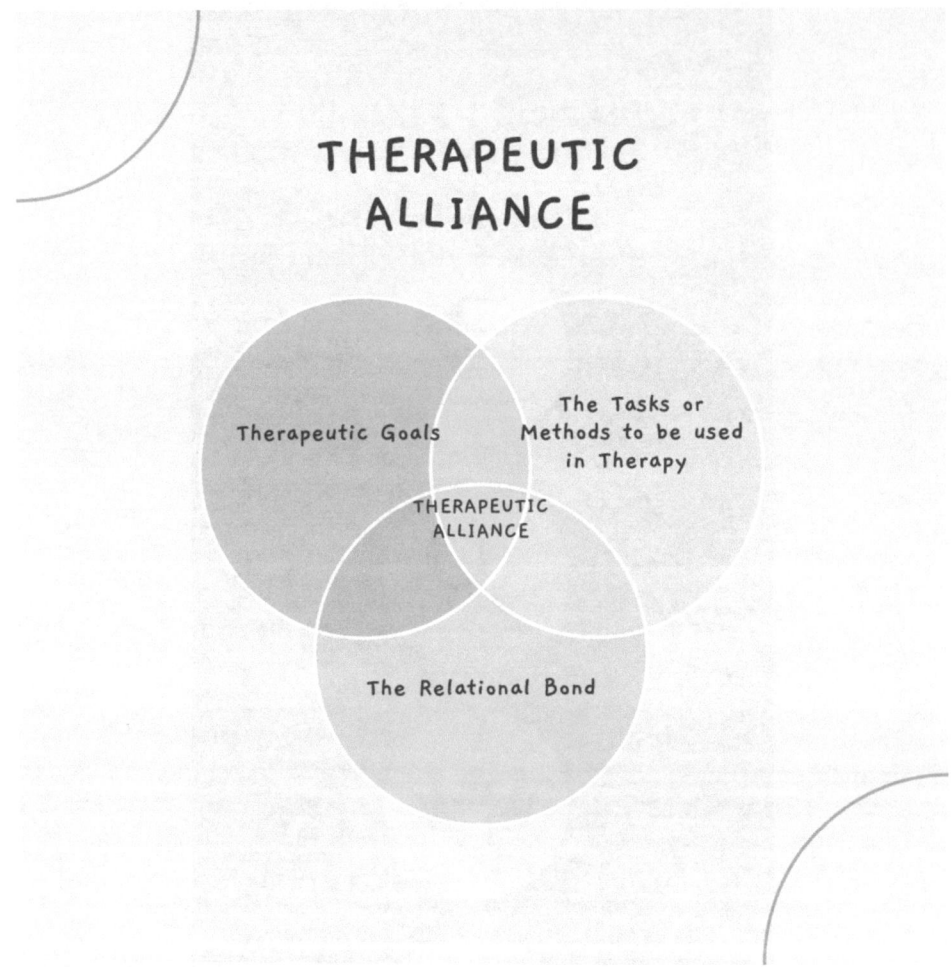

Figure 6.2 Infographic 8: Three dimensions of a therapeutic alliance.

In the practice of relational therapy (therapy with couples and families), forming strong therapeutic alliances is especially important and is more complicated, because we are forming relationships with multiple people at once (Sprenkle, Lebow & Davis, 2009).

Moreover, the alliances among the family members (not just with us as the therapist) also matter, as do the balances among the parties involved (e.g., a strong connection with one client, but a weak connection with another, reflects an imbalance in the alliance and could be a problem). Common Factors research specific to couple and family work indicates positive outcomes are associated with such a systemic view of the alliance, as well as goals and interventions that are systemic or relationally framed. Here again, we see that forming a strong alliance is interconnected with the rest of the therapeutic process, and that theory (including both systems theory and specific therapy models) can be incredibly helpful in navigating the joining process.

Although the Common Factors research suggests that many models of therapy can be effective and that forming alliances is a shared feature across effective therapies, being intentional (a product of being guided by theory) is crucial for forming a strong alliance. As Sprenkle et al. (2009) point out, "Good intervention that makes sense to families feels helpful and engages and therefore leads to better therapeutic alliances, just as such alliances lead to better outcomes" (p. 105). In other words, therapist intentionality (being guided by theory) and strong alliances go hand in hand. Being intentional with what you do in therapy builds alliance, and a strong alliance makes what you do in therapy more beneficial.

Hopefully, it becomes clear just how important a therapist's self-aware use of theory is: thoughtful use of theory and intentionality go hand in hand. When there's a logic to what we do with our clients, this carries over into how we connect with them, how we collaboratively problem-solve and plan the therapy process, and how they in turn connect with the therapy process.

"It is the theory that decides what can be observed." (Albert Einstein, as cited in Tomm, St. George, Wulff & Strong, 2014).

Core therapy process 2 – assessment: a practical and philosophical look at how we learn with our clients in therapy

Throughout our work on treatment planning and the core processes of therapy, we have emphasized the influence that our personal and professional assumptions have on how we conduct therapy. One of the main reasons that professional theory is so important is that it enables professional therapists to conduct therapy according to assumptions that are both explicit and carefully considered. Perhaps nowhere else is the use of theory more important than when we are going through the assessment process with our clients. As the opening quotation states, "It is the theory that decides what can be observed." If our minds are closed to certain possibilities, then we are effectively closing off those possibilities for our clients. Using the journey metaphor, if we will go down only certain paths and not others, then we are imposing those same limits on our clients. Thoughtful use of theory is about being conscious of our maps.

The purpose of this particular chapter on assessment is to look both practically and philosophically at how theory guides our process of learning with our clients about the situations that bring our clients to therapy. In this section, we will consider:

- terminology related to assessment
- the fundamental conceptual, practical and written processes involved with assessment in MFT
- how foundational MFT theories, including systems theory and social constructionism, inform the ways that MFTs approach assessment
- how a therapy model is involved in assessment
- how theory relates to our use of formal assessment tools

Terminology associated with assessment in therapy

For those new to the practice of therapy, the terminology can be confusing.

Certain terms – like the term **assessment** itself – can be used to mean a number of different things. Plus, parts of the assessment process happen in the therapist's mind, while part of assessment happens in interactions with clients, and part in writing. Thus, the terminology related to assessment has to do with conceptual, practical and written aspects of therapy. This means that terms are used in a variety of ways.

The term **assessment** can be used to refer to a process of learning about the client and their situation. A therapist might say, "I've just started working with this couple and we're still in the assessment phase" or "I'm still assessing the problem". In this regard, assessment or assessing is something that the therapist does. The therapist is actively learning with the client and about their situation in order to best address whatever needs have brought the client to therapy. While it is most common to associate assessment with the beginning of therapy, when the therapist is most actively learning with the client and about their circumstances, assessment (as a learning process) happens throughout therapy.

We should always be open to learning alongside our clients, even if we've been working with them for a while.

The term assessment can also be used to refer to a product, often a written document, that organizes and summarizes the information we've gathered from our client. A therapist might say, "I'm just about finished with writing my assessment for this client." In this context, the term "assessment" refers to an organized presentation of information about a client and the situation bringing them to therapy. In this regard, an "assessment" involves making some judgments about what information is important and about how various pieces of information fit together. In some contexts, therapists will use the term "evaluation" as a synonym for "assessment".

It is worth taking a moment to think about this aspect of assessment. What does it say about the therapy process if the therapist is "evaluating" the client? How do the therapist's views about human behavior and human relationships factor into the assessment process? How might clients feel about being "evaluated"? In the spirit of being aware of our assumptions, it is important to consider how the attitude that you bring to assessing or evaluating a case is a product of your own assumptions about people and therapy. It is also important to remember that the assessment process needs to be a positive experience for clients and needs to contribute to joining and to forming a strong therapeutic alliance. How we approach the assessment process will inevitably affect how our clients feel about us and about therapy.

There is one additional meaning of the term "assessment" that is worth mentioning. The term "assessment" can also be used to refer to a specific type of questionnaire that the therapist uses to gather information from the client about some aspect of the client's life. In this regard, an "assessment" is a carefully designed set of questions that are intended to measure some aspect of how clients interact, think, feel or behave. A therapist might say, "I'm working with a family who is concerned about their son's behavior and I'm considering using an assessment to get an objective measure of behavior. I think the Child Behavior Checklist might be a good option." In this context, we sometimes refer to a "formal assessment" or an "assessment tool" in order to distinguish this from the other two meanings of the term "assessment". Later in this chapter, we will talk a little more about the use of formal assessments and how this relates to theory and professional assumptions.

As we are discussing terminology, there are some other important terms to consider: case conceptualization and diagnosis. To understand and appreciate the importance of these terms, though, it is helpful to take a step back to consider what is happening during the assessment process in therapy.

"Case conceptualization", or just "conceptualization", refers to a process of organizing relevant information about a client's situation in order to provide a meaningful explanation or understanding of the client's presenting concern (Gehart, 2017a). "Conceptualization" is a part of assessment, but is distinct from assessment in that, in conceptualizing a case, we are not just learning about a client and their situation; we are adding in our own interpretation of what we've learned about the client in order to develop a useful way of viewing the client's situation (Patterson et al., 2018). Often a therapist's written assessment document will include a section where the therapist conceptualizes the presenting concern. This is typically a concise paragraph where the therapist highlights key pieces of information from the assessment in order to explain the issue bringing the client to therapy.

Conceptualization doesn't just happen in writing, though. As the word itself suggests, conceptualization is something that happens conceptually and is very much in the mind of the therapist, as well. As we'll discuss in more depth later, theory is important throughout assessment, but it is absolutely crucial in conceptualization. Different aspects of a client's experience are highlighted by different theories and will guide a therapist to focus on different pieces of information (Patterson et al., 2018). Each therapeutic model also comes with its own underlying assumptions, which are the determinant of how the therapist will explain or understand the issue that is bringing the client to therapy. Take another look at the quotation that appears at the beginning of this section:

"It is the theory that decides what can be observed" (Albert Einstein, as cited in Tomm et al., 2014). The thoughtful use of theory is what opens up helpful possibilities in your work with a client. This is a good point to mention one of the defining assumptions of systems theory and social constructionism: the idea that all people have strengths.

When going through the assessment process with people, we want to make a conscious choice to think in terms of strengths rather than deficits. Even if clients are really struggling in a certain area (e.g., a parent has a hard time setting limits with a child), we want to be mindful not to label people as being completely incapable (e.g., saying something like, "this parent has no boundaries with their child").

If we see people in an all-or-nothing way ("there is zero consistency" or "the couple shows no affection"), it makes it hard for us to have something to build on. No one is always anything. Rather than seeing clients as having a complete lack of something, it can be helpful to make a slight shift in our thinking and language, so that we're seeing areas that are low in something, but not completely lacking. When we, as therapists, make this shift in our thinking, it shapes the way that clients see themselves, ultimately making the change process a little easier. This reflects social constructionism and the strength-focused professional value of the MFT field.

Having defined **conceptualization** as a process of organizing information into a meaningful understanding of the client's presenting concern, there are a few additional terms that should be defined as part of our look at assessment. One is the term "**diagnosis**".

Consider Merriam Webster's (2020) definitions of this term. As a verb in medicine, **diagnosis** is "the art or act of identifying a disease from its signs and symptoms". As a noun, diagnosis is defined as "the decision reached by diagnosis", as in "the doctor's diagnosis".

In a more general context, not specific to medicine, diagnosis is the "investigation or analysis of the cause or nature of a condition, situation, or problem" or "a statement or conclusion from such an analysis". For example, a mechanic makes a diagnosis of engine trouble.

In mental health professions, including MFT, "diagnosis" (either as a verb or as a noun) typically reflects the medical definition of the term, which involves identifying and organizing a list of symptoms and associating a medical label or disease with those symptoms. There are two widely accepted methods for labeling mental health symptoms: *The Diagnostic and Statistical Manual of Mental Disorders* (DSM) (American Psychological Association, 2013) and the International Statistical Classification of Diseases and Related Health Problems (ICD). By and large, the DSM approach to diagnosis dominates mental health practice in the U.S.

Having heard these definitions of diagnosis, hopefully the parallels between conceptualization and diagnosis are apparent. Both are efforts to organize assessment information in a meaningful way so as to provide a basis for addressing the problem in question. In some regards, we could consider medical diagnosis a type of problem conceptualization. But, there are some very important differences to note.

Throughout, we have repeatedly emphasized the role that a therapist's assumptions play in how therapy is carried out. In this particular chapter, we noted earlier that our assumptions are especially influential when it comes to assessment.

Assumptions provide a basis for what questions we ask or don't ask, what information we choose to highlight and how we interpret the meaning of our client's experiences. Making a medical diagnosis of a mental health problem involves focusing only on symptoms and on grouping together these symptoms using a disease classification framework (most often the DSM).

In this regard, a diagnosis does NOT tell us what factors have contributed to a particular set of symptoms, nor does a diagnosis tell us what factors may be leading those symptoms to continue. Let's take a moment to contrast this with a conceptualization, the purpose of which is to provide a basis for how to effectively treat a problem in therapy. A diagnosis is one way of making sense of a particular subset of information (symptoms): by clustering a set of symptoms and associating these with a disease label. A diagnosis alone is not sufficient for informing therapy. Perhaps more significantly, if we're not careful, a diagnosis can limit our thinking, and we may end up only seeing a diagnosis rather than a whole person.

Thus, even when you are asked to make a DSM diagnosis as part of your assessment process, you will always need a more thorough conceptualization of a problem in order to provide effective therapy. Taking a closer look at our use of theory, specifically systems theory and social constructionism, will help provide greater clarity about how the conceptualization process both encompasses and is distinct from making a diagnosis. We'll say more about this in a moment.

Leading into our discussion of systems theory and social constructionism and their relevance to assessment, there is one final term to define: "**systemic hypothesis**". This is another term you may hear in the context of talking about assessment. Earlier we explained that the assessment process involves both gathering information and also organizing this information. Conceptualization refers to the process of organizing the information in a way that is guided by theory. For therapists whose work is guided by systems theory, their conceptualization process often involves developing a systemic hypothesis or explaining a presenting problem in a way that looks at that problem in the context of the relationships and mutually reinforcing patterns surrounding the problem (Metcalf, 2011). A "hypothesis" is an educated guess about something. A "systemic hypothesis" is an educated guess that uses systems theory to help explain a problem. As an MFT, your assessment process should always involve a systemic hypothesis, even if you are also expected to make a DSM diagnosis, too.

What we are going to do next is look at how the assumptions of systems theory and social constructionism influence how we approach assessment in MFT. This idea of developing a systemic hypothesis will come up again later on.

How systems theory and social constructionism inform assessment

Let's quickly review some of the defining assumptions of systems theory and social constructionism and consider their implications for assessment in MFT.

1. *Learning about interconnections, patterns of interaction, and context*

A definitional concept in systems theory is the idea of a system itself. In systems theory, the term "system" refers to an interconnected group of parts that is capable of exchanging information and adjusting behavior on the basis of that information (Minuchin, 1982). A group of parts that interacts over time is going to develop patterns of interaction. Human beings are fundamentally social, which means they are always sending and receiving information with those around them. A group of people that interacts repeatedly over time is going to develop patterns of interaction. What are the implications of this for assessment in therapy?

To understand a person and their experience, we must learn about their social context, that is, the people and other entities that the person interacts with on a regular basis. To understand an issue, we must understand the social context surrounding the issue. This means that when we gather information about a problem, we are not just listing symptoms, but rather we are viewing "symptoms" as part of a larger interpersonal context. What people and things influence the problem, and what people and things are affected by the problem? Our goal is to understand the patterns surrounding a problem, not to simply define the problem as a list of symptoms. Earlier, we explained diagnosis and systemic hypothesis as two ways to "make sense of a problem". Therapists who are guided by systems theory approach assessment with the goal of developing a systemic hypothesis, even if they are also expected to identify symptoms and associate a diagnostic label with those symptoms.

2. *Understanding problems in terms of circular causality and equifinality*

The systems theory assumption that truly distinguishes MFT assessment and conceptualization from that of other mental health professions is the belief that the vast majority of human issues are best explained by circular causality, rather than linear causality. Circular causality involves recognizing that causes can also be effects, and effects can also be causes (Bohecker & Kleist, 2017). In most situations, many things are happening simultaneously and they all mutually influence each other. For example, a spouse who loses trust in their partner may sometimes make unfair accusations, leading the partner to become defensive. Meanwhile, the partner's defensiveness prompts the spouse to further lose trust. If this couple sought out therapy, focusing only on one person's loss of trust or the other person's defensiveness is not an adequate explanation for the problem. The assessment process must go beyond just noting these two sets of symptoms; systems-theory informed assessment would involve identifying the mutually reinforcing pattern.

3. *Benevolent, strengths-focused way of viewing people*

One of the most powerful contributions of systems theory to the practice of therapy is the very simple idea that all behavior makes sense when viewed in the appropriate context. No matter how troubling or odd or socially unacceptable a behavior may be, the behavior somehow makes sense to the person or somehow serves a function within their relational system. What this means is that the assessment process involves understanding symptoms in terms of the function that they serve. This systems theory assumption also influences the attitude that MFTs bring to assessment in that there is a belief in people's inherent strengths and good intentions. We approach assessment with the idea that people are doing the best that they can. As we try to understand a situation, it is just as important to assess the client's perspective on the problem as it is to document the "symptoms". This aspect of systems theory relates to another foundational theory, social constructionism, which also influences how MFTs approach assessment.

4. *Assessment is not just recording the client's story, it is writing the client's story*

Human beings are meaning-making creatures. We are always in the process of making sense of things. We put experiences into stories. How we make sense of things is personal, but also socially influenced. This means that there are always multiple perspectives on a situation and that how we make sense of experiences is influenced by our contexts and the language that we use to describe and share those experiences (Mercadal, 2019). How we inquire about a client's experiences during the assessment process matters. Assessment is not just an objective process of gathering information. It is an interpersonal process of writing or rewriting a story. How you ask questions, what information you or the client emphasize or do not emphasize, what words you use to describe things, all of this matters. By recognizing that assessment is a social construction process, you have the opportunity to positively influence the way that the client narrates their experience of the problem in therapy.

Although clients generally arrive at therapy already telling a particular story about the problem, your process of inquiring about the problem matters and can end up being one of the earliest ways you help your clients' situations to improve. In fact, some scholars argue for the use of therapeutic assessment, which aims to move past simple information gathering to provide therapeutic benefit to clients (Finn, 2015).

5. *Assessment is an important experience in clients' relationships with each other and with the therapist*

Another thing that social constructionism teaches us about assessment is that perspective matters. When you're learning about the issues bringing clients to therapy, you're not just learning about what's happening; you're also learning about how each member of a couple or family sees the situation. What this means is that assessment is a process of gathering multiple perspectives on a problem. Regardless of what model or models of therapy you use, it is essential to gather information in a way that carefully incorporates each person's perspective on the problem.

Paying attention to **multiple perspectives** can be really powerful. This ties in with the systems theory ideas we discussed earlier, particularly the ideas of circular causality and patterns of interaction. By assessing the presenting problem from the perspective of each person in the system, the nature of the problem starts to shift, from one of linear causality (for example, blaming statements like "He does X" or "She does Y") to one of circular causality ("We are stuck in a vicious cycle of blame and defensiveness").

Assessing with multiple perspectives in mind provides us with a foundation for everyone defining the problem in a new, more useful way (in a systemic way).

One distinctive, common element in all larger system therapies is conceptualizing human difficulties in relational terms. This element stands in sharp contrast to the DSM view that mental disorders are conditions that occur "within a person". If Jamaal (age 35 years) is depressed, relationship therapists would not deny "within-person" elements like reduced serotonin (biology) or cognitive distortions (psychology) since they value a biopsychosocial (Engle, 1977) approach. However, Kayla, his relationship therapist, would be much more likely to view Jamaal's malady within the context of his social network, paying particular attention to the complex web of reciprocal influences contributing to the complaint. This view would lead Kayla to keep the whole system (or systems) in view when interacting with any part of the system. So, for example, Kayla might pay attention to Jamaal's problematic relationship with his employer, while at the same time paying attention to patterns or expectations about work that derived from his family of origin, where occupational success was highly valued. Kayla, herself an African American, would certainly take into account the race of her client (also African American) and what it was like for him to work in a predominantly White company. Jamaal's cognitive distortions (for example, his perfectionism) would also be conceptualized as both influenced by and influencing his social interactions and cultural environment. Moreover, Kayla would attempt to relate in a positive way to all elements of the system(s), irrespective of who happens to be in the therapy room. So, for example, if Jamaal's wife, Samantha, happened to refuse treatment (which she did not), Kayla would still consider her to be very much "present" in the treatment, as she would also with Jamaal's boss and colleagues at work since they were part of the relationship therapy conceptualization of Jamaal's depression (Sprenkle, Blow & Dickey, 1999). Pinsof (1995) calls the "cast of characters who are important to treatment and yet not physically present the 'indirect' treatment system. Another way of stating this unique common factor is that relational therapies pay special attention to the interactional cycles among the various subsystems that constitute the larger system in which the problem is embedded" (Sprenkle et al., 2009, pp. 35–36).

To see how these systemic and social constructionist ideas are relevant in assessment, let's consider the following example from Sprenkle et al.'s (2009) book, *Common factors in couple and family therapy*. This example illustrates many (although perhaps not all) of the systemic and social constructionist assumptions reviewed above.

Take a moment to think about this example in light of what we have discussed in terms of assessment. How did Kayla's assumptions, as a therapist, influence the information she gathered about Jamaal's situation? How did these assumptions influence her conceptualization of the case? Informed by systems theory and social constructionism, the MFT assessment process involves:

1. learning about interconnections, patterns of interaction and context
2. understanding problems in terms of circular causality
3. benevolent, a strengths-focused way of viewing people
4. not just recording the client's story, but writing the client's story
5. an important experience in clients' relationships with each other

These implications are relevant regardless of what specific style of therapy you use.

Using a therapy model during assessment

In our earlier overview of assessment, we explained it as a process of both gathering information and organizing that information into a useful understanding of the client's presenting concern. Assessment is the broader process of learning about a client (Gehart, 2017b), while case conceptualization refers to the more focused process of developing a useful view of the client's situation (Gehart, 2017a), so that we can proceed with a helpful therapy process. Having a clear set of guiding assumptions is important during the assessment process and it becomes crucial when it is time to develop a clear conceptualization of the case. Writing a treatment plan and actually carrying out therapy will be very difficult without a coherent understanding of the problem.

This is where using a therapy model is absolutely crucial. A model gives both you and your clients a common set of concepts for understanding the presenting problem and for planning a useful process to resolve the concern. During the information gathering process, a model operates as a sort of map of different "areas" that you'll want to "visit" in order to better understand the clients and their presenting problem. Having this map is essential because it guides you in what to inquire about. It is essential for the therapist to guide the assessment process, not just for the purpose of gathering information, but also to establish a therapeutic environment. Clients often come to therapy in distress; without support from the therapist in managing this distress, they'll tend to let the distress guide the conversation. This might seem cathartic at the time, but it is usually not helpful. An intentional, well-prepared therapist – guided by a therapy model – can help turn the assessment process into a positive experience for clients, one where they feel heard and where they feel hopeful about the prospect of improving their relationships. This is an instance where it's useful to think back to the earlier section on joining and also to those systemic and social constructionist assumptions we discussed above. Assessment is an experience that affects the therapeutic relationship!

Another way that using a specific model is important is with conceptualization specifically. One of the most important contributions of a therapy model is that it provides a set of assumptions about how and why problems develop in people's lives (Patterson et al., 2018). These assumptions are essential for conceptualizing the problem, that is, for having a coherent view of the problem that allows the clients and us to see a way forward.

When you're working with real clients (something that may not happen for a little while, depending on where you are in your career), conceptualization is very practical in the sense that your main objective is to figure out how to help clients in therapy. As a therapist in training, working on conceptualization also has a different purpose that has to do with learning to be a therapist. Conceptualization is something that you'll practice in order to expand your theory tool kit. Learning to conceptualize problems using different models of therapy is a valuable way to expand your options for how you think about your work with clients. Different models of therapy are to therapists what different styles of music are to a professional musician: while an accomplished musician may eventually settle on a favorite style, great musicians typically learn many different styles of music in order to develop well rounded skills. It's similar for therapists; practicing with different models will help expand your options for how you think about and work with your clients.

What does model-specific case conceptualization look like? Let's consider a situation that might bring people to therapy and explore how a therapist guided by a particular MFT model might approach the assessment and conceptualization process.

What follows is a case study, The Case of the Aversive Adolescent, which was originally included in a famous family systems theory book called *Tactics of Change* (Fisch, Weakland & Segal, 1982). The authors of this book developed one style of strategic therapy. In the original text, you can read at length about how a strategic therapist approached this case. Here we will use the same case to consider how a therapist using structural family therapy might approach assessment and conceptualization with this case. This example is not intended to provide a complete account of structural family therapy. Instead, it is designed to illustrate how a model guides the assessment and conceptualization process. This example will also provide the opportunity to consider how some of the systemic and social constructionist assumptions reviewed in an earlier lesson are relevant in assessment, regardless of the particular therapy model being used.

In The Case of the Aversive Adolescent, (Fisch et al., 1982) the parents of 15-year-old Suzie contacted a therapist at the suggestion of their daughter's probation officer. She had run away from home and had temporarily been placed in a juvenile detention facility but was now home again. The parents, Lydia and Tom, are in their early 40s and Suzie is the oldest of four children (the younger siblings are 12, 10 and 8 years old).

Latisha, who uses structural family therapy as her primary model of therapy, gets a call from Suzie's mother, Lydia, who explains the situation and asks when they can be seen. Latisha offers a few appointment times and Lydia selects a time when she and Suzie can come. Latisha asks when both parents might be available to come with Suzie, and explains that it can be helpful to get each parent's perspective. Lydia calls her husband to confer and then leaves a message for Latisha to confirm the appointment time. At the beginning of the first session, Latisha warmly welcomes the parents, greeting Lydia first, since they've spoken on the phone already. Latisha also thanks Tom and Suzie for coming and invites the family to sit down. Suzie plops down on one side of a two-person sofa. Tom sits next to her, and Lydia takes a chair in between Suzie and the therapist. Latisha asks the family members some simple questions to get to know them, before asking them how they think therapy can be helpful. Latisha addresses the question to Lydia first, explaining that since she and Lydia had already spoken, she wanted to ask Lydia to share her concerns so that all of them could develop a common goal for how therapy might be helpful. Lydia is forthcoming with information about the constant conflict between her and Suzie. Tom and Suzie both sit quietly; Tom sits up stiffly, while Suzie slouches over with arms crossed. Lydia explains that the conflict with Suzie goes back several years and has seemed to escalate over time. The mother also comments that she is worried about her daughter's moodiness and wonders whether she might be depressed. At the mention of depression, Suzie joins the conversation in her own defense, commenting that her mother needs to "get a life and stop putting all of her problems onto me". At this point, Tom steps in, partly to defend Lydia, but mostly to calm Suzie down.

Let's pause for a moment and consider Latisha's assessment process so far. Latisha's assessment process begins well before the first session. Learning about a client involves paying attention to how the family members relate, both with each other and with the therapist, even before we see them in therapy. In systems theory, we talk about the difference between **process** and **content**. Who makes the first phone call, who sits where during the first session, body language, who speaks first and so on… all of this provides clues about the interactional patterns in the family (note the systems theory assumptions here: all behavior is communication)? Latisha would also take into account, though, that she is seeing the family in a very specific circumstance. How the family operates in the therapist's office is not going to be exactly the same as they are at home (social constructionism is relevant here). As a structural therapist, Latisha's observations about the interactional process are especially relevant for guiding the process of joining with the family. All therapists must build rapport with clients; however, structural therapists are especially careful to pay attention to interactional patterns so that the therapist can connect with the family in a way that will give the therapist maximum therapeutic influence (the structural model is influencing Latisha here).

Besides noting the interactional process happening in the therapy room, Latisha also records some key pieces of information that Lydia and Suzie provide verbally. Lydia identifies the following concerns: legal problems, family conflict and possible depression. Suzie also alludes to Lydia being preoccupied with Suzie's behavior, a possible additional concern. An important part of all therapy is carefully listening to what the clients perceive as the main problems or concerns. These are the things that bring people to therapy and that will motivate people to engage in the therapy. The assessment and conceptualization process needs to keep the presenting concerns as a focal point, even if the therapist identifies other issues that might warrant attention.

Systems theory in general, and structural family therapy specifically, views presenting problems as pieces of a larger puzzle that involves interactional processes. The systemic assumption that "all behavior makes sense in context" reminds Latisha to be curious about how the main symptoms or problems, no matter how troubling, may make sense somehow, given the family organization. Structural therapists assess the role or function of the symptom. What this means is that they are considering how the symptom may be a part of an ongoing pattern of interaction that somehow keeps the symptom going. In the case of Suzie and her family, this question about the function of the symptom is likely something that Latisha would be wondering about from the beginning. While a structural therapist would want to look at the context surrounding a symptom like depressed mood, Latisha might still consider using a formal assessment tool, such as a youth depression inventory. A formal assessment measure could be helpful in documenting changes over time. Additionally, providing a DSM diagnosis may be required, depending on how the family has been referred for therapy. As a structural family therapist, Latisha would be very careful about how such assessment activities were presented to the family. Without first understanding the interactional processes and the meaning of Lydia labeling Suzie as "depressed", Latisha might accidentally reinforce a family pattern that is part of the problem. From a structural therapy standpoint, we might say that Latisha could form an unintentional coalition with Lydia as a result of how a formal assessment measure like a depression inventory or DSM diagnosis is incorporated into assessment. This would not rule out using such assessment tools, but rather would make it necessary for Latisha to be thoughtful about how they're incorporated.

While no two structural therapists are the same, it is likely that Latisha's next assessment steps would involve learning more about the family structure. Are the parents on the same team? Are they connected as a couple? Are they in an effective leadership position within the family? What are the boundaries like among the family members? Structural therapists typically assess family structure using the process of the session and through indirect observation. For example, we have already seen a few clues about structure based on where the family members sat and based on who spoke when.

Structural therapists also use enactments or in-session interactions to assess structure. Latisha might ask Lydia, Tom and Suzie to reenact how their conversation went following the last time Suzie came home after running away.

Structural therapists also use the process of therapy – for example, the scheduling of appointments with certain members of therapy – as both an assessment tool and as an intervention. At the close of the session, Latisha might propose that she meet with Lydia and Tom alone for the next session. The structural model would motivate this action on Latisha's part. Meeting with Suzie's parents is a way of drawing a boundary around the parental subsystem. By proposing this for the next session, Latisha is learning about the parents' tendencies with regard to working together as a team. Latisha might also consider inviting the younger siblings to therapy in order to learn more about how they see the concerns bringing the family to therapy. These practical scheduling decisions, guided by the structural model, are an important part of the assessment process.

Moving forward, Latisha could proceed in a number of ways, depending on what she learns from the family and how the family members respond to the process. As early as the first session, she is noticing areas that might require urgent attention (for example, Suzie running away could involve immediate concerns related to safety), and she is also probably starting to formulate a conceptualization of the problem in her head. This conceptualization would be very tentative and would be open to revision based on new information. In subsequent sessions, Latisha would continue to learn about the family's typical interactions and how the presenting concerns, including Suzie's behavior, can be better understood in the context of the interactional patterns in the family. Looking through the lens of structural family therapy, Latisha would consider whether the symptoms might be calling attention to the need for adjustment in the structure of the family so that the family structure can best support the wellbeing of individual family members and of the family as a whole. This would essentially be her systemic hypothesis. During this process, Latisha will be paying very careful attention to how the family members respond to her and to her efforts to gently reframe the problem in new ways that take into account interconnections among all of the family members of the family system. Within the first few sessions, structural therapists carefully and strategically share their systemic hypothesis with the family in order to help the family shift the way that they are seeing the problem. This forms the basis for setting goals that the whole family supports, paving the way for writing a collaborative treatment plan with goals that involve the whole family.

This brief case study, although oversimplified, provides a look at how the assessment process in MFT is guided by theory, including foundational ideas of systems theory and social constructionism and the assessment concepts from a specific model of therapy. In your course work and later in your clinical work with clients, you will use theory (including systems theory and a specific therapy model) to learn about your clients and to develop helpful conceptualizations of the issues that bring them to therapy.

Before concluding this section on assessment, there is one final important topic to consider: the use of formal assessments. Toward the beginning of this section, we explained that the term "assessment" refers to an overall information gathering process, or it can refer to a specific organized set of questions that a therapist uses to gather information about a specific issue. A "formal assessment" can be a written questionnaire, a specific set of questions that a therapist asks verbally or a particular task that a client is asked to carry out while the therapist observes. A formal assessment tool (sometimes called a "measure") is carefully developed so that the information that is gathered can be compared to a set of standards that are grounded in research.

Often, therapists use formal assessments to measure particular aspects of a client's presenting problem. Using formal assessments, we can identify needs early, objectively measure areas targeted for change and provide a convenient means for gathering information repeatedly throughout therapy (Huff, Anderson & Edwards, 2014, citing Cromwell, Olson & Fournier, 1976). For example, a therapist might use the Conflict Tactics Scale in order to assess for the presence of violence in a relationship. Using formal assessments to measure aspects of the presenting problem can be helpful in noticing issues that reach an objective threshold of concern (for example, using the Conflict Tactics Scale may help a therapist determine whether a relationship includes abuse that could present a safety risk).

Using formal assessments can also help us track progress over time. For example, with a client whose presenting concerns involve symptoms of depression, using the Beck Depression

Inventory every few sessions could help the therapist and client both notice progress. Formal assessment can be especially valuable in providing clients with feedback about their progress (Huff et al., 2014, citing Lambert et al., 2001). Moreover, using formal assessments to evaluate progress fulfills the therapist's ethical responsibility to evaluate the effectiveness of their services (Shaw & Murray, 2014). Monitoring client progress using formal assessment tools is increasingly seen as a requirement in competent mental health care. For example, in January 2018, the U.S. Substance Abuse and Mental Health Services Administration (SAMHSA) and The Joint Commission (one of the largest independent accreditors of health care organizations) announced that organizations would be required to use standardized assessment tools to measure progress. This is a sign that documenting progress using formal assessment tools is becoming the norm.

Besides using assessments to learn about different aspects of a client's life and to document progress, we can also use assessments to monitor the therapy process, particularly the therapeutic alliance. Asking the client directly about their perceptions of the therapeutic alliance can be incredibly helpful (Shaw & Murray, 2014). As noted elsewhere, the Common Factors research teaches us that therapeutic alliance is one of the most important factors in determining the success of therapy (Sprenkle et al., 2009). The client's perception of the therapeutic alliance is a particularly good predictor of whether therapy will succeed (Shaw & Murray, 2014). Moreover, making it a habit to assess the therapeutic alliance can actually improve the therapeutic alliance (think about how encouraging it would feel to have someone formally check in to ask, "Is this process helpful for you? Are we working on what's important to you?" etc.

When thinking about the use of formal assessments, we can't forget the importance of theory and awareness of assumptions. "It is the theory that determines what may be observed." In the context of looking at formal assessments, we might as well say, "it is the assessment tool that determines what may be observed". When using formal assessments, it is essential to keep theory always in mind. The assumptions of systems theory, social constructionism and specific MFT models all come into play when using formal assessments. Think back to earlier consideration of how systems theory and social constructionism are relevant in assessment. If we choose formal assessments that focus only on symptoms within a person (e.g., the Beck Depression Inventory), how might that frame or limit the way that we (both therapist and client) think about the client's presenting concerns? How might that affect the therapeutic relationship? Think back to the example of Jamaal and Kayla (Sprenkle et al., 2009) and the value of maintaining a relational perspective, even when working with individual clients. Being aware of the assumptions we're making about a client and their presenting concerns is absolutely essential when using formal assessments, because those tools reflect someone else's assumptions! As systemic therapists, we need to be particularly aware when using assessments that view problems as something that comes from within a person. This can counteract all of our best efforts to collaborate with clients in seeing problems in systemic ways. On the other hand, using systemic assessments (assessments that target interpersonal patterns) specifically can support clients in seeing problems in a systemic way (Huff et al., 2014). Such systemic reframing is identified as one of the common factors of effective relational therapy (Sprenkle et al., 2009), and your careful choice of assessment tools can aid in this.

Remember that assumptions guide all of our decisions in therapy. How does your selection of formal assessments influence the therapy process? It's essential to be intentional in thinking about why you choose a particular formal assessment and how your use of this tool may influence the client's experience and the way that the client and therapist are both viewing the problem.

Albert Einstein said, "If I were given one hour to save the world, I would spend 59 minutes defining the problem and one minute solving it." Time spent carefully assessing can pay off tenfold. A thoughtful assessment process, guided by theory, helps therapists and clients collaboratively identify information that can end up being invaluable for solving or resolving the issues bringing a client to therapy. In many ways, the assessment process flows seamlessly into goal setting, which we will consider next. Assessment conversations involve obtaining a clear description of the presenting problem. When therapists and clients collaboratively agree on the focus of therapy (defined in terms of what clients don't want), this paves the way for important conversations about the goals of therapy (defined in terms of what clients **do** want).

Core therapy process 3 – goal setting

One of the most important points in therapy journey is the formulation of goals. Whereas assessment involves a collaborative process of learning about aspects of a client's situation relevant to the problem, goal setting involves defining the destination for the therapeutic journey. What do clients want to achieve as a result of their work with you? Defining goals for therapy is the ultimate collaborative process because the clients' desires and the therapist's expertise are both incredibly important. The client's desires are paramount in that therapy is the client's journey; we may serve as a guide, but the client ultimately determines the destination. The Common Factors research consistently supports the importance of therapist-client alignment around goals as a key ingredient in successful therapy (Sprenkle et al., 2009). At the same time, it is important to note that clients typically come to therapy unsure about where to go.

While they may know what they don't want, defining positively what they do want is often the biggest hurdle. This is why a therapist's thoughtful use of theory and a specific therapy model is essential during goal-setting conversations. Guided by theory, we can work with clients to identify new territory so that the client can ultimately say, "Yes! This is where I want to go!"

Why does the client's perspective matter so much in goal setting? In their book, *Common factors in couple and family therapy*, Sprenkle, Lebow and Davis (2009) drive home the point that "Clients are the ones who choose what to pay attention to and how to make it work" (p. 70). They go on to explain, therapy facilitates naturally occurring healing aspects of clients lives.

Therapists function as support systems and resource providers. "This view contrasts with most of the literature on psychotherapy. There, the therapist is the 'hero' who, with potent techniques and procedures, intervenes in clients' lives and fixes their malfunctioning machinery" (as cited in Sprenkle et al., 2009, pp. 70–71). This insight from the Common Factors research reminds us that therapy is helpful to the extent that it connects with clients' lives in meaningful ways.

Consider what Perry (2016) observes about identifying the focus of therapy:

Conventional wisdom in psychotherapy is that the presenting problem – what the client comes in wanting to see changed – is seldom the real problem. There are at least three reasons why this may be true. First, clients may be applying a lot of effort at the wrong place. In other words, they may be actively trying to solve the wrong problem. For example, the client may believe the problem is their spouse's "unexplained" emotional distance, when the real problem is their own unacknowledged depression. Second, clients may be hesitant to reveal the real problem for fear the therapist will reject them in some manner. For example, never, in this author's experience, has an adult client come in with a presenting problem of having been sexually abused as a child. That real issue emerges only later, when trust is established. Third, the therapist may be so eager to 'get to the root of the problem' that the therapist misses the main issue entirely. Abraham Maslow is quoted as saying, 'to the man who only has a hammer in the toolkit, every problem looks like a nail (Perry, 2016, p. 26).

Perry's (2016) comments here show why goal-setting conversations are so important: as we talk with clients about what they want from therapy, the nature of the problem often transforms in helpful ways that allow the client and therapist the chance to move forward. When clients begin to name what they do want, the way forward becomes much more accessible (in this regard, think about how the goal-setting process can affect the therapeutic alliance and the clients' hopefulness).

This idea that goal setting transforms the problem is complex and is worth thinking about carefully. There is A LOT of knowledge and skill that a therapist brings to the table during goal-setting conversations. Our foundations in systems theory and social constructionism and our use of a therapy model are all important in formulating useful therapeutic goals. As you set goals with clients, your awareness of your own assumptions is crucial! The assessment process, reviewed earlier, is the foundation for goal setting… think back to the ways that systems theory, social constructionism and specific models relate to conceptualization. This serves as a springboard for productive goal-setting conversations.

There are some particularly important shifts that happen as MFTs set goals with clients. The early sessions in therapy involve subtle, but powerful shifts in the way that everyone is thinking about and talking about the problem. As the therapist and client collaboratively learn about the problem and what the client hopes to accomplish in therapy, the meaning of the problem usually evolves. Goal setting is not just a practical step that leads to a treatment plan. Goal setting is a delicate, collaborative process wherein the initial reasons the clients came to therapy morph into a productive focus for the therapeutic process. During this process, the therapist's knowledge and skills are essential. Asking questions and exploring the goals of therapy in particular ways can not only lead to useful goals, but can also move the clients closer.

Often the view of the problem shifts from one that is individually framed to one that is systemic. There is a systems theory assumption about circular causality – that problems are usually affected by many things, not just one thing, and that people are usually mutually influencing each other, as opposed to there being a single, one-directional cause-effect relationship (Metcalf, 2011). What this means is that helpful goals are often framed in ways that incorporate relationships and interconnections, rather than just individual thoughts, emotions and behaviors. Even when goals are framed in terms of individual changes, the relationship context is a part of the picture.

In shifting to a more systemic perspective, goal setting can be one of our earliest interventions. Helping clients be invested in a systemic conceptualization of their problem builds further alliance (a common factor) and expands the treatment system (a systemic common factor); goal setting can be therapeutic in itself (Baker & Chang, 2013). With couples and families in therapy, conversations about goals (what do **we** want) can offer therapeutic opportunities to understand differences in perspective and to identify common ground.

Another important shift that therapists can help foster during goal setting is the move from framing things in a negative way (what we **don't** want) to a positive way (what we **do** want). Well-formulated goals need to be positive and concrete (Baker & Chang, 2013, p. 89; Gehart, 2017b). They are expressions of what **will** be happening, phrased in ways that are easy for clients and therapist to identify. There are a number of different frameworks available for guiding the formulation of clear, objective goals.

These shifts – from individual to systemic and from negative to positive – involve a lot of therapist skills and theory, which are incredibly important. This is one of the most important places that theory can be our guide. Rooted in systems theory and/or social constructionism, the MFT models each offer insights relevant to formulating systemic, positively defined goals.

For example, consider a contextual therapist who is working with a mother and adult daughter around substance abuse and issues stemming from childhood trauma of the adult daughter. While the problem may be defined in terms of substance abuse and trauma symptoms, the goals for therapy might be defined in terms of interactions that build trust and provide opportunities for forgiveness. Guided by the contextual model (which ties in systems theory and social constructionism), the therapist can contribute to goal-setting conversations by weaving ideas regarding justice, trust and forgiveness. Simply talking about these things during a goal-setting conversation could end up being therapeutic, even if longer term healing is needed.

As another example, imagine a solution-focused therapist working with a young adult client who has struggled with symptoms of depression and suicidal thoughts.

During goal setting, the therapist is guided by the core assumptions of solution-focused therapy – that the client is the expert, that they have the resources they need to develop solutions and that collaborative conversations harness the power of meaning-making to reinforce solutions. Talking with this client about times when they felt stronger and happier and about what they want for their life, the therapist and client collaboratively identify that increasing closeness with the client's parents is associated with those times when the problem is less of a problem. The client defines goals that have to do with interacting with their parents in ways that fit with a life where the problem is reduced to a manageable level.

In each of these examples, consider how the assumptions of systems theory and social constructionism are apparent, in addition to specific concepts from particular therapy models.

These are just a few examples of how therapists can draw on theory – including specific therapy models, systems theory and social constructionism – in order to collaborate define goals with clients.

Although this section has focused on goal setting as a conversation, actually writing goals is essential, and this is one of the many reasons that formal (written) treatment plans are important. Before moving on to discuss the development of formal treatment plans, we will look at the planning of therapeutic interventions using theory. We'll end by considering documentation and evaluation, giving specific attention to written treatment plans.

Core therapy process 4 – intervention

While goals and objectives are the heart of a treatment plan, identifying interventions is probably the part of treatment planning that challenges new therapists the most. When you have never moved a client through the therapeutic process before, it is hard to know what you will actually **do** with clients in order to help them achieve their goals. This is where your use of theory (particularly a therapy model) is absolutely essential. Therapy models provide therapists with strategies for resolving problems and for facilitating growth and development. Each model includes its own set of assumptions about the sorts of experiences and activities that will lead to positive change. Earlier in this lesson, we talked about therapy models involving a "**theory of change**". As you become more experienced as a therapist, you will become more and more able to articulate your own personal theory of change. Early in your career, though, the use of a model is essential for having a sound theory of change. Let's look at a couple of therapy models, giving particular attention to their theories of change.

We'll consider how each model's theory of change translates into specific interventions that therapists use to help clients meet their goals. The following discussions of specific models are not meant to be comprehensive reviews of the model. Instead, they provide brief overviews of the model's theories of change, illustrating how the model's assumptions about change relate to the interventions a therapist might list in a treatment plan.

Example of intervention planning using the structural family therapy model

In a classic structural therapy book, Minuchin and Fishman (1981) said the following about structural therapy's theory of change:

> The structural approach sees the family as an organism: a complex system that is underfunctioning. The therapist undermines the existing homeostasis, creating crises that jar the system toward the development of a better functioning organization. Thus, the structural approach has elements of both the existential [Whitaker's experiential] and strategic frameworks. Like the strategist, the structuralist realigns significant organizations to produce change in the entire system. And like the existentialist [e.g., Whitaker in experiential therapy], the structuralist challenges the family's accepted reality with an orientation toward growth. Structural family therapy partakes of the existentialist's concern for growth and the strategist's concern for cure. The techniques of structural therapy lead to family reorganization by challenging the family organization. The word challenge highlights the nature of the dialectic struggle between family and therapist within the therapeutic system. The word does not imply harsh maneuvers, or confrontation, though at times both may be indicated. It suggests a search for new patterns, as well as the fact that, as in the work of Siva, goddess of destruction, the old order must be undermined, to allow for the formation of the new. There are three main strategies of structural family therapy, each of which is served by a group of techniques. The three strategies are challenging the symptom, challenging the family structure, and challenging the family reality. (p. 67)

Structural therapy's theory of change focuses on making changes to the organization or "structure" of a family system. Changes in structure can happen in a variety of ways. Therapists can support clients in changing their thinking. Structural therapists may challenge certain aspects of a family's worldview or may reframe the problem in helpful ways. These conversational techniques are interventions that a structural therapist might list in their treatment plan in association with particular therapeutic goals.

Changes in structure can also happen when families are supported in interacting with each other in new ways. Structural therapists are known for asking families to enact common conflict situations; during these enactments, therapists can coach clients on relating to each other in new ways, which can foster shifts in the boundaries, hierarchy and subsystem functioning of a family. An enactment is a classic structural therapy intervention that a therapist would list in a treatment plan, both for the purposes of assessment and for the purposes of encouraging specific changes in the family structure.

Example of intervention planning using the experiential therapy model

Emotionally-focused therapy (EFT) founder Sue Johnson (2004) explains EFT's theory of change:

> EFT is a synthesis of experiential and systemic approaches to therapy… The human-istic experiential perspective focuses upon how to help partners to reprocess and expand their experience and the systemic perspective focuses upon how to help partners modify their interaction patterns… Change in EFT is associated with the accessing and reprocessing of the emotional experience underlying each partner's pos-ition in the relationship. The creation of new elements of emotional experience and new ways of expressing that experience tend to modify the positions partners take with each other, and allow for key new interactions to occur that then redefine the bond between partners.
>
> Change does not occur primarily through insight, through some type of catharsis, or through negotiation. It occurs through new emotional experience and new inter-actional events. As Einstein suggested, " "All knowledge is experience: everything else is just information."
>
> (pp. 41–52)

Experiential forms of therapy – including Satir's Human Growth Model, Whitaker's Symbolic-Experiential and contemporary experiential approaches like Emotionally-Focused Therapy – are named after the word "experience", which refers to the fact that change happens through what people experience. Experiencing a meaningful interaction is different from reflecting on that interaction. In experiential styles of therapy, interventions involve working with what clients are experiencing during the therapeutic session (McDowell, Knudson-Martin & Bermudez, 2018). A therapist applying EFT would select interventions that involve working with clients' in-session experiences. For example, a therapist might ask a couple to talk about a difficult time in their relationship, practicing being aware of pri-mary and secondary emotions. This might be one of several interventions associated with a goal of increasing the frequency of interactions that involve emotional intimacy.

Example of intervention planning using the solution-focused therapy model

Solution-focused therapists Walter and Peller (1992), explain what makes solution-focused theory of change different:

> We like to think that therapists develop therapy models out of some initial struggle or question. The question may arise from the therapist's particular experiences with a certain population of clients or with certain types of problems… These therapy models

begin to take shape as the developers speculate and then articulate answers to their initial questions about their clients and their clients' problems... The questions that developers of therapy models ask contain presuppositions within them. Therefore, by their very asking the questions, developers pre-select directions toward particular answers or classes of answers. The evolution of ideas and trends of therapy models can thus be traced through the assumptions within the original questions of the therapy modelers. For example: WHAT IS THE CAUSE OF THE PROBLEM? In the early part of this century, science was shaped by the objectivism of the traditional scientific method. The chief question modelers usually asked was: What is the cause of the problem? ... WHAT MAINTAINS THE PROBLEM? This question presupposes that a problem is being maintained and stresses its maintenance rather than its cause. As with "What causes the problem?" the therapy modeler accepts that there is a problem, but presupposes that the problem is being maintained and that there is a relationship that can be found and described between the maintenance and the problem. Most of the answers to "What maintains the problem?" explain the maintenance as taking place within interactional patterns that can be mapped in different was... HOW DO WE CONSTRUCT SOLUTIONS? Within recent years, there is another, different, and new question being asked: How do we construct solutions? The presuppositions within this question are: 1. that there are solutions, 2. that there is more than one solution, 3. that they are constructable, 4. that we (therapist and client) can do the constructing, 5. that we construct and/or invent solutions rather than discover them, and 6. that this process or processes can be articulated and modelled... One, define what the client wants rather than what he or she does not; two, look for what is working and do more of it; three, if what the client is doing is not working, then have him or her do something different.

(pp. 1–6)

As the name indicates, solution-focused therapy involves a very deliberate shift in the attention of both the therapist and the client, from problem-focus to solution-focus. Solution-focused therapy's theory of change is heavily influenced by postmodern theories of knowledge (social constructionism and constructivism), which suggest that our realities are created through the process of putting experience into narratives or stories we tell about life (McDowell et al., 2018). These stories are fundamentally relational, meaning that our life stories are not just written by us as individuals, but by important social connections in our lives. Solution-focused therapy's theory of change also includes unique assumptions (relative to other therapy theories) that preferred ways of living can be intentionally chosen, that no problem is universal or permanent, and that solutions to problems can be intentionally constructed. Therapeutic interventions in the solution-focused approach involve things like helping clients to define, clearly and positively, what they want and deliberately noticing both exceptions to the problem and progress. The interventions in solution-focused therapy involve strategies for guiding the way that clients and therapists talk about and think about the problem.

Core therapy process 5 – documentation and evaluation

Documentation refers to how you record, in writing, what happens in therapy. Evaluation refers to making judgments about how the therapy process is going and about the effectiveness of therapy. Although it is possible to separate these two things, in today's professional practice of therapy, documentation and evaluation are virtually inseparable. When you are documenting what is happening in therapy, questions such as "How am I doing as a therapist?" and "How is the client doing relative to their goals?" should always be involved.

Therapists have both ethical and legal responsibilities to document the process of therapy in writing (AAMFT, 2015). In particular, therapists are expected to document the clients' progress or improvement relative to the goals of therapy. Documenting your work with clients keeps you accountable, both to yourself and to your clients.

Appropriate documentation helps you carry out therapy in an intentional way (there is a logic behind what you're doing; there is a clear plan from one session to the next). In this regard, documentation, evaluation and your use of theory go hand in hand, as theory is also an essential part of carrying out therapy in an intentional, competent way. Documenting therapy also helps you be accountable to your clients. How you document therapy in writing will influence how you talk about the therapy process with your clients. In this regard, your documentation process supports the formation of a therapeutic alliance (see Sprenkle et al., 2009). In addition to promoting accountability to yourself (checking your own competency) and to your client, documenting therapy also allows your work in therapy to be reviewed by other professionals, when ethically or legally appropriate. For example, if a client is referred to therapy by the court system, by child protective services or by another type of professional such as a physician, these entities may request to see certain information about how therapy is being carried out. With the client's consent, you may share information with other professionals. Or your clients may seek therapy services as a benefit covered by their health insurance. With the client's permission, you will share information with the insurance company about the service you're providing. In all of these cases, documenting therapy in a clear, professional way (a way that others can understand) is really important. Being aware of your own assumptions about how therapy works, having a clear theory of change and being solidly grounded in a therapy model are an essential part of documenting therapy and evaluating progress in a way that other professionals can understand.

Therapy is documented in several ways. You'll need to record basic information about who the client is. You'll need to document that you've taken essential ethical steps as part of initiating therapy, obtaining the client's consent to the therapy process, reviewing confidentiality policies, etc. You'll need to document your assessment or information gathering process. This includes documenting your client's reasons for seeking therapy (sometimes called the "presenting problem" or "presenting concern"). This also includes other information you gather in order to understand the presenting problem and in order to evaluate other needs that the client might have. Depending on how you approach your information gathering process, you may be documenting the results of formal assessment you give your clients to learn about them. Part of documenting the information gathering process involves developing a tentative explanation or "picture" or conceptualization of the client's presenting concern. Think back to what we discussed earlier about the importance of the assumptions you bring to therapy. Your beliefs about people (including about how/why problems happen in people's lives) are going to influence how you learn about your clients, what questions you ask, how you "frame" the presenting problem, etc. And when it comes to documenting what you've learned about your clients, your assumptions are going to be an essential part of the way that you document this information in writing.

Another important place that you document therapy is in something called a **treatment plan**. While all forms of documentation are important, the written treatment plan has special significance for several reasons. As a written document, your treatment plan captures the problem or problems that are the focus of therapy, the goals of therapy and your basic strategic for helping your client address their reasons for coming to therapy. When you put this information in writing, you are helping to solidify the focus of therapy both for you and for your clients. The process of developing a treatment plan is not a mere administrative step; it is pivotal in helping you and your client have a clear, shared focus for your work together. When doing couple and family therapy, specifically, developing a treatment plan is arguably even more important, because writing shared goals for therapy helps the members of the couple or family come together around a unified purpose. More often than not, this is an important first step in the healing or change process. You need to be intentional and thoughtful in how you go about defining the problem that therapy is addressing, and how you develop written goals. As noted elsewhere in the section on joining, forming shared goals is a crucial part of the therapeutic alliance. Developing a written treatment plan in a collaborative way helps support the alliance in this regard. This is supported by Common Factors research (Sprenkle et al., 2009). On top of clearly defining the issue that therapy addresses and clearly identifying the goals of therapy, the written treatment plan also includes information about the things you'll do with your clients in therapy in order to accomplish the goals. Your theory of change and your model of therapy are going to be your guiding force during the development of your treatment plan. While all treatment plans address these three basic things – the presenting concern, the goals for therapy and what you'll do to meet the goals – written treatment plans can take on many different formats. The next section looks more closely at the development of written treatment plans, including why they are important and options for how they can be formatted.

Why do therapists write (formal) treatment plans?

In today's therapy world, written treatment plans are a standard of competent therapy. Treatment plans are like a map that aids therapists and clients on their journey together. Consider what Perry (2016) says here about the importance of treatment plans:

> The treatment plan functions like a road map on the journey the counselor and client are taking together – the journey from where the client is at the beginning of therapy to where the client wants to be at the conclusion of therapy. While it is true that many managed care companies require treatment plans before reimbursing for therapeutic services rendered, that is probably the worst reason to do them. Simply constructive treatment plans to satisfy an insurer's requirements can result in the plan being a meaningless exercise in paperwork. A far better reason to consider the treatment plan is to further express the therapist's ethical duty to provide the best possible care for the client.
>
> However, the counselor does the diagnostic work, the treatment plan serves the invaluable function of keeping the therapist from chasing every new issue the client happens to present. Each new issue is measured by the questions, 'How does this issue relate to our agreed upon focus of therapy? How will solving this issue help us reach our agreed upon goals?' Unless the client and counselor explicitly contract for an additional focus of treatment, if the new issue does not meet the pragmatics of the treatment plan, the therapist must simply let the issue die from lack of attention.
>
> (Perry, 2016, pp. 78–79)

Treatment plans are important for you (the therapist) and for other stakeholders who may be involved in therapy (for example, an insurance company or Child Protective Services), but, more than anyone else, the treatment plan exists for the client. Although the plan for therapy will often evolve as therapy progresses, having a plan is essential in that it guides you and the client together through a process that could otherwise become aimless. Having clear goals and a plan for accomplishing those goals is essential! This cannot be overstated. Even if the goals and the intervention plans change, your clients will be much better off as a result of having started with a clear plan. Let's consider how a treatment plan helps the client, the therapist and other stakeholders involved in therapy.

Developing the treatment plan helps the client identify their goals and become invested in the therapy process

More than any other entity, it is the client who benefits the most from the development of a good treatment plan. **It is their journey!**

More often than not, clients have tried to solve their own problems for a long time before seeking therapy. Frequently, clients have thought about the problem a lot, but often they don't have a clear picture of what the opposite of the problem is. One of the most helpful things you can do early in therapy is to help clients define what they **do** want. This is a key place where therapeutic skill and professional theory come into play. As you talk with your clients about their presenting concern or presenting problem you will make use of professional theory in order to expand and adjust how the client is talking about the problem and in order to identify what life will look like for the client when/if therapy is successful.

A treatment plan guides the therapist: having a clear plan for the therapy process is necessary for competent therapy

Earlier in this lesson, we explained the therapy process as involving the following: forming a relationship, gathering information, setting goals, intervening and documenting. Depending on how you approach writing a treatment plan, your written treatment plan may explicitly plan out this entire process or it may only focus on the goals and interventions. The treatment plan can help guide you through the therapy process; it allows you to organize your thinking and to plan from one session to the next. In particular, a written treatment plan is essential for helping therapists be intentional in connecting the conceptualization, goals and therapeutic interventions.

A treatment plan conveys to third parties (e.g., insurance companies, Medicaid, Child Protective Services, the legal system) what will happen in therapy

Carefully written treatment plans are necessary for making it clear what the purpose or aim of therapy is and what methods are being used to accomplish the aims of therapy. If therapy is being paid for by a managed care entity or is mandated by the legal or child protective systems, then these entities may have expectations about what problems will be addressed by therapy. These entities may also have expectations about what types of therapeutic methods are used to address these problems. In some instances, insurance companies or other entities will only pay for services that use therapy methods with a certain amount of research support. In these cases, a clear treatment plan demonstrates how these evidence-supported methods will be incorporated into a course of therapy.

A major focus of this chapter on treatment plan writing is on how we talk with clients about problems, how we introduce new and helpful ways of thinking about the problem and how we work with clients to define the goals that the client hopes to achieve through therapy. During the assessment phase of therapy, you're learning about the problem and about the client's circumstances in order to expand the understanding of the problem in helpful ways and to positively define what therapy is aiming for. This conversational process, which happens during your interactions with your clients, is the foundation for writing a treatment plan.

The components of a written treatment plan

Treatment plans always include a clear statement of the problem or problems being addressed by therapy. The description of the problem should incorporate the client's perspective of the problem and should also reflect the therapist's expertise in helping the client turn vague descriptions of the problem into clear, observable descriptions (Patterson et al., 2018). As systems-theory informed therapists, MFTs also use their professional expertise to help clients move from individual descriptions of the problem (which often involve blaming) to systemic descriptions that capture the patterns of interaction that are a part of maintaining the problem. Describing the problem systemically helps clients shift their way of looking at the problem, which can help all members of the client system be more engaged in the therapy process.

Describing the problem systemically also paves the way for setting systemic goals.

Clear goals are the heart of any treatment plan. Every treatment plan will include some statement of what therapy is helping the client to accomplish. Some treatment plans include goals that are problem-focused and only frame goals in terms of reducing or eliminating problems. For example, if a couple presents for therapy complaining about conflict, then a problem-focused goal might involve reducing the conflict to an acceptable level. While problem-focused treatment plans may "pay the bills" (literally, in that they may satisfy insurance companies), they tend not to be the most helpful to clients. A wise MFT colleague of mine made this comparison: imagine getting into a taxicab and telling the driver, "Don't drive me to the beach!" Other than saying where you don't want to be, this instruction is not very helpful in getting you to your destination.

Terminology note: goals versus objectives

What are we aiming for in therapy? The terminology "goals and objectives" in therapy, used in treatment plans (and guidance about writing treatment plans), can be really confusing. A variety of terms are used to describe what we're aiming for in therapy. What therapy is aiming for is generally described in two ways within a treatment plan: a more general, global description of what we're aiming for, and a more specific, observable description of how we'll know that therapy has been successful. More often than not, the term "goal" is used to refer to the more global aim of therapy, whereas as the term "objective" is used to refer to very specific, observable indications of progress. When you're writing a treatment plan, ideally you will include both. You'll have statements of the broad aims of therapy and you'll also have statements of measurable, observable changes that will indicate progress toward the client's goals. In some treatment plan formats, the global statements of what we're aiming for are accompanied by several specific objectives that provide observable indicators of progress toward a goal. In other treatment plan formats, you'll provide only the specific, measurable indicators of change.

Therapy can aim at resolving problems, restoring or establishing individual and relational health, and promoting growth and development (Makover, 2016). While eliminating problems may be the goal in some cases, therapeutic goals are generally much more helpful when they are stated in positive terms about what the client does want, and this often involves defining how the client hopes to be operating, either individually or relationally or both. Defining goals in positive terms also involves describing progress, growth and development that may subsume the resolution of the problem. As mentioned above, the therapist's professional expertise is incredibly important when working with clients to define meaningful goals. The therapist's theoretical assumptions and preferred model(s) will be an important part of defining the aim of therapy.

So far, we've talked about two essential components of a treatment plan: a description of the problem and goals. The third essential component of a treatment plan are interventions. **Interventions are specific actions that a therapist takes in order to encourage positive change in a client.** When writing out a treatment plan, it wouldn't be much of a plan unless we included some description of what we're actually going to **do** with the client in order to help them reach their goals.

Interventions can be described in varying levels of detail within a treatment plan. Some treatment plan formats involve describing interventions in very broad ways. For example, for a presenting problem of "depression", the goal of "resolving symptoms of depression" might be accompanied by listing a particular type of therapy (e.g., cognitive therapy) as the intervention intended to address this goal. This very general description of the intervention plan is not very helpful to you as the therapist, nor does it help the client know what to expect from therapy. More often than not, you'll want to be fairly specific in listing interventions to accomplish treatment goals.

Specifying interventions is challenging, especially when you're first beginning as a therapist. This is both the art and the science of being a therapist. Until you've gone through the therapy process with real clients many times, you won't have first-hand knowledge of what the therapeutic change process involves. This is one of the many reasons that studying therapy theory and research is important, particularly for beginning therapists. Studying theory and research about how therapy helps people, and specifically studying a therapy model, will help you identify interventions to address the goals you and your client have developed. During your first few weeks with a client, make sure that you schedule yourself some time, outside of session, to think about the client's goals and what experiences (and interventions) could be helpful. You will need this time to plan treatment and to write the treatment plan. Put this time in your schedule, just as you would an actual meeting with a client.

In addition to describing the problem, stating goals and listing interventions to meet goals (these describe the "what" of therapy, as in "what is going to happen"), treatment plans should also provide basic information about "who" and "when", that is who is attending therapy, how frequently and for about how long. A treatment plan should identify who the client is, making it clear whether the client is an individual, a couple or a family. It should be apparent whether the therapy will be carried out in individual meetings, couple meetings, family meetings or a combination of these. Many therapists also state in the treatment plan how frequently they plan to meet with clients (for example, weekly, twice weekly, every other week, once a month, etc.). When you write a treatment plan, you should have in mind an approximate length of time therapy will last. While this is just a guess, it is important for you, for the client and for any other stakeholders to be on the same page as far as how long therapy is expected to last. Moreover, when thinking about the length of therapy, you'll also want to consider when you'll need to review the treatment plan to determine progress toward the goals and to see if the goals are still appropriate. We'll talk more about reviewing the treatment plan a little later.

A discussion of formal treatment plan writing would not be complete without emphasizing the importance of **having the client's ongoing buy-in**. Part of writing a good treatment plan involves reviewing it with your client. This is important for informed consent purposes and for strengthening the therapeutic alliance. Reviewing the treatment plan, and particularly talking about the goals of therapy, helps build consensus about the purpose and methods of therapy.

Formatting written treatment plans

It is important to be deliberate when deciding on the format for the treatment plan. As you're getting started in therapy with a client, you'll want to have some idea of the format you'll use for your treatment plan. Deciding on the format involves taking into account a number of factors. The format of a treatment plan is practical in that it simply allows you to organize information, however, the format of the treatment plan also involves some deeper philosophical questions.

Where you are practicing may determine the format you'll need to use. If you are working for an agency or organization, they may have a treatment plan template that their therapists are expected to use. This template or format may be based on:

- the specific types of services the organization offers (for example, an agency may focus on serving families involved with the foster care system)
- whether certain stakeholders (insurance companies, court systems, child protective services) are involved in therapy
- whether certain ways of approaching problems (e.g., making a DSM diagnosis or using an evidence-based therapy model) are expected within that organization

Organizations will vary in terms of what factors influence the format of their treatment plan. An organization may operate according to a particular therapeutic therapy (e.g., Ecosystemic Structural Therapy) or they may be more influenced by the practical considerations having to do with payment for therapy. Elsewhere in this chapter, we have emphasized the importance of being aware of our own assumptions and how these assumptions influence the therapy process. When using a treatment plan format developed by an organization, it is important to examine the assumptions inherent in the treatment plan format. For example, if the treatment plan only describes the problem in terms of a DSM diagnosis and does not provide a space for conceptualizing the problem in a contextual, relational way, the treatment plan format reflects more individually-oriented assumptions about the problem. As an MFT, you will want to consider the extent to which the treatment plan format allows you to define the problem, the goals and the interventions in a systemic way. Here are a few questions to consider:

- Can the "client" be more than one person? Does the treatment plan inherently focus on an individual or can a system (a couple or family) be the focus of your services?
- Can the presenting problem be defined in terms of a systemic hypothesis? If a DSM diagnosis or symptom-based statement of the problem is required, is there the opportunity to also describe the relational context for the problem?

- Does the treatment plan name client strengths and resources in addition to detailing the problem?
- Can goals be written such that they target interpersonal patterns, in addition to individual behaviors?
- To what extent do the intervention descriptions allow for describing relational interventions?

Depending on the format you're expected to use in your setting, you may decide to prepare a supplemental treatment plan where you map individually framed problems, goals and interventions onto a systems-theory-informed treatment plan. Below, we'll offer more guidance about incorporating the core assumptions of the family therapy field into treatment plan writing.

Who is paying for therapy may also influence how you format your treatment plan. The managed care system (including insurance companies and government payers like Medicaid) are dominated by a biomedical paradigm, which largely approaches health care from a problem-focused perspective. A specific problem is identified through a diagnostic process, a diagnosis is identified, and then a treatment plan is largely determined by the standard protocols for that diagnosis/problem. Many sectors of the mental health field view this biomedical framework as insufficient for capturing how mental health and mental health care operate, and yet managed care companies have driven the expectation that treatment plans follow this problem-focused format. Consequently, in cases in which a treatment plan will be shared with a managed care entity, your written treatment plan may need to follow a problem-focused format. The treatment plan would feature a statement of the problem that mainly consists of a DSM diagnosis. The goals of therapy would correspond to the primary symptoms that qualify the client for the diagnosis. As an MFT, you will be thinking of these symptoms as just that: symptoms or clues about a bigger picture. Your work with the client will hopefully be guided by a systemic conceptualization of the problem, which tries to make sense of individual symptoms in terms of interpersonal interactions.

In an ideal world, your treatment plan format would align perfectly with your assumptions as a therapist. For example, as an MFT grounded in systems theory, ideally your treatment plan format would allow for defining the problem in a systemic way and would be conducive to defining goals that are relational (focused on interpersonal patterns rather than on individual thoughts, feelings and behaviors). In practice, though, there may be competing interests in terms of the expectations for a treatment plan. If you work in an organization where services are funded by Medicaid, for example, there are certain assumptions (driven by the Medicaid system) that will affect treatment plan writing. For example, the Medicaid system must verify that services are addressing the needs of the individual who is authorized to receive help. In the interest of reducing fraud, Medicaid funding encourages an individual-oriented approach to therapy (where services target one person). When writing treatment plans for clients receiving Medicaid funds, marriage and family therapists navigate conflicting assumptions. The requirements of Medicaid encourage a treatment plan focused on one person, whereas the systems theory assumptions of the MFT profession encourage a treatment plan that addresses relationships and thus more than one person. There are a few areas that all treatment plans should address (Patterson et al., 2018), which are addressed below.

All treatment plans should address who, what, when, where, why and how

Who is the client? Identify the individual, a couple or a family involved in therapy.

Who is the therapist? You will typically identify yourself as the person providing the therapy.

What type of services? Individual therapy? Couple therapy? Family therapy? Some combination? In addition to providing therapy, a therapist may also refer clients for other assistance. This may also be discussed in a treatment plan.

When will therapy happen? What is the approximate frequency of the therapy? Weekly? Every other week? Estimate for how long?

Where is therapy happening? In an office setting? In the client's home? At school? This may not be relevant for all treatment plans, but it will be important in some cases, for example, therapists doing in-home work.

Why is therapy needed? In other words, what problems and goals are being addressed? This is articulated in a clear, concise statement of presenting concern (includes clients' perspective(s) of problem and therapist conceptualization, which may include DSM diagnosis when appropriate)

Depending on the format, the treatment plan may be organized around a list of problems or there may be one section where the presenting concerns are listed. Essentially, treatment plans document the need for the therapy. They will vary in terms of how much information the plan provides. An assessment document, something separate from the treatment plan, is often used to provide much more thorough assessment information about the presenting problem and the client's background. The treatment plan generally provides a briefer summary of the problem (the why).

Goals. What are the goals of therapy? How goals are written is going to vary depending on your specific practice context. Broadly speaking, the expectation will be that goals are phrased in clear statements that can be measured. Some treatment plan formats involve more abstract goals and then measurable objectives, which are concrete, measurable steps toward the goals.

How will therapy address the problems and goals? In other words, what interventions, methods or strategies will be used to address the problems and goals. Treatment plan formats will vary a lot in terms of how much detail is provided about how therapy will be carried out. Nonetheless, treatment plans need to provide some indication (no matter how brief) of how therapy will address each problem and goal.

Options for treatment plan formats

The formatting of the who, what, when and where information typically doesn't vary a whole lot from one format to the next. Where treatment plans tend to vary widely is in how they approach the why (the problem and goals that therapy addresses) and the how (how therapy is actually carried out and what interventions are used). Here we provide a couple of different examples of how this "meat" of the treatment plan may be formatted.

One approach to writing a treatment plan involves a step-by-step overview of the therapy process that includes the therapeutic tasks the therapist carries out, in addition to the clients' early, middle and late phase goals. Elsewhere, we have talked about the difference between planning therapy and writing a treatment plan. The most comprehensive written treatment plan formats involve a chronological plan for each phase of therapy. This approach to writing a treatment plan involves laying out the tasks or steps the therapist will take in order to carry out therapy, in addition to highlighting the client's goals and the interventions used to address these goals. For example, this approach to treatment plan writing might specifically name joining as a task and might list strategies for joining with the particular client. Here is a consolidated example of a chronological treatment plan with tasks. This example draws from Gehart's (2014) text, *Mastering competencies in family therapy* (pp. 241–242) and incorporates information from a treatment plan for a real client. One of the nice things about Gehart's approach to writing a treatment plan is that it uses theory (a specific model) to guide each step of the process. The example provided here reflects the Bowen Family systems model, and you can see how this model's assumptions are incorporated in both the therapeutic tasks and the goals.

Many treatment plan forms do not incorporate therapeutic tasks. In these treatment plans, the focus is solely on the problems, goals and interventions in therapy.

Sample treatment plan listing tasks, goals and interventions

Presenting problem: AF(48) and AM(50) sought therapy at AF's request. Both partners report frequent, ongoing arguments over parenting issues.

Initial phase tasks:

1) Develop working therapeutic alliance. Be sensitive to cultural background, gender differences and couple's life cycle stage.

   a) Engage with each client from a differentiated position, conveying a nonanxious presence.
   b) Introduce Session Rating Scale as a tool for getting client feedback on working alliance.

2) Assess individual, systemic and broader cultural dynamics.

   a) Use three-generation genogram to identify multigenerational patterns.
   b) Assess both partners' levels of differentiation in current problem situation and in the past.

3) Define and obtain client agreement on treatment goals.

   a) Work with couple to define goals that relate to differentiation and decreased systemic anxiety in order to reduce couple conflict and reduce AM's use of alcohol to a level that both partners find acceptable.

4) Identify needed referrals, crisis issues, collateral contacts and other client needs.

   a) Referrals/resources/contacts: make referrals and collateral contacts as appropriate.

Initial phase client goals:

1) Reduce triangulation between AF and oldest daughter to reduce conflict avoidance within couple.

   a) Detriangulate in session by maintaining therapeutic neutrality, supporting partners in communicating concerns directly to each other and refocusing each person on their portion of problem interactions.
   b) Use process questions to increase awareness of how triangulation is used to unsuccessfully manage conflict.

Working phase tasks:

2) Monitor quality of working alliance.

  a) Monitor therapist responses to ensure differentiated position.
  b) Monitor ongoing use of Session Rating Scale with both partners to get client perspective on alliance.

3) Monitor client progress.

  a) Assess each client's ability to use a differentiated position to relate to therapist, to each other and to those outside of session.
  b) Assess frequency of conflict over parenting.

Working phase goals:

4) Decrease chronic anxiety and reactivity during couple interactions to reduce parenting conflict and increase positive interactions between partners.

  a) Encourage differentiated responses to common anxieties, including instances involving disciplining children.
  b) Use relational experiments to practice responding to parenting challenges rather that reacting to perceived anxieties and stressors.

5) Decrease repetition of couple interactions stemming from multigenerational patterns passed down from each partner's families of origin.

  a) Use genogram to identify family-of-origin expectations influencing each partner.
  b) Process questions to help clients identify how family-of-origin experiences and present-day anxieties influence conflict over parenting decisions.

Closing phase tasks:

6) Develop aftercare plan and maintain gains.

  a) Identify specific couple bonding activities that couple considers most important opportunities for intimacy.
  b) Identify relationships and habits that help clients maintain differentiation. Partner A identified yoga practice as important for her. Partner B identified developing more supportive friend relationships.

Sample treatment plan organized around problem statements

Presenting concern: AF(38) and AM(40) sought couple therapy to address conflict stemming from both partners' past divorces and over-discipline of their children, including AF's two daughters (ages 8 and 10) and the couple's daughter together (age 2).
  Behavioral Statements of Problem:

1) Frequent arguments between parent and stepparent over child discipline differences.
2) Frequent arguments between the partners over favoritism for biological versus non-biological children.
3) Financial pressures and resentment about the financial aspects of divorce settlements.

Long-term goals:

4) All members of the combined family treat each other with mutual respect, equality and fairness.
5) The partners trust each other's loyalty, love and commitment, and work cooperatively on child-rearing.
6) The partners resolve jealousy, hurt and anger toward their ex-partners.
7) Each partner develops understanding about the dilemmas and conflicts that the other experiences with his/her ex-partner.

Short-Term Objectives Therapeutic (corresponding goal) and Interventions

8) Describe conflicts with the ex-partners. (1)

   a) Ask the partners to describe their feelings about, and conflicts with, their ex-partner.

9) Describe the guilt about the ex-partner and about the dilemmas their children face because of a separation or divorce. (2, 3)

   a) Have the partners relate the ways in which they experience conflict about dealing with their ex-partner.
   b) Encourage the partners to openly discuss their guilty feelings about the "failure" of the former relationships, and how these feelings affect their present relationships with their ex-partners and children.

10) Review any implicit or explicit divorce or separation financial agreements and discuss their implications. (3, 4)

   a) Discuss the respective divorce and separation agreements, and have the partners discuss the short- and long-term implications of these agreements.
   b) Guide the partners in discussing how they will cope with problems that may result from respective legal and/or financial agreements (e.g., a husband having to pay a large percentage of his salary to his ex-wife, leaving relatively little money for the combined family, educational expenses of the children).

The second example of a treatment plan format reflects a problem-focused treatment plan. This treatment plan is largely drawn from The Couples Psychotherapy Treatment Planner (O'Leary, Heyman & Jongsma, 2015).

This problem-focused treatment plan includes some advantages in that it is much more direct in highlighting why therapy is needed and how the therapist plans to address each specific problem and the corresponding goals using specific therapy activities. Compared with the chronological treatment plan, though, this treatment plan is less explicit in laying out the actual process the therapist will go through. Notice that the tasks (joining, assessment, goal setting, etc.) are not explicitly stated. Additionally, the second treatment plan doesn't necessarily tie in a specific theory as the guiding force for therapy.

These two examples of treatment plans are far from being the only options. They are offered here not because they reflect the right way to write a treatment plan, but rather to illustrate key ways that treatment plans can vary. Whether you are already seeing clients now or you are preparing to do so in the future, keep in mind that the treatment plan format you end up using will need to be tailored to your specific practice context.

Theory and me: what does it mean to "choose a model"?

We started out this chapter asking you to think about your existing beliefs about therapy and the therapy process. In doing this, we mention that training to be a therapist, and specifically learning to use theory, involves taking your existing beliefs and laying them out to examine them. It also involves comparing these beliefs with the theories that are out there. Not all theories are the same, and learning theory is partly about a personal choice. This choice also needs to be informed by the existing knowledge (including research), but it is a choice. So, what is involved in this choice? **What does it mean to choose a theory?** I find many students wonder whether they can choose multiple theories and use them together or choose one or the other, depending on who their client is. The purpose of this section is to consider questions regarding how the use of theory syncs with the unique viewpoint of the therapist.

In a way, the model that you choose becomes like a teacher; as you learn the model, the model teaches you various aspects of therapeutic practice. Even if you later switch models, you'll still have learned a great deal that can be applied while using other models.

Therapist self-knowledge and selection of therapy model

In a way, the "Which theory do I choose?" is a two-pronged question. Part of selecting a model is learning how you fit with that model by challenging yourself to think about who you are as a person and what kinds of information and approaches interest you (Goodell, Sudderth & Allan, 2011). It also is about developing your own personalized theory of change. **Theory of change** is a therapist's comprehensive framework for organizing how they work in therapy. A theory of change is related to a model, but it is not synonymous with a model. A beginning therapist can start to uncover their own theory of change by studying one or more models and trying them out to see what feels comfortable (Goodell et al., 2011). The idea is that you will take an active role in learning about and experimenting with these models as you learn about who you are as a therapist (Piercy & Sprenkle, 1988). Studying a particular model deeply can also be incredibly useful in helping therapists to expand their knowledge and skills. In the real world, many therapists describe their practice as integrative in that they incorporate ideas from several models of therapy.

Choosing a model is also about the client, too. Clients differ according to both their presenting concerns and their personal qualities and what suits them best in terms of a change process. Ideally, a therapist's theory of change will include ideas about how to tailor therapy to the unique needs of particular clients. Once therapists have an established theory of change, then they can thoughtfully select from different models and techniques based on what they think best suits their client. In today's therapy world, an important part of this decision-making process involves being informed about research support for different ways to approach different problems. Therapists need to know themselves (their own philosophical orientation and their own areas of competency), know the research and then make informed decisions. As far as competency goes, your course work in this program will provide a foundation for competently practicing the models you're being exposed to in your theories courses and in later courses (e.g., you'll look at certain models that are designed for couples). But your exposure in your classes will only get you part of the way. When you start seeing clients as part of your clinical training, you'll need to continue learning about your preferred models and techniques, and you'll have support from clinical supervisors in doing this.

Reflecting on the limits of theory

We began this section on theory and treatment planning with a consideration of assumptions and the importance of therapists being self-aware and conscious of their assumptions. An important aspect of being aware of assumptions is seeing the limitations of certain theories or models.

Some of the original developers of family systems theory noted that "The map is not the territory" (Bateson, 1972). In other words, the models that we use to make sense of experiences are not identical to real experience. Maps are representations of the world. There are an infinite number of ways that we can draw a map of any particular territory. Some maps will be more helpful than others, but no map is a perfect presentation of reality.

It is especially important to recognize that human beings within specific cultural contexts have developed models and theories. The assumptions of a given model (how it views people, how it defines health, how it approaches problem-solving) reflect cultural assumptions about these same things. As you study various models and theories, ask questions about the cultural influences on the model.

Reflection: How does a given model of therapy reflect the social "location" of the person who developed it? How was Symbolic Experiential Therapy reflective of Carl Whitaker being a White male medical doctor, living at a particular time in history in a particular part of the U.S.? How might Satir's model reflect her being one of the only well-known women in the family therapy field? Virtually all of the MFT models were developed by European American (White) people. What cultural perspectives may be missing from certain models of MFT? In what ways do some MFT models overlook the experiences of couples and families who are not legally married? Who involve same sex relationships? Who are connected through kinship relationships rather than blood relationships?

Being intentional in our use of theory involves thinking about the biases or "blind spots" that might be a part of certain models. Being able to think critically like this involves self-awareness just as much as it requires an understanding of theory. When we learn about and challenge our own blind spots, this is what prepares us to recognize that a particular theory is missing something important about our clients' experiences.

Consider what we said at the beginning of this lesson:

If our minds are closed to certain possibilities, then we are effectively closing off those possibilities for our clients. Using the journey metaphor, if we will go down only certain paths and not others, then we are imposing those same limits on our clients. Thoughtful use of theory is about being conscious of our maps.

References

AAMFT (2015). AAMFT Code of Ethics from: www.aamft.org/iMIS15/AAMFT/Content/Legal_Ethics/Code_of_Ethics.aspx on June 19, 2019.

American Psychiatric Association. (2013). *Diagnostic and statistical manual of mental disorders* (5th ed.). Washington, DC: Author.

Asay, T. P. & Lambert, M. J. (1999). The empirical case for the common factors in therapy: quantitative findings. In M. A. Hubble, B. L. Duncan & S. D. Miller (Eds.), *The heart and soul of change: what works in therapy* (pp. 23–55). Washington, DC: APA.

Baker, P. & Chang, J. (2013). *Basic family therapy* (6th ed.) Hoboken, NJ: Wiley- Blackwell. https://ebookcentral.proquest.com/lib/ncent-ebooks/detail.action?docID=4206558 [Full-text through NCU library]

Bateson, G. (1972). *Steps to an ecology of mind: collected essays in anthropology, psychiatry, evolution, and epistemology*. Lanham, MD: Jason Aronson.

Blow, A. J. & Sprenkle, D. H. (2001). Common factors across theories of marriage and family therapy: a modified Delphi study. *Journal of Marital and Family Therapy, 27*, 385–402.

Bohecker, L. & Kleist, D., (2017). Circularity and Linearity. *The SAGE encyclopedia of marriage, family, and couples counseling*. Thousand Oaks, CA: SAGE Publications, Inc.

Bordin, E. S. (1979). The generalizability of the psychoanalytic concept of the working alliance. *Psychotherapy: Theory, Research & Practice, 16*, 252–260. doi:10.1037/h0085885.

Cromwell, R. E., Olson, D. H. & Fournier, D. G. (1976). Tools and techniques for diagnosis and evaluation in marital and family therapy. *Family Process, 15*(1), 1–49.

Engle, G. (1977). The need for a new medical model: a challenge for biomedicine. *Science, 196*, 129–136.

Fife, S. T., Whiting, J. B., Bradford, K. & Davis, S. (2014). The therapeutic pyramid: a common factors synthesis of techniques, alliance, and way of being. *Journal of Marital and Family Therapy, 40*(1), 20–33.

Finn, S. E., (2015). Therapeutic assessment with couples. *Pratiques Pscyhologiques, 21*, 345–373.

Fisch, R., Weakland, J. H. & Segal, L. (1982). *The tactics of change: doing therapy briefly*. San Francisco, CA: Jossey-Bass.

Gehart, D. (2014). *Mastering competencies in family therapy* (2nd ed.). Belmont, CA: Brooks/Cole.

Gehart, D. (2017a). Clinical case conceptualization with couples and families. In J. Carlson & S. B. Dermer (Eds.). *The SAGE encyclopedia of marriage, family, and couples counseling*. Thousand Oaks, CA: SAGE Publications, Inc.

Gehart, D. (2017b). Treatment planning with couples and families. *The SAGE encyclopedia of marriage, family, and couples counseling: S-V, 2017*, 1734–1739.

Goodell, K. A., Sudderth, B. G. & Allan, C. D. (2011). In L. Metcalf (Ed.), *Marriage and family therapy: a practice-oriented approach*. New York, NY: Springer Publishing Company.

Huff, S. C., Anderson, S. R. & Edwards, L. L. (2014) Training marriage and family therapists in formal assessment: contributions to students' familiarity, attitude, and confidence. *Journal of Family Psychotherapy, 25*, 200–315. doi: 10.1080/08975353.2014.977673

Johnson, S. (2004). *The practice of emotionally focused couples therapy* (2nd ed.). New York, NY: Brunner Routledge.

Lambert, M., Whipple, J., Smart, D., Vermeersch, D., Nielsen, S. & Hawkins, E. (2001). The effects of providing therapists with feedback on patient progress during psychotherapy: are outcomes enhanced? Psychotherapy Research, *11*, 49–68.

Makover, R. B. (2016). *Treatment planning for psychotherapists: a practical guide to better outcomes* (3rd ed.). Arlington, VA: American Psychiatric Association Publishing.

McDowell, T., Knudson-Martin, C. & Bermudez, J. M. (2018). *Socioculturally attuned family therapy: guidelines for equitable theory and practice*. New York, NY: Routledge.

Mercadal, T. (2019). Social constructionism. New Jersey, NJ: *Salem Press Encyclopedia*.

Merriam-Webster Dictionary, (2020). Retrieved from https://www.merriam-webster.com/dictionary/diagnosis.

Metcalf, L. (2011). The practice of marriage and family therapy. In L. Metcalf (Ed.), *Marriage and family therapy: a practice-oriented approach*. New York, NY: Springer Publishing Company.

Minuchin, S. (1982). Reflections on boundaries. *American Journal of Orthopsychiatry, 52*(4), 655-663.

Minuchin, S. & Fishman, H. C. (1981). *Family therapy techniques*. Cambridge, MA: Harvard University Press.

O'Leary, K. D., Heyman, R. E. & Jongsma, A. E. (2015). *The couples psychotherapy treatment planner, with DSM-5 Updates*. Hoboken, New Jersey: Wiley.

Panichelli, C. (2013). Humor, joining, and reframing in psychotherapy: resolving the auto-double-bind, *The American Journal of Family Therapy, 41*(5), 437–45.

Patterson, J., Williams, L., Edwards, T. M., Chamow, L. & Grauf-Grounds, C. (2018). *Essential skills in family therapy: from the first interview to termination.* New York, NY: Guilford Publications.

Perry, W. (2016). *Basic counseling techniques: a beginning therapist's tool kit* (3rd ed., Kindle Edition). Bloomington, IN: Author House.

Piercy, F. P. & Sprenkle, D. H. (1988). Family therapy theory-building questions. *Journal of Marital and Family Therapy, 14*, 307–309.

Pinsof, W. M. & Wynne, L. C. (1995). The efficacy of marital and family therapy: an empirical overview, conclusions, and recommendations. *Journal of Marital and Family Therapy, 21*(4), 585–613.

Shaw, S. L. & Murray, K. W. (2014). Monitoring alliance and outcome with client feedback measures. *Journal of Mental Health Counseling, 36*(1), 43–57. doi:10.17744/mehc.36.1.n5g64t3014231862.

Sprenkle, D. H. & Blow, A. J. (2004). Common factors and our sacred models. *Journal of Marital and Family Therapy, 30*(2), 113–129.

Sprenkle, D. H., Blow, A. J. & Dickey, M. H. (1999). Common factors and other nontechnique variables in marriage and family therapy. In M. A. Hubble, B. L. Duncan & S. D. Miller (Eds.), *The heart and soul of change: what works in therapy* (pp. 329–359). American Psychological Association. https://doi.org/10.1037/11132-010

Sprenkle, D. H., Lebow, J. & Davis, S. D. (2009). *Common factors in couple and family therapy: the overlooked foundation for effective practice.* New York, NY: The Guilford Press.

Tomm, K., St. George, S., Wulff, D. & Strong, T. (2014). *Patterns in interpersonal interactions: inviting relational understandings for therapeutic change.* New York, NY: Routledge.

Walter, J. L. & Peller, J. E. (1992). *Becoming solution-focused in brief therapy.* New York, NY: Brunner/Mazel.

7 Clinical Practice
Preparing for Day 1

Michael Knerr

The employment system

Chapter 6 introduced you to thinking about therapy as a larger process of helping clients seeking change. Joining with new clients, assessing their relational systems, and developing goals and interventions all guided by your chosen MFT theory, is the basis for a successful therapy outcome. In order to support you as you develop your therapy skills, there are several key resources at your disposal. In this first section, you will be introduced to some of these resources so that, as you begin your clinical practice, you will have some ideas about where to go when you need some help. A foundational skill to develop as a new therapist is the ability to recognize when you need help and to take the initiative to ask for that help. At times, this requires finding a specific person and asking them for the help you need, but, just as often, there are resources you can use at any time.

Employee handbooks and policy manuals

Most employers have policy manuals or employee handbooks available for your benefit. Now, you may sigh deeply at the thought of reading through a thick stack of policy and procedure documents – but, remember, these exist for your benefit. Many of the policies and procedures at clinical sites represent the various mistakes someone made in the past, resulting in a policy designed to prevent you from making similar mistakes. While reading through the employee handbook, or the procedures manual provided by your site, can seem dull, please do not dump these documents in the bottom of a drawer and forget about them. In order to become a great therapist, you also need to understand and benefit from learning how the site operates and where you fit in the overall goals of the site.

While employer handbooks or orientation guides will provide you with a baseline of information, they are rarely comprehensive enough to cover every possible topic. So, as you read through these guides, it is also good practice to make some notes in the margins about questions that occur to you that may not be in the manual. This approach will allow you to have some thoughtful responses when your supervisor asks if you read the documents and if you have any questions. (Supervisors are another resource, which is covered in further depth below.)

In order to get your thinking started, here are just a few topics that often appear in an employer's policy manual or that you could ask about during orientation to the site:

DOI: 10.4324/9781003382621-9

Use of social media?

Contacting Clients via Text? Email? Phone? Online? Driving clients in your car?

The type of technology I need

What type of computer system do I need? Will I need a laptop? How do I record sessions?

How should I store/safeguard recordings? What are policies regarding using my phone?

What are the expectations for timeliness? Returning client calls? Completing documentation?

How should I dress? Look? What is the professional expectation here? What do I do if there is an emergency?

How do I contact my supervisor?

Besides my supervisor, who else should I talk to if I have questions? If I have questions about?

What forms are used most often and how do I access them?

What is the policy around clients who may be suicidal? Is there a safety planning form?

Who else works here and what are the various roles people have? How does intake work and how will I know I have a new client?

What is the typical treatment process like from beginning to end? What meetings do I need to attend?

What happens if I make a mistake? A BIG mistake?

Ethics code and state laws

Two other resources that are available to you and are similar to employment policies are the AAMFT Code of Ethics (AAMFT, 2015) and the laws in your state. The ethics code applies to all MFTs, from interns to fully licensed clinicians, so you will want to keep it handy for when a question arises. Ethical issues can crop up at any point when working with clients and sometimes they appear in the form of a nagging feeling that "something doesn't seem right". You probably cannot memorize the ethics code, but you can learn to pay attention to that feeling and train yourself to explore the code for help. You may not even be sure if the ethics code applies at all, but reading through the code and noting any specific segment that might apply is a good habit to develop. Following this up by talking through your questions with a supervisor is a great way to make sure you are practicing ethically, and to make any necessary changes you might discover.

Just like employer policy manuals, the AAMFT Code of Ethics is also not a comprehensive document that covers all possible situations you may encounter. So, in addition to the ethics code, you also want to locate the various state laws that most directly apply to your clinical practice. Sometimes, your state licensure board will post these laws or links to sections of the state legal code you can follow. However, you may need to find these laws on your own. (Often these are easily found online by searching "Laws" and the name of your "State".)

Before looking at specific sections of your state laws, one other thing that is useful to know is how the legal code is generally organized. (Terminology may be different by state, but the concepts are similar.) Usually there is a section of laws and a section of rules – often referred to together as the Laws and Rules of the State. **The laws** are the exact words of the legal code – what the state legislature passed and the governor signed – and these can only be changed by that process. **The rules** are descriptions of procedures around the laws – the "how to section" – so people know the process for applying the law. For example, the law says to be an MFT you must complete the following _____then you can be licensed. The rules often pick up from there and describe "how" you get that license: *you must complete Form X, Pay Y Fees and send your form and the fee payment to Z address.*

Once you have located the site where your state laws are listed, you might suddenly feel a little overwhelmed or queasy. So, take a breath. You will not need to go to law school to understand this information; you just need to find a few key sections in the state laws. Also, you do not need to read all of the laws and rules regarding topics like "Agriculture" or "Driving". In fact, there are really only two places you need to identify at this point. The first is to find the laws regarding your **clinical practice as an MFT.** You may have already seen these previously because these are the rules that describe the qualifications for licensure, what MFTs can and cannot do and, in many states, additional rules about ethical practice. Once you find this section, bookmark it in some way so that when you need it you can get there directly.

The second section of state laws you want to identify are those related to **"family law".** These may appear in more than one section of the code, depending on your state. Typically, this section of the legal code is where you will find laws regarding child abuse and mandated reporting, as well as laws about marriage, divorce, child custody and more. This is also a good site to bookmark for future use. At the moment, you may not need to read through each of these sections of your state laws, but it is helpful to know where to find them and to be aware that, just like checking the ethics code, checking the laws of your state may be beneficial.

In addition to the resources discussed above, you also will likely have some key people around to help you understand the site, their expectations of you and your new role as a working therapist. Depending on your location, you may have several peers working alongside you in various capacities. In a larger treatment setting, you might work together with counselors, social workers, psychologists, school counselors, drug and alcohol counselors, case managers, administrative staff, psychiatrists, teachers, hospital staff and more. All of these peers can help you understand how the treatment site operates and where you fit in the process. On the other hand, your location may include only two people – you and your supervisor.

CONSIDER THIS

Your site is a system

As you become oriented to your new role as an MFT, it can be helpful to remember that, while many of the people listed above may provide therapy to clients just like you, your perspective on clients may differ in some key ways. As an MFT, you are learning to think systemically to understand even individual clients as people living in a relational system; so, as you consider how to help that client, you are thinking about both the individual and the system at all times. Not all clinicians are trained this way, which means they may not always see clients the way you see them. As you develop your MFT skills, you will discover some

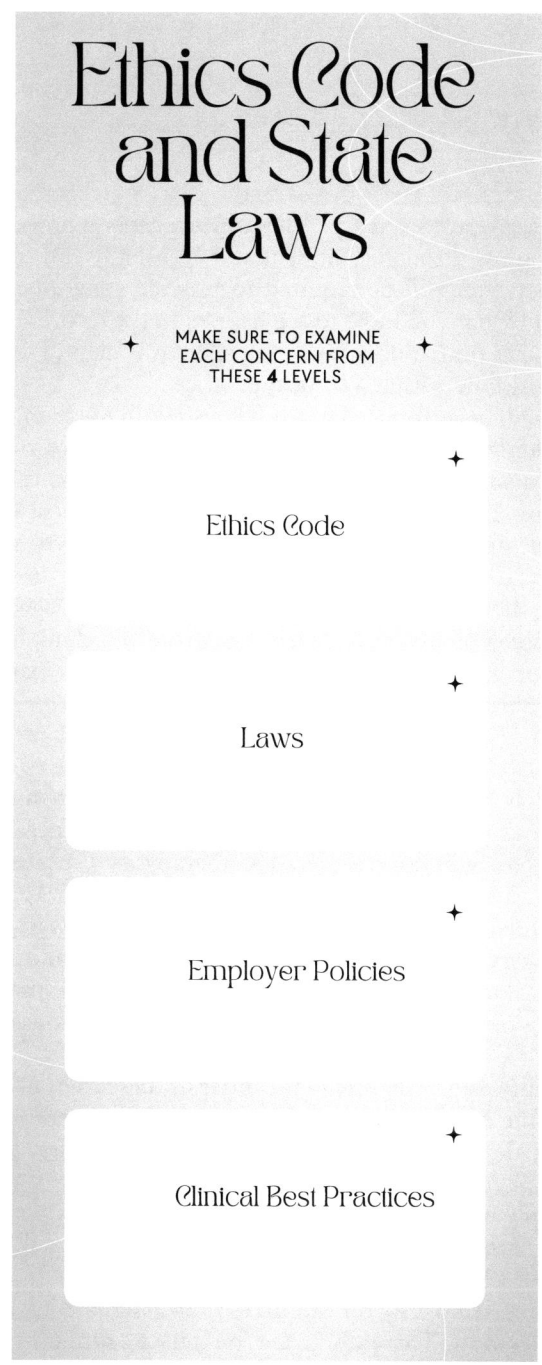

Figure 7.1 Infographic 9: Ethics Code and State Laws 4 Levels.

of your questions may not always "fit" with the answers you get back. Take these moments as a time to learn.

The work process

General workflow

Clinical practice, like many professions, has developed a general process for how new clients come into therapy, progress through treatment and eventually end therapy. At most points throughout this journey, you will be required to provide some documentation regarding what has happened and what you hope to see happen in the future. Each treatment facility develops their own system for handling these steps, but it is helpful to know what to expect generally about the workflow within a clinical practice.

In this section, you will be introduced to the main steps in the therapy process, along with information about where to go to learn about the specifics where you work. As you work with clients, you will also need to learn about the typical forms used to document what is happening in therapy. Later, you will be introduced to the most typical types of forms used in clinical practice and learn about their purpose and how to use them effectively. It can sometimes be hard to complete these documents, which occasionally leads therapists to complain about all the "paperwork" involved in therapy. However, the purpose of the paperwork is not to force you fill out forms, it is to make you think hard about your client, their needs and how you will help them improve. In that sense, the paperwork is your friend if you are willing to embrace it.

Intake Procedures – Every treatment setting has some kind of intake process where potential clients contact the site and determine if they would like to receive therapy. These processes can vary widely depending on the types of clients seen, the most common treatment problems and the various paths by which clients are referred to therapy. The intake process is different if a client has been court ordered to therapy as a means of avoiding jail time from if a parent finds the therapist online and calls to make an appointment. Still, many of the steps are the same. Each site will have a procedure for taking new client information, discussing their services, scheduling a first appointment and assigning someone as the client's therapist. Likewise, once you have a client assigned, there are procedures for scheduling, completing intake documents, providing informed consent and signing all the required documents.

Each treatment facility differs slightly in the order of these steps as well as who is responsible for each part of the intake process. At some clinics, the therapist may manage everything from answering the first phone call all the way to the first appointment. In other settings, perhaps two or three different people will manage part of the intake process and the therapist may simply meet the client at the first appointment.

Systemic Progress Notes – After each therapy session, you will be expected to complete a progress note or a case note to be stored in the client file. In the Appendix, there is a systemic progress note template you can access for assignments, so that you can begin practicing writing notes now. There are a few matters to recognize regarding a progress note: **it is a legal document**; and it is the official record of what occurred during the therapy session. It takes practice to learn how to write these notes, striking a proper balance of providing not too much, but not too little information. The progress note serves several functions: **it reminds you of what you have done and plan to do next**; it is helpful to the site and supervisors if, for some reason, the client needs to transfer to a new therapist; and **it**

protects both you and the client if challenges arise around payment, the outcome of therapy or who is allowed access to the records.

Assessments – Assessment is another key step in the therapy process that often occurs at the beginning of therapy, but can be reviewed throughout all of treatment. When MFTs talk about assessments, they can discuss two different tasks even though they use the same term. One way to talk about assessment is when referring to a specific assessment tool, such as the Beck Depression Inventory (APA, 2020b). Many clinical sites have some standard assessments like this that clients are asked to complete at the beginning of therapy. Some are **formal assessment** tools with a scoring and numerical result, while others may be less formal such as paperwork collection, demographics and having clients state what brought them to therapy. When you start clinical practice at a new site, it can be helpful to go through all of the assessment tools that clients typically complete at the start of therapy. Be sure you understand what each one is supposed to measure, why it was chosen, how it is scored and what the results mean. (One easy way to learn all of this is to take them all for yourself, score them and then see if you can correctly interpret your results. This approach will also help you view the assessments through the client's eyes.)

A second way MFTs talk about assessment is by looking at the client and their presenting problems through the lens of your systemic MFT theory. This involves asking yourself – and the clients – questions that help you think about the client using your systemic theory. While many of these overlap by theory, the kinds of questions a structural therapist might consider differ from the ones a Narrative therapist might consider. Both models explore the client system, but they are focused on viewing that system in different ways, which leads to different types of interventions – but you will get to that later. Sometimes, MFTs call this type of assessment "**conceptualizing**". This is a fancy way of saying, how does your MFT theory help you to "make sense" of all of the information clients drop on you during that first session?

Session planning – Every time you meet with a client, you will want to enter that session with a plan. The plan may change as you learn more about the client, as they describe problems differently or become more specific about their goals, or if a crisis of some kind happens. So, the session plan is not a strict formula to follow, but it is at least a good **outline** of what you plan to do or discuss in the particular session. Your assessment, systemic conceptualization and MFT model will help you to devise this plan, as will your supervisors. For now, it is key to remember to **always enter with a plan; therapy is too important to enter and simply try to "wing it"**. For example, imagine you are preparing for your first session with a new client. The client has already completed all of the intake and consent forms before the session; so, you are free to greet them and get started. How will you proceed?

One concept all therapists are likely to focus on is "**joining**" **with the client.** Finding ways to build rapport, learn about the client and start developing a trusting relationship to set the table for the work ahead are examples of *joining*. Establishing a therapeutic alliance like this is considered a "common factor"; it is known to be helpful regardless of the client's presenting problem or your approach to therapy. However, how you decide to build this therapeutic alliance can be different depending on the MFT theory you choose to employ. In narrative therapy, part of the joining process would be to first "meet the person" and only later "meet the problem". So, the narrative therapist would make a point of meeting and getting to know whoever attends the therapy session – and would put off hearing about the presenting problem until later. On the other hand, a Bowen therapist might begin the joining process by working with the clients to construct a genogram so that everyone has a clear sense of the relational system clients bring to therapy.

Treatment Plan – In addition to planning out individual sessions, you will also be required to develop a plan for treatment as a whole. Clients are often coming into therapy feeling overwhelmed, with multiple relationship conflicts, several specific problems and a sense that they are stuck and cannot see a good path forward. As a therapist, it is easy to become overwhelmed and start to feel that perhaps the client is right – there is no good path forward!

A good treatment plan pulls together all of the client information gathered from the intake, assessments and previous sessions, and begins to project a path toward change. As client goals become clarified, you can begin to plan out more than a single session, instead looking at the big picture and thinking about what you will do across multiple sessions to help clients reach their goals. The next section of this chapter will introduce you to the Systemic Treatment Plan and how to make use of it with clients. It breaks down the treatment planning form into segments, so that you can see how to complete the document and what the purpose of each section is toward developing a useful plan.

Supervision plan – You may not yet have considered this, but you will also want to **enter your supervision time each week with a plan**. Sometimes supervisors may provide you with a format or document to help you structure the time and learn to present cases in ways that are most helpful to your learning. At other facilities, there is no formal plan other than to meet on specific days and times for supervision. No matter how your time with a supervisor is set up, you will want to think about what you want to get out of the time. Before you show up for supervision, think about what questions you have; what you need the most help with now; and what kind of feedback you are looking for from the supervisor. This is a precious time set aside for your growth and learning, so take some time and come prepared.

Case presentations – Eventually, all MFTs will make case presentations. These may be formal presentations, with PowerPoint slides and session videos, or informal presentations where you discuss your work one-on-one with a supervisor. To make the most of these presentations, it is helpful to do some work in advance so that what you present is easily understood and the bulk of the time can be spent on learning, rather than describing every detail about the client or session.

Documentation tools

Systemic treatment planning – step by step

One of the things that makes putting together a written treatment plan frustrating for many clinicians is the realization that what you write down is static/fixed; but the people you work with everyday are not static, rather they are constantly changing. Another aspect of the written treatment plan therapists sometimes complain about is the fact that they are **required** by someone – a supervisor, agency, funder, insurance company – and many of us do not like doing things just because we have to. Finally, therapists sometimes resist having to write a treatment plan in reaction to the form itself.

Clearly, having some kind of plan for therapy seems like it will serve both the therapist and the client more than having no plan at all. Therapists who enter sessions with plans like, "I'll just see where it goes" or "I'm going to kind of wing it and see what the client wants to do" are not serving their clients and are bordering on being unethical in their clinical practice. Since treatment planning is more comprehensive than other clinical documentation, in

Treatment Planning Flow Chart

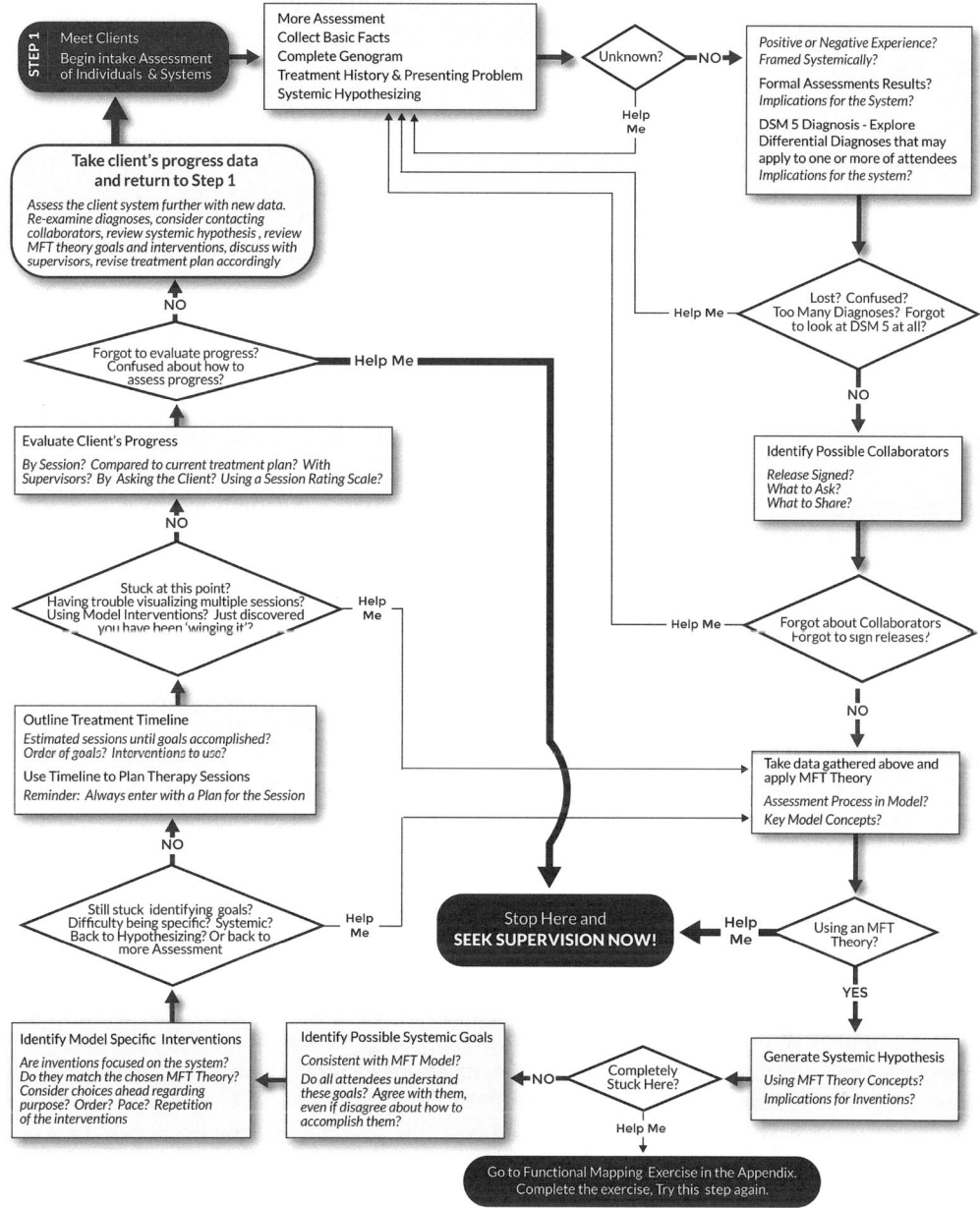

Figure 7.2 Image of the Treatment Plan Workflow.

this section you will get to walk through a treatment planning (and writing) process step by step.

You will be introduced to the systemic treatment planning form in snapshots, so that you can understand what is included in each section and how each section fits into the whole plan.

Ultimately, the result should be a document that is understandable and serves both you and your clients. So, the emphasis here is on the "how tos" of writing out a treatment plan, so that you can begin thinking about the process even before you begin working with actual clients. By its very nature, completing a form is a linear process. We literally go line by line through the form, answering questions and filling in boxes, which can lead to unintentionally thinking about clients in the same linear fashion. The chart should help you to see how all of the various steps are interconnected. The treatment planning form is linear, **but actual treatment planning is systemic** – it never stops, there is always more to consider because the client system is fluid. The diagram is meant to help you see that, even when you have "finished" the treatment planning form, you have not finished the process. After you have had a chance to look at the flow chart, continue reading about each of the sections of the treatment planning form. Keep the flow chart handy, so you can begin to visualize how all these pieces fit together.

Treatment planning forms

As noted in the previous chapter, there are many uses for the written treatment plan that go beyond the benefits to just the therapist and their clients. At any time in your clinical practice, you may find yourself collaborating with professionals both within your employment setting and outside of it. A treatment plan can help you to be articulate about clients' needs and goals when interacting with collaborators in schools, hospitals, courts or conferring with insurance providers, agency regulators and funders, and your own direct supervisor. One result of all of these intersecting interests is that some assessment or treatment planning forms can become quite lengthy. Most employers either have guidelines for writing a treatment plan or they have their own forms for you to complete and you will likely notice differences immediately.

The form presented here is simply one approach to developing and articulating a treatment plan. You are free to use it at your clinical site, assuming it meets the site's requirements, or to adapt it as needed. The goal is to help you become familiar with the process and try to have some "how do I do this" experiences before you start working with specific clients. The systemic treatment planning form has been specifically developed to help you to focus planning in two key ways – thinking about clients systemically and using your selected MFT treatment model appropriately.

Finally, before looking at the treatment planning form template in detail and discussing how to complete it, one last item to note. Forms, by design, are static and linear; they often are arranged so you can either answer specific questions or fill in the blank spaces. One consequence of this is that the form can lull you into the misguided perception that your job is to fill out the form. If you find yourself falling into this perception, **stop immediately!** Then, go take a walk, get something to drink, clear your head and remember the job is not to fill out the form; you are filling out the form so that you are as prepared as possible to help your clients get better.

Rather than trying to digest the whole process at once, the goal of this chapter is to help you understand the various components of a written treatment plan while also seeing how each section fits together to form a plan. It is hoped that this will also make it easier to understand the "how do I do it" part of preparing a treatment plan. That said, it takes practice, feedback, and more practice – which is why MFTs spend as much time as they do in training with a supervisor. In the next few sections, you will be introduced to various sections of the treatment planning form and given some explanation of what you would include if you were completing the process with your clients.

The facts

Start slowly by including the basic facts regarding the clients, including the date they started coming to therapy, today's date and how many sessions they have had up until this point. Written treatment plans may be required by your supervisor at different times depending on where you are working. In some locations, clients may complete two, three, four or more sessions before a written treatment plan is completed, allowing you time to reflect about how you will work with these clients. At other sites, the therapist may be required to write out a treatment plan at the end of the first therapy session. Either way, it is helpful to know the time span between the start of therapy and the writing of this treatment plan. It is also helpful to know, if possible, who referred the clients or who called for the appointment if they were self-referred.

Drawing the picture

As an MFT, you are interested in the client's relational system, even if the client comes for individual therapy. As part of the intake process, many sites have clinicians develop a genogram as a means of exploring some of the client system. Even if this is not required, for the purposes of the treatment plan, it is helpful to include an abbreviated version of the genogram here. Include the primary, day-to-day relationships to identify the people the client will likely interact with repeatedly while seeing you for treatment. Include some basic facts – ages of adults/children, marriage/divorce dates, work or school status, whether or not a particular person is the Identified Patient (IP). All of this information reminds you of key factors in a quick glance, which helps you to account for them in developing your plan.

The variables

No matter who the client is or what problem they bring to therapy there are always variables. Most of the time, there are so many variables that it is easy for both the therapist and the

Table 7.1 Treatment Plan – Client's Information

Client First Names	Current Date	Intake Date	Sessions to Date

Referral Person	

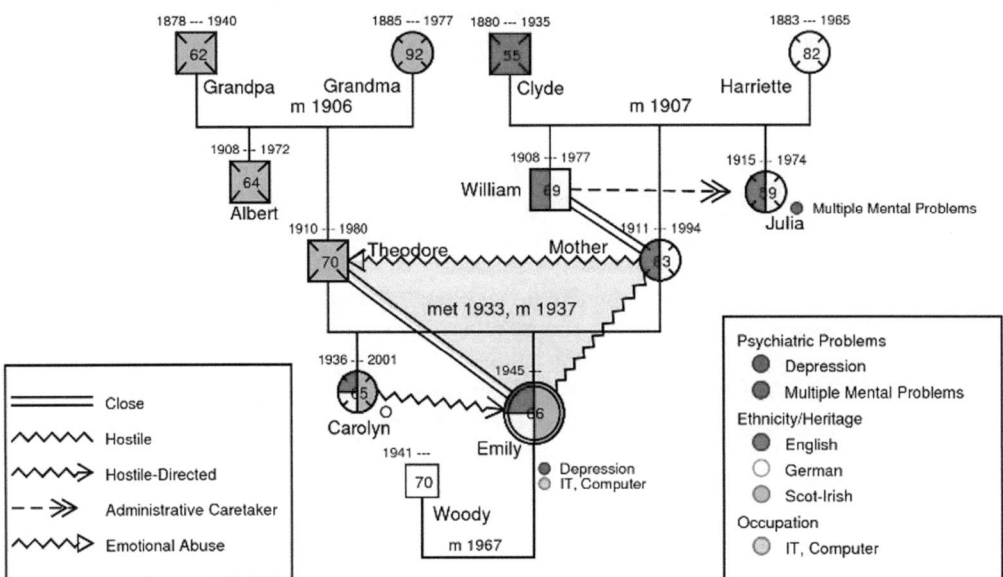

Figure 7.3 Brief Genogram – Current Primary Relationships, Ages, Work/School Status, Key Dates (Marriages/Divorces/Crisis Events), Identified Patient (Ip) Highlighted.

client to become quickly overwhelmed. There is no way to track them all – which turns out to be good since tracking every possible variable is not very helpful when it comes to clients getting better. Your treatment plan is a way to highlight some of the most important variables when it comes to these specific clients.

Your chosen MFT therapy model and a commitment to viewing clients through a systemic lens are two key factors in determining what variables are deemed important. One of the primary benefits of using an MFT model to guide you as a therapist is that it helps you focus your attention, rather than being distracted variables that may seem urgent but turn out not to be all that important.

Here, you are making note of a few key items: a brief (one or two sentences) description of the presenting problem; ask clients what prompted them to seek therapy now; and another brief description of any previous therapy the clients have had (dates, the name of the provider and any diagnosis they were given are useful here). The risk of harm is always important to note – the one to ten scale is quick and clear. Be sure to also include a brief list of medications clients are taking or have taken in the past (along with the dosage and prescriber name) and a brief statement indicating if the client has benefited from taking these medications.

This portion of the treatment planning form is designed to give a quick summary of the clients, their family system, what brought them to therapy, and their past experiences with therapy and/or medications. After this section, there are two more pieces of data to report, before you begin the hard part of thinking about how your approach to therapy will help you take all of this information and develop a plan to support the clients' change. The next two data points to cover are information regarding possible DSM (APA, 2020a) diagnoses and making a list of other professionals that could become collaborators with you as you help your clients.

Formal assessments and diagnosis

Many clinical sites use formal assessment tools, often as part of their intake process with clients; so, it is helpful to report what you have learned from these assessments. For example, sites may have clients complete the Beck Depression Inventory (BDI) (APA, 2020b) or the Dyadic Adjustment Scale (DAS) (Busby, Christensen, Crane & Larson, 1995) or use a simple one to ten scale to indicate how Satisfied or Committed each partner is to their relationship. There are many different assessment tools for specific DSM disorders that can be helpful in exploring symptoms of anxiety depression, ADHD, trauma, etc. In this section, list any assessments completed along with the results and a brief description of what the results mean. (For example, reporting that the client has a BDI score of 9 is not very helpful unless you know what that number means – is it 9 out of 10? 9 out of 100? 9 symptoms of depression?)

Table 7.2 Treatment Plan – Client's History

Presenting Problem at Intake

Previous Treatment History

Current Risk for Harm

Risk is Low 1   2   3   4   5   6   7   8   9   10   Risk is

High Current Medications if any

Medication Benefit to Client

No Benefit   1   2   3   4   5   6   7   8   9   10   Great Benefit

Table 7.3 Treatment Plan – Assessment and Diagnostic History

Formal Assessment Tool Results (If any)

```
┌─────────────────────────────────────────────────────────────┐
│                                                             │
│                                                             │
└─────────────────────────────────────────────────────────────┘
```

Current DSM-5 TR Diagnosis   As evidenced by (primary symptoms)

```
┌─────────────────────────────────────────────────────────────┐
│                                                             │
│                                                             │
└─────────────────────────────────────────────────────────────┘
```

```
┌─────────────────────────────────────────────────────────────┐
│     A word about assignment tools                           │
└─────────────────────────────────────────────────────────────┘
```

In addition to the results of assessment inventories, include a description of current DSM-5 TR diagnoses for all clients. In addition to the basic diagnosis and code (Separation Anxiety Disorder F 93.0), it is also good practice to list the qualifying symptoms – describe the client's symptoms and severity and use the DSM-5 TR criteria to make it clear how the client fits this particular diagnosis, rather than another possible category. You can also list possible diagnoses you think might be present, but you have yet to "rule out". As you consider possible diagnoses that might apply, be sure to get some input from the list of collaborative professionals you make in the next section. And, of course, discuss your thinking with your local supervisor to help you make decisions.

Consider this:

Diagnosis and systems

A DSM-5 TR diagnosis for clients is often required in many treatment facilities. You will need to understand the site's process for reaching a diagnosis. You also want to be able to think about where this information fits within a systemic conceptualization of presenting problems.

One baseline you can start with is to use the DSM-5 criteria to help you distinguish the specifics of client symptoms and search for the best description. This can help you move into the role of detective/explorer with the client, rather than someone who "announces their diagnosis" to them. You can use your own uncertainty to join with clients as you explore together to determine if a diagnosis fits and what it means.

First of all, a diagnosis is a description of symptoms – and just like descriptions of other variables, like age or work history, it can help you think about how their system currently operates.

Second, often the easiest way to conceptualize a client diagnosis as a factor within the system is to ask your clients this question: How can we make sense of this diagnosis in regards to your relationships?

Your collaborators

Part of the work of MFTs is to work together with other professionals who may provide services to your clients. Below is a partial list of possible professionals you might decide to work with on behalf of your clients. (Of course, you would follow the AAMFT Code of Ethics and make sure you have clients' written permission before contacting any of these professionals.) If you have already had some contact with any collaborators, this is a good place to provide a brief summary of what you learned (one to three sentences). If you have others you still hope to work with, you can identify that person and what you hope to gain by working with them.

Here comes the hard part

Now that you have a summary of what you know about the client so far – history, presenting problems, medication and/or diagnosis, family system, it is time to put your thinking cap on. In order to create a plan for change, you will need to take the variables above and "conceptualize" – that is be able to see – how they keep the client stuck and where you have opportunities to help them create change. The reason this is the "hard part" is because you are now past the part where you can fill in the blanks; to create a plan for treatment now requires you to put it all together. You will need to think about the client variables, the client system and your preferred MFT model in order to see a path forward and to articulate what you plan to do to help your client change.

Choosing an MFT model

So, start with the easy part. Which MFT model are you using to guide your treatment for your clients? Having identified your MFT approach, list a few key concepts this model would

Table 7.4 Release Forms Checklist

Potential Collaborators to Contact	Name/Contact	
Release Signed?		
Previous Therapist		☐
Primary Care Doctor		☐
Psychiatrist		☐
School Court/Probation		☐
Extended Family Others		☐
		☐
		☐

Table 7.5 Treatment Plan – MFT Theory and Model

MFT Theory You are using

MFT Model Assessment Concepts

have you assess. For example, if you chose Structural Family Therapy, you would likely assess the clients' current hierarchy, subsystems, boundaries and coalitions. If you chose Solution-Focused Therapy, you might consider whether or not the clients are customers, visitors or complainants.

Now, take these concepts and the data you have above and write out an *initial* systemic hypothesis. The emphasis is on initial – even though you are committing your treatment plan to paper, it is not final. It is never final because, as clients change, you will also need to adjust your plan. But, like a good outline for writing a paper, your written plan guides you in the direction of change. Your systemic hypothesis should include several parts: each of the key people in the relational system; a representation of how the client's interactions keep the problems in place (their homeostasis currently); and a picture of how they experience circular causality. If your hypothesis is linear – Client A does and Client B is mad, keep working at it. Sometimes the easiest way is to draw out a circle, insert all of the various key people in the loop and then write down next to their names what they do that keeps the loop going around.

If you find yourself getting stuck at this point – which is a common experience for beginning MFTs – try using the Functional Mapping Exercise. This short exercise may help you to think about your client and the information you have so far, so that you can begin to see patterns and connections. Should you find your initial attempts to generate a systemic hypothesis are frustrating or you find yourself just staring at a blank page and not knowing what to do next, the Functional Mapping Exercise should help get you jump started.

Once you have a simple systemic hypothesis, take what you have and look at it through the lens of your MFT model. Take the basic descriptions and add in the key concepts from the model that apply and draw out this version in the box. For example, a basic systemic hypothesis might be:

Client A bickers with Client B. The more this happens, the more Client B whines about it to Client C; and the more this happens, the more Client C yells at Client A to 'knock it off'. Of course, the more Client C yells, the more Client A blames and bickers with Client B.

You can use your map to begin generating circular questions to use with clients, which will help you develop a circular/systemic hypothesis to guide your treatment and session planning with your clients.

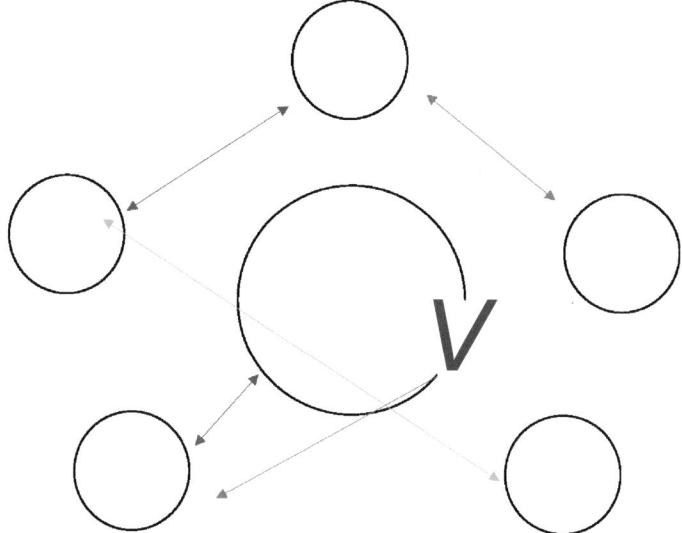

Figure 7.4 provides you with a simple example of a possible function map. However, the real value of the exercise is in developing your own map, rather than trying to create one that matches the example.

Case Scenario - *George has come to see you for therapy. George has been married for 28 years, he has two grown children who are now living on their own. After completing all of the intake forms and meeting George for two sessions, here is a list of all of the various problems George has raised:*
• *On the intake form, George reported that his wife had moved out of the house two weeks ago and he is afraid she may be preparing to divorce him.*
• *During the first session, George added that his children always seem too busy to talk to him - though they seem to keep up with their mother. He also mentioned that his own mother died a little over three months ago after a long battle with cancer.*
• *At the second session, George complained that he is under a lot of pressure at work. His license was suspended because of a DUI that his lawyer told him was going to be dismissed. He does not want work to know about this, but it is hard to keep up with required travel for work.*

Figure 7.4 Functional Mapping Exercise.

Table 7.6 Treatment Plan – Initial Systemic Hypothesis – Circular Diagram

Initial Systemic Hypothesis – Draw a circular diagram to illustrate your hypothesis; include all primary relationships of the clients.

How might you view this through a Solution-Focused lens?

The more Client A tells Client B what they appreciate about them, the more calm Client B is when they have a conflict. The more calm Client B is, the less they need to whine to Client C; and the less Client C is interrupted by whining, the more Client C engages and encourages Client A.

You can now examine your circular hypothesis, your MFT theoretical viewpoint and the client details to generate possible goals for therapy. Goals describe the big picture, the outcome of successful therapy. They help you and the clients to visualize what the client system would be like if they received all that they wanted from therapy.

Two key areas to keep in mind as you consider therapy goals

- Be sure to focus on system level (not just symptom level) goals. The goals should incorporate changes to the client's relational system, not just to a single individual within that system.
- Make sure your goal setting is a collaborative experience, rather than a task you complete alone.

Now that you have identified some possible goals, think about interventions you might use that are consistent with your MFT therapy model. Interventions are the "How tos" of therapy – they answer the question, "How will you accomplish these goals?" For now, it is enough to identify interventions that fit with your MFT model. Later on, you will be asked to map out which interventions you plan to use over the course of each session.

The final step in producing your treatment plan is to map out how you anticipate therapy might proceed over the course of multiple sessions. Of course, even as you design this plan, you will continue to further assess your clients, revise your systemic hypothesis and specify, in more detail, the goals and interventions.

A good way to start this process is to consider the treatment plan in groups of three sessions at a time. In the first box, you can list general goals, interventions and session outcome measures (how you will determine if the session you planned moved you closer to the goals). This will help you think across three sessions – so you can envision the plan session by session, but also be clearer about how sessions connect to each other. Once you have done this, you can use the smaller boxes to specify what you hope to do in each particular session. In your full treatment plan, you would continue this process for sessions 4–6, 7–9 and so on.

Having mapped out goals, interventions and what you plan to do over multiple sessions, there are just a few questions that remain in order for your treatment plan to be as effective

Table 7.7 Initial Hypothesis –MFT Theory Concepts

Describe Initial Hypothesis Using Your MFT Theory Concepts

Table 7.8 Goals Based on MFT Theory

Possible Goals based on Systemic Hypothesis/MFT Theory

Table 7.9 Possible Model Interventions

Possible Model Interventions

as possible. Remember, the purpose of treatment planning is not to complete an assignment, it is to help you and your clients work together successfully. This means you would do well to consult with an editor. Writing of any kind is challenging; therefore, everyone benefits from having someone review what you have written by providing them with a chance to offer some revisions.

There are two great editors waiting to help you with this – your supervisor and your client. While your supervisor may want to read the entire document – providing edits regarding your writing, suggestions for other variables to consider or provide helpful questions about your hypothesis – your client offers a different type of editing. Your clients may have little interest in reading the treatment plan in written form, but they probably have great interest in understanding what you think is ahead of them during the therapy process. Reviewing the big picture and asking what clients project as the future path for therapy is helpful to both of you.

Now what?

Now that you have worked all the way through the process, what will you do with the results? Unfortunately, all too often what happens is the treatment plan gets shoved into the client's file and no one looks at it again. Please, do not do this to your treatment plan. Instead, here are two ways you can use your treatment plan immediately to benefit yourself and your clients.

First, use your treatment plan to prepare for supervision. When you consult the treatment plan, you will see places where you are stuck and questions that you have – these are exactly what you want to bring into supervision. Supervision is best used when you arrive with questions, topics you want to discuss, ready to ask for help. The process of developing and utilizing a treatment plan will help put you into this position so you can get the most out of your supervisory experiences.

Table 7.10 Projected Treatment Timeline

Projected Treatment Timeline

Sessions 1-3	Goals	Interventions	Session Outcome Assessment

Session 1 Plan	Session 2 Plan	Session 3 Plan

What is group therapy?

Second, you can use your treatment plan to prepare your "session plan". The treatment plan provides you the big picture and an outline of where you hope to see therapy go; so, use it to prepare for the next session. Before you see the client for the next session, review the treatment plan to determine where you are. Are you ahead of the plan, behind the plan or are there steps you missed? Can you identify new data you picked up during the previous session? The treatment plan will help you stay on track and avoid providing "drama of the day" therapy sessions that are intense, but never seem to go anywhere.

NCU Systemic Treatment Plan

Client First Names	Current Date	Intake Date	Sessions to Date

Referral Person

Brief Genogram – current primary relationships, ages, work/school status Key dates (marriages/divorces/crisis events), Identified Patient (IP) highlighted

Presenting Problem at Intake

Previous Treatment History

Current Risk for Harm

Risk is low   1   2   3   4   5   6   7   8   9   10   Risk is High

Current Medications if any

Medication Benefit to Client

No Benefit   1   2   3   4   5   6   7   8   9   10   Great Benefit

Figure 7.5 Treatment Plan.

Formal Assessment **Tool Results (If any)**

Current DSM 5 Diagnosis

As evidenced by (primary symptoms)

Potential Collaborators **to Contact**	Name/Contact	Release Signed?
Previous Therapist		☐
Primary Care Doctor		☐
Psychiatrist		☐
School		☐
Court/Probation		☐
Extended Family		☐
Others		☐

MFT Theory You are Using

MFT Model Assessment Concepts

Figure 7.5 (Continued)

Initial Systemic Hypothesis – Draw a circular diagram to illustrate your hypothesis include all primary relationships with the IP

Drawing box

Describe Initial Hypothesis Using Your MFT Theory Concepts

(Be sure your hypothesis is circular, rather than linear.)

Possible Goals based on Systemic Hypothesis/MFT Theory

Figure 7.5 (Continued)

Possible Model Interventions

Projected Treatment Timeline

Sessions 1-3   **Goals**   **Interventions**   **Session Outcome Assessment**

Session 1 Plan   Session 2 Plan   Session 3 Plan

Figure 7.5 (Continued)

Sessions 4-6	Goals	Interventions	Session Outcome Assessment

Session 4 Plan	Session 5 Plan	Session 6 Plan

Sessions 7-9	Goals	Interventions	Session Outcome Assessment

Session 7 Plan	Session 8 Plan	Session 9 Plan

Figure 7.5 (Continued)

Additional Factors **to Consider**

```

```

List questions to bring to Supervision

```

```

Figure 7.5 (Continued)

References

American Association for Marriage and Family Therapy. (2015). *AAMFT Code of Ethics*. Retrieved from https://www.aamft.org/Legal_Ethics/Code_of_Ethics.aspx

American Psychological Association. (2020a). *DSM-5 Online Resources*. Retrieved from https://www.psychiatry.org/psychiatrists/practice/dsm/educational-resources/assessment-measures

American Psychological Association. (2020b). *Beck Depression Inventory*. Retrieved from https://www.apa.org/pi/about/publications/caregivers/practice-settings/assessment/tools/beck-depression

Busby, D. M., Christensen, C., Crane, D. R., & Larson, J. H. (1995). A revision of the dyadic adjustment scale for use with distressed and nondistressed couples: construct hierarchy and multidimensional scales. *Journal of Marital and Family Therapy, 21*, 289–308. doi:10.1111/j.1752-0606.1995.tb00163.x

Part II

Modern or Classic Models of Family Therapy

8 Milan Systemic Family Therapy

Valerie Q. Glass

Introduction

Milan Family Therapy originated in Milan, Italy and is one of the originating modernist models in the field of marriage and family therapy (MFT) (Barbetta & Umberta, 2021). The Milan approach branched off from the MRI strategic approach and the two models share some similarities in how they view the systemic maintenance of problems. Founders of both MRI strategic and Milan embraced Bateson's epistemology that understood families as working like a system (Penn, 1982). The MRI approach highlighted the importance of considering the "problem" within the context of the system and interrupting the homeostasis that the family is in that is maintaining that problem. Milan therapists took these ideas a step further and identified specific ways to consider that systemic context when looking at families. The Milan model conceptualized elements (e.g., context and family roles) that further allowed therapists to better understand the way that the system was maintaining the problematic homeostasis. This recognition of systemic functioning is one of the key reasons that Milan is recognized as critical to the history of the field of MFT. This chapter will underscore how the Milan method viewed problem formation and maintenance, techniques that further explore and create changes within systemic interactions, and how the tenets of the model have been both criticized and expanded upon as the field of MFT has continued to develop.

History and philosophical underpinnings

Milan Systemic Family Therapy evolved in 1971 out of the MRI strategic approach (Barbetta & Umberta, 2021). Mara Selvini Palazolli founded the model along with colleagues Luidi Boscolo, Gianfranco Cecchin and Giuliana Prata. The founders were trained in psychoanalysis and began to integrate systemic thinking into their work, highlighting the role of systemic symbolism to explain what they saw happening in family dynamics, prior to the development of the Milan model. Selvini Palazolli specifically had worked extensively with individuals with Schizophrenia and individuals with Anorexia. She recognized that family involvement in treatment created systemic change that seemed more sustainable than individual psychoanalysis. Selvini Palazolli and her colleagues founded the *Center for the Study of Family* in Milan to work with families as a whole. Their work sparked what became known as the Milan method (Barbetta & Umberta, 2021). In 1979, the Milan team shifted, Selvini Palazolli and Prata went one direction and focused on research while Boscolo and Cecchin continued to provide clinical training on the Milan method (Simon, 1987).

DOI: 10.4324/9781003382621-11

The Milan model is infrequently utilized (in its original format) by therapists in present day; however, one could argue that the initial ideas and interventions created roots for the modernist and postmodernist models that followed it. The Milan model highlights the importance of family change rather than focusing on individual behavior (Selvini Palazzoli, Boscolo, Cecchin & Prata, 1974); this is the foundational epistemological stance of all MFT models to this day (Breunlin & Jacobsen, 2014; Kaslow, 2010). Additionally, certain techniques, such as circular questioning and the reflecting team, are ever present in MFT training programs. Many ideas developed by the Milan team produced a framework for MFT theories and techniques that followed.

Systemic foundation

Milan therapies are grounded in systemic thinking (Campbell, Draper & Huffington, 1989). For example, if a person enters into therapy and begins to cry, the Milan therapist recognizes that the presence of tears (e.g., sadness, fear, anger, etc.) cannot be viewed independently from the context where they arise. Milan thinkers may ask the questions: "How do the other parts of the family system interact when that crying occurs?" or "Does this crying help other parts of the system from feeling what they need to feel?", or "What interactions contribute to this person feeling this feeling?" Systemic understanding means recognizing that the emotion is both influenced by and also influences the other parts of the system. Another assumption from systemic thinking that Milan brings to the model is an understanding that one's behavior is dictated by thoughts and beliefs, almost as if beliefs are reinforced behaviors that exist in a system. Here is an example that explains this process.

Assume that there is a father and their teenage child in therapy. The father has been increasingly strict with the child as the child was maturing, or so it seems to the child. The child reacts emotionally and will yell at their father when they feel this strictness. The child has their own context of the world around them and feels that, when their father is holding them back from activities, the father does not like them or does not want them to enjoy life. This is the child's understanding of the world and the belief that they have come to in their actions. The father, on the other hand, has heard messages that the stricter you are with teens, the safer they will be. This "causes", in a sense, the father's decision to be strict with the child, based on their belief system. Because these belief systems cause emotional intensity (e.g., the child may feel like the father does not care, which brings in deep primary emotions and the father may feel fear for safety, which is a separate primary emotion). These beliefs, the emotions evolving out of the misunderstanding of these beliefs and the resulting behaviors associated with these beliefs are causing a rift in the system. The family can get into a rut over time because there might be relief at times (e.g., maybe the father did not let the child go to a big party and felt relief in his sense of safety and security). These behaviors can begin to reinforce each other and cause a continuation of the cycle, even intensity in the cycle over time. This is the problematic homeostasis that the family is stuck in.

Milan therapists will take this information and make a conclusion about what they feel is happening and create a situation that shakes up the system. Campbell et al. (1989) stated that "the aim of a family therapist is to interact in a way that introduces differences into the belief/behavior" (p. 13). For example, in this scenario, the therapist might bring in different ways of looking at child development as a way for the father to consider the importance of freedom. The therapist may help the child to see some of the behaviors of the father are rooted in his love for them. By introducing this new vision of previously held beliefs, change can occur. Keep in mind that second-order cybernetics recognizes the therapist as part of the system and part of the change process. The therapist enters the therapy room with their own belief system and these beliefs could become part of the systemic interactions. Being aware of that role and one's own set of beliefs can be a critical part of the therapeutic process.

Problem formation

Milan therapists recognize the intricacies of problem behaviors or what brings people to therapy exists through interactions within their systems (Barbetta & Umberto, 2021). Problems occur, according to the Milan model, as families start to engage in a pattern that may have adapted over time or may be the result of a specific change (Rhodes, 2013). These patterns often increase in intensity over time and the family is stuck in the cycle, the homeostasis. Families create rules that (even unconsciously) keep the family at the homeostasis.

Main concepts and interventions

The Milan model can be best considered through the ways the model views problems, the maintenance of problems and what creates the change process within the system (Barbetta & Umberto, 2021). This section will explore major interventions and conceptualizations introduced by the Milan model.

Hypothesizing

One of the key interventions of the Milan approach is systemic hypothesizing (Barbetta & Umberto, 2021). Milan therapists generate a loose and malleable hypothesis of what they perceive is happening in the family system. This hypothesizing is based on the discussion, behaviors and experiences the therapists are observing. Hypothesizing occurs outside of the therapy room and without client collaboration. Milan therapists recognize the subjectivity in observing family dynamics and encourage a deeper look into the hypothesis (or assessment) by connecting to colleagues or supervisors to further discuss and narrow down the hypothesis. The hope is that a clear picture of the "real" hypothesis develops through this discussion process, through a deeper alliance and connection with the family, and through continued work and interaction. Selvini Palazzoli, Boscolo, Cecchin and Prata (1980) shared that:

> The formation by the therapist of an (sic) hypothesis based upon the information he (sic) possesses regarding the family he (sic) is interviewing. The hypothesis establishes a starting point for his (sic) investigation as well as his (sic) verification of the validity of this hypothesis based upon specific methods and skills. If the hypothesis is proven false, the therapist must form a second hypothesis based on the information gathered during the testing of the first.
>
> (p. 3)

Hypotheses can begin at the time of referral or intake, as often much information is available at a first phone call or referring party. Think of hypothesis building like building a theory, you have a theory, test the theory, take the parts that work and develop a more specific theory, then test the new theory and so on.

Graphic 1: Hypothesis testing

The hypothesis can be uncovered through what the client shares, what they do not share, what their body language suggests, how they present information in their tone and their actions (Selvini Palazzoli et al., 1980). In the Milan model, the hypothesis must consider the systemic elements of the family. Hypotheses can explore alliances between members of the system, myths about rules or expectations, or communication patterns. A Milan therapist would not state "client has depression", rather the hypothesis would include the system and these interactions. The Milan therapist might hypothesize:

> family has developed a difficult homeostasis, as mother is often withdrawn and does not seem to connect her body language to her son, the son's behavior seems to be working to gain attention from his mother, when she gets angry, that seems to be the only time she provides him with attention. Son is experiencing a sense of isolation and fear because of witnessing his mother's frequent crying and her difficulty completing daily tasks, previous partner never played an active role in the family; however, emotions are present in mother since the partner left.
>
> (Selvini Palazzoli et al., 1980, p.8)

Let us consider an example of what this might look like with clients. Assume that a Milan therapist received a phone call from a mother who indicated that her 7-year-old son was acting out recently at school. He has been disturbing other children in the school setting and is talking back to his mother. When the therapist asks who will be attending the therapy session, the mother shares that it will be just her, her son and a younger daughter. She shares that her partner left the home about a year ago and has very little to do with the family. Immediately, the therapist can begin creating a loose hypothesis that at least some of the son's behaviors may be related to the other adult in his life not staying connected to him. Once the three arrive to session and more information is given, it is possible that hypothesis could shift. Consider that the son is reacting to his mother's recent depressive behaviors and maybe the perceived negative behaviors had little to do with the other parent not engaging with him. It might be observed that the younger daughter is constantly over-achieving and the therapist might be able to assume this plays into the hypothesis in some way.

Milan therapists work to identify the strengths or positive elements in the hypothesis; this is known as a reframe or positive connotation (Selvini Palazzoli et al., 1980). A positive connotation may look at the example above and consider that the girl is over-achieving because she loves her mother so much that she is working hard to make her happy, or they may bring up that the mother is really caring by seeking out therapy services to make things better for her children. Hypothesizing in the Milan model creates hypotheses that do not pathologize or blame any one person or diagnosis, rather it explores systemic behaviors as a whole, the patterns of interactions. Several elements are considered throughout the hypothesis formation process.

Therapeutic perspectivism highlights that idea that many elements of the therapist's life and experience can play a role in understanding the dynamics of the family (Barbetta & Umberta, 2021). Milan therapists are encouraged to better understand their own context and the role that this could be playing in their hypothesizing.

Interventive interviewing is the first point of contact the therapist has with the system. Milan therapists request to see entire families initially (Campbell et al., 1989). This intervention allows the therapist to best consider the many dynamics, beliefs and behaviors that are occurring among the family members. The therapist hones in on who is doing what during conflict, how the family is believing in these moments and who is responding. The therapist can start to piece together the multitude of challenges that might be occurring (for example, is there a scapegoat in the family? Is there a fused type of relationship? Where did the beliefs come from?)

Formulation occurs when the therapist has an initial understanding of the hypothesis after interventive interviewing (Campbell et al., 1989). This is sort of a hypothesis that the therapist can attribute to the many dynamics and beliefs that have been observed during interventive interviewing. "The formulation ought to try to connect the problem or symptomatic behavior to the contradictions between the beliefs and behavior demonstrated in the interview" (Campbell et al., 1989, p. 63). The "symptom" (the reason the family came to the therapist) can be described as the "attempt to resolve contradictions between the family's beliefs and behavior" (p. 63).

Milan therapists work to better understand the context and the belief system of each family member (Campbell et al., 1989). They work to break down belief systems that have contributed to behaviors. Understanding and formulating the hypothesis can create space to challenge the homeostasis.

Reflecting teams

The reflecting team has been utilized by many different modalities in the systemic therapy. In a reflecting team, one therapist, or sometimes co-therapists are designated as the primary therapist(s), works directly with the family, while a team of therapists observe through a one-way mirror (Mitchell, Rhodes, Wallis & Wilson, 2014). In the Milan model, the primary purposes of the reflecting team are to refine and consider the family hypothesis, consider appropriate interventions and aid the therapist in establishing neutrality (Barbetta & Umberta, 2021; Mitchell et al., 2014). The therapist will meet with the family as the team observes the session and the therapist will have check-ins with the reflecting team to consider the case, the hypothesis and possible interventions.

The Milan model reflecting teams included a five-state process (Mitchell et al., 2014):

1. Presession – Prior to sessions, the team of therapists arrive at a loose hypothesis for what they think is going on. This is based on referral information or what was gathered from the initial contact.
2. Session – In this stage, the therapist(s) meet with the family and asks curious questions about the family system to deepen their understanding of what is happening.
3. Intersession – After meeting with the family, the therapist will take a break from the session about halfway through and confer with a team behind the mirror. The therapist and the team may tweak the hypothesis based on their observations. Additionally, interventions will be discussed.
4. Intervention – In this stage, the therapist returns to the session after the intersession and applies an intervention.
5. Discussion – After the session is over, the family is dismissed and the therapist meets again with the team to further refine the hypothesis and consider future clinical direction.

Reflecting teams can occur for each session and continue to narrow down what is happening in the system that can be addressed.

Circularity and circular causality

Circularity and circular causality are like, well, a circle, just like it sounds. The system is interacting and there is not a beginning or an ending, simply, the homeostasis is stuck in one spot and the same things are happening over and over again (Selvini Palazzoli, et al., 1980). This circular process is what is being uncovered by the hypothesis. Essentially, the hypothesis is refining the language around this circularity and describing, as closely as possible, what is exactly happening in the circle.

Penn (1982) discusses the way that circularity works. They state circularity is:

> A system being made up of patterned circuits and populated by differences that produce information. A circuit can loop in many directions including more or less components depending upon whether it is a lower or higher-level circuit, i.e., a simple or complex cybernetic loop. It can be as simple a loop as a man out for a stroll or as complex as the 'corrective loop,' consisting of the therapist, family, symptom, and intervention.
>
> (p. 270)

This brings us to circular questioning. The purpose of circular questioning is to change these circuits and the way that information is being processed (Penn, 1982).

Circular questioning

The Milan model highlights the role circular questioning has in uncovering the hypothesis and shifting the homeostasis (Penn, 1982: Selvini Palazzoli, et al., 1980). The therapist is very much a part of the systemic process because they have their own perspective and background that feeds into their understanding of the hypothesis (Penn, 1982). Simply put, circular questioning recognizes the role of the "investigation" (p. 4) that occurs during hypothesis consideration. It is asking questions of the family in a way that highlights new thinking around the "problem" (Penn, 1982). Early Milan therapists believed in the role of language and re-languaging to create insight and change. In circular questioning, the inclusion of second-order cybernetics plays a role in this change process. The therapist and the insertion of new interjections lead to change. Circular questioning involves diving in to consider feedback when ideas are presented.

What does this process look like? Circular questioning starts with asking each member of the family to explain their experiences with the family, how they see their relationship with each of the other family members and how they perceived the relationships to be between other family members. Then, as the answers unfold, the therapist continues to ask questions that challenge the way that the patterns are evolving by considering other ways to have the system interact. For example, if two people are arguing, the therapist asks a third person a question about that interaction (e.g., "When your Dad and sister argue, who takes Dad's side?") One purpose of these questions is to gather details about all parts of that "circular" hypothesis as possible.

Another important purpose of circular questioning is about the change process. Milan therapists believed that circular questioning distorted the natural flow of the (problematic) homeostasis in a way that progressively led to change (Penn, 1982). If two people are having a conflict and constantly are engaging in this conflict, it is the perspective of a third that might shift this established homeostasis. The idea is that these questions insert a new interaction or a new way of looking at an interaction, which ultimately messes up the current problematic homeostasis.

Additionally, circular questioning could create a space that allows a return to a healthier homeostasis. Penn (1982) stated:

> The aim of circular questioning is to fix the point in the history of the system when important coalition underwent a shift and the consequent adaptation to that shift became problematic for the family. The information sought by circular questions are the difference in relationships the family has experienced before and after the problem began.
>
> (p. 272)

Questioning in circular causality is about uncovering. When one element of the family pattern is uncovered, questions from that pattern build on this in a way that dives deeper. Family members are questioned on how the other family members react and if they feel those responses fit their experiences. All of this helps the therapist uncover the most accurate a hypothesis of what the family system is doing.

There are different types of circular questioning that can be implemented to meet these goals

Paradox and counterparadox

Milan therapists recognized the interventions of paradox and counterparadox (Selvini Palazzoli, 1989). When a therapist intervenes with a paradox, the purpose is to create a scenario where the therapist instructs the family to do something that seems opposite to what would be expected. For example, when siblings are constantly arguing, a counterparadox might be to tell them to argue more often. A paradox could challenge the system by saying or doing things that interrupt the flow of what is happening. Some examples might include: presenting positive language around something that is seen as problematic, putting the family in a double bind (e.g., telling them to "feel more" when they desire to "feel less"), suggesting they do something for a problem that seems obscure (e.g., when your parents are arguing, you and your sister must sing), or even telling them not to change something that they feel is problematic. The purpose of these interventions was partly to observe how the homeostasis fluctuated as a result of these obscure interventions. Additionally, these interventions lead to shifts in homeostasis because of their obscurity – the family was interacting in a different way.

Invariant prescription

Selvini Palazzoli (1989) introduced a specific intervention she coined invariant prescription. This method seeks to rebalance coalitions and appropriate subsystems by helping parents achieve appropriate hierarchy in the system. One well-known example of how Selvini Palazzoli utilized this technique was in their work with children with Schizophrenia. They prescribed the parents to make plans that the children did not know the details of. The parents would go off "on a date" and not share with the children where they were going, what they were doing or when they would be back. The idea behind this was that the parents would establish an appropriate coalition and subsystem. This intervention frequently came under scrutiny because many felt this intervention was unfounded and manipulative (MacKinnon & Miller, 1987; Simon, 1987) and is not utilized in present day. Selvini Palazzoli herself questioned this intervention and stopped using it in her later years (Simon, 1987).

Table 8.1 Circular Questioning Interventions

Name of Intervention	Definition	Examples of this intervention in the therapy room:
Diachronic Investigation (Selvini Palazzoli, 1980)	The therapist explores the way people are interacting with the "symptoms" rather than looking at the symptoms.	The therapist might respond to a statement like "I am feeling sad" by asking another member of the family how they interact with the "sad" person when they get like that. This helps the therapists better understand dynamics around the behavior. Rather than getting into the details of an argument, the therapist might turn to the person not in the argument and ask what they do when the other two are arguing like they are." This focus assists the therapists in locating the cycles in the dynamic and what is causing the system to maintain itself in a problematic space.
Dividing up Subsystems (Selvini Palazzoli, 1980)	Therapists recognize subsystems within the family dynamic and ask questions that divide up these subgroups to reflect in a way that explores that subsystem (Selvini et al., 1980)	In a family with two parents and two children, where the children are constantly bickering, the therapist may ask one child, "what does your father do when you say that to your sibling?"
Verbal and Analogic Information (Penn, 1982)	The therapist pays attention to ti. The therapist observes a family using the word "angry" often in their dialog about different people and events and asks different family members about their experience with this emotion or ask them to reflect on how they observe other people interacting with this emotion.hemes that are occurring in the family and constructs ways (e.g., asking questions or being curious) to better understand these themes. This can be related to what the family is saying (for example, using a similar word to describe their pattern) or their body language around topics or themes (including eye contact, facial expressions, and tone).	A child rolls their eyes when their father brings up one of the child's recent behaviors and the therapist asks another child "who notices first when your sibling rolls their eyes?" When the therapist is speaking to the stepparent, family member's all have a shift in tone. The therapist might ask a child, "who does your stepparent get along with most?"
Problem Definition (Penn, 1982)	The therapist asks the family about their present day problem. The intention behind this is to explore the problem as it exists in the family in the moment (often, later in therapy this will be asked again and the initial answer will be used for comparison).	Simply, this is asking a family, "tell me about what the problem is that is occurring in your family right in this moment." Milan therapists would likely intentionally ask all members of the family this question to consider all perspectives.

Technique	Description	Examples
Coalition alignments in the present (Penn, 1982)	When the therapist explores the different family members' relationship with the problem that is being presented. The goal is to consider the problem that is noted by the family and ask questions that will highlight the different parts of the system and how they are interacting with the problem.	"Who gets the most angry when Jay acts out in public?" "Who is the first to notice when mom starts to feel sad?" "When Katie is frustrated, what does Dad do?"
A Different Sequence (Penn, 1982)	The therapist begins to really track what is happening when the problem occurs. They seek to best define the sequence of events and how the problem is maintained by who is doing what and when in the problem behavior.	"When Katie is frustrated and Dad yells at her, what does Jay do next? Then, what does Papa do?" "Last night when Jay acted out in public, what did the family do? What happened first? Second? How did Jay respond to these things?"
Questions of Classification and Comparison (Penn, 1982)	As the sequence of events has been identified, classifying and comparing events further explores the therapists' hypothesis about the family dynamic. Classifying further dives into the roles that people are playing in the problem maintenance and comparing looks to better understand how sub-systems are broken down.	Classification: "Who gets the most overwhelmed when Papa retreats to his room? Who is next, for being most overwhelmed? Who is least overwhelmed?" Comparison: "Which behavior is least frustrating, when Papa retreats or when he yells?" Comparison: "Who is the best at calming Jay down when he acts out in public?"
Agreement questions (Penn, 1982)	In this form of circular questioning, the therapist filters through the family to consider the coalitions within the family and which ones are stronger. The therapist will ask all members to consider these possible coalitions.	Assume that Papa and Katie are noted as very close in the family. The therapists will ask Papa "is it true that you and Katie have a strong relationship?" They may ask Jay "would you also say that Katie and Papa are the closest in the family?"
Gossiping in the presence (Penn, 1982)	This questioning takes agreement to another level by asking more details from one person about the relationship between two other people.	The therapist asks "Katie, tell me a little more about the relationship between Dad and Papa."
Subsystem Comparison (Penn, 1982)	In this line of questioning, the therapist compares the problem and the dynamics of the problem with other subsystems.	Assume that Dad is always yelling at Papa. The therapist might ask Katie "which one of your Dad's is most likely to be calm with you when they are frustrated with you?"
Explanation Question (Penn, 1982)	These questions can take any of the presented information a bit further, asking for elaboration.	"Was there a time that Dad and Papa were not yelling at each other?" "When did Katie and Papa develop such a great bond?" "Was what is like when Jay wasn't acting out in public?"

Neutrality

Milan therapists stress the importance of therapist neutrality (Campbell et al., 1989). When the therapist is neutral to the family members, they do not take sides in the issue or with the problem. Additionally, they do not let their own background influence their understanding of what is happening in the system. Maintaining neutrality is a key in Milan Family Therapy (Campbell et al., 1989). One way that Milan therapists work toward neutrality is being held accountable by reflecting teams. Reflecting teams share various perspectives and also challenge therapists at times if there seems to be something from their own life or perspective clouding their understanding of the hypothesis.

Multipartiality

On the flip side of neutrality is multipartiality, which is the goal of the Milan model. This is when the therapist focuses on everyone's thoughts and perspectives equally (Campbell et al., 1989). Multipartiality is taking everyone's side and creating space where all members feel like the therapist honors them individually.

Curiosity

Curiosity is a critical element in the Milan model and is integrated into all interventions (Campbell et al., 1989; Selvini Palazzoli et al., 1974). Curiosity in the Milan model is about creating space for really diving deep into what each person has to say and how they understand their dynamics and to better refine the hypothesis. In this curiosity space, the therapist honors each individual's view of the problem. Much like in postmodernism, curiosity recognizes that there is not one truth and that multiple perspectives will lead to a better understanding of the systemic pattern that has evolved; however, unlike postmodern models, curiosity has a specific goal of better understanding the hypothesis.

Positive connotation

One key intervention in the Milan model is putting the family in a space where strengths, resiliencies and positive elements are explored and brought into sessions (Selvini Palazzoli et al., 1974). This is referred to as positive connotation. The idea behind positive connotation is to not focus on behaviors that are considered pathological. For example, if a family comes in and a child has Anorexia, the Milan therapists focus on the entirety of the observable behaviors of all family members and the patterns (rather than a specific intensity on the Anorexia or the person with Anorexia). Using positive connotation, the therapist will highlight and further explore what strengths they are seeing in the interactions. For example, in the family mentioned where the child has Anorexia, a therapist might mention how responsive and caring the father has been or how patient and loving the sibling has been over the past couple months. These things ultimately cause shifts in the homeostasis, which has been built around the perceived "pathology" (Selvini Palazzoli et al., 1974). Respect and appreciation of the family, by the therapist, creates a stronger alliance and softens more difficult interventions. Selvini Palazzoli et al. (1974) explained the process of change utilizing positive connotation:

> We do not consider positive connotation a ploy or trick... we consider the observable behavior of a family in therapy as self-corrective and thus tending to maintain

the equilibrium of the system. A family who comes into therapy is usually a family in crisis, frightened by the possible loss of homeostasis and therefore anxious to maintain it at all cost. If we were to tell them explicitly that they must change, it would make them enter into a virtually monolithic coalition in order to ward us off. To be accepted into the family system, it is necessary for us to approve their behavior, no matter what it is, since it is directed at a more than understandable goal: the cohesion of family... through positive connotation we implicitly declare ourselves as allied of the family's striving for homeostasis. By thus strengthening the homeostatic tendency, we gain influence over the ability to change that is inherent in every living system.

(pp. 5–6)

Ultimately, locating these positive aspects of family can help "unite" (p. 58) the family. Looking for and pointing out aspects of the family dynamic that are positive can help the family envision what they do well and how they have functioned well.

Use with a diversity of clients

As the Milan model grew in the 1970s, the model did not elaborate on diverse experiences or the efficacy of Milan techniques with various populations. There has, however, always been recognition that family background, history and context are critical to understanding the hypothesis (Selvini Palazzoli et al., 1974). One tenet of the Milan model highlighted that hypotheses could not be accurate without the recognition of the context (which included culture, social injustices and experiences). In addition, Milan therapists worked to both compartmentalize the therapist's self and the recognition that the therapist's context also played a role in their understanding.

Current Milan therapists advocate for transitions within the Milan approach to include attention to the role of discrimination, marginalization and social justice (Barbetta & Umberta, 2021). This includes building on the interventions in a way that include these recognitions, for example, including questions that integrate the client's experiences with power and social issues.

Research support

Early research studies identified that the Milan method focused on the efficacy of systemic treatment (Carr, 1991; Scheel & Conoley, 1998; Simpson, 1990). These early studies did suggest that the way that the Milan approach is applied in that it takes into account the system, rather than the individual, and seeks to shift homeostasis, does create systemic shifts (Carr, 1991). One example in the research, Simpson (1990) researched outcomes with children in a psychiatric unit and found that those utilizing traditional (e.g., behavioral) approaches had similar outcomes (individually) as those who had participated in Milan approaches. The difference was that those that had participated in the Milan approach had notable changes in the family dynamics post-treatment, compared to those in behavioral treatments.

The Milan approach is not often represented in research in its entirety; however, many of the foundational ideas and interventions that originated from Milan have paved the way for current clinical research. For example, the role of considering family dynamics within their context is frequently evolved in research (e.g., Anslow, 2014). Sometimes Milan approaches and interventions are explored as ways to create shifts in family homeostasis (Mitchell et al., 2014). Circular questioning and circular causality have been supported ideas in the area of helping families consider the systemic nature of interactions (Pinelopi & Tseliou, 2016). Additionally, reflecting teams, became part of many clinical settings and training programs (from both modernist and postmodernist perspectives) and were found to have notable benefits to both clients and clinical students (Willott, Hatton & Oyebode, 2012).

Criticism and ethical considerations

Over time, there have been notable criticisms of the Milan approach (Mitchell et al., 2014; Treacher, 1988). As postmodernist models evolved, there was increasing discussion around the expert stance of the Milan approach. The arguments highlighted that the approach held views of family that did not allow for variation in experience, culture and family dynamics, essentially, that there was one "way" to family (Mitchell et al., 2014). Other adversaries felt that the way Milan therapists approached reflecting teams and creating hypotheses, in a way that does not uncover thoughts and ideas to the client, to be a disservice to the clients involved (Mitchell et al., 2014; Treacher, 1988). Treacher (1988) goes so far to say that this is "dehumanizing" and compares the process of Milan therapy to the therapist being a scientific observer that is creating a hypothesis without feedback from the client perspective. Similarly, the concept of neutrality has been criticized (Treacher, 1988). The MFT field evolved to recognize that neutrality is an impossible construct and detrimental to the therapy process. Therapists, in the Milan model, worked to maintain neutrality, rather than recognize that each therapist does come from their own place of experience (culture, history, family dynamics, etc.) and that social influences do influence their perspectives.

Ethical response

Adversaries of the Milan approach argued the model was both directive and presented manipulative interventions that could be seen as unethical (e.g., invariant prescriptions and positive connotations) (Mitchell et al., 2014). These are seen as manipulative and invoke a power dynamic within the therapist-client relationship. Similarly, Treacher (1988) challenged the Milan model's lack of attention to the clients' stories and hearing their perspectives. They argued that the Milan model is more of a game and less of a recognition of peoples' voices, experiences and perspectives. Criticisms for this model questioned power dynamics and the therapists' lack of being aware of this power and/or manipulating the power that they had.

Summary

It could be argued that the direct criticisms of the Milan approach (and other directive and manipulative approaches) sparked new directions in the field that contributed to the growth of ethical understanding, the recognition of power dynamics in therapeutic relationship, recognition of value of the therapist self in the room and the importance of understanding the client's perspectives and contexts (Breunlin & Jacobsen, 2014; Kaslow, 2010; Treacher, 1988). Much like the evolution of research, the core aspects of the Milan model and other modernist models and the criticisms around them allowed for growth in the field as a whole, including adaptations of both modernist and postmodernist models (Kaslow, 2010: MacKinnon & Miller, 1987). Rhodes (2013) identified that the Milan model viewed the therapist in "an expert role" (p. 136) where they view their work with families much like a "mechanic works on a car" (p. 136). Similarly, scholars found the Milan approach did not address social context, including culture, bias, marginalization and basic rights (MacKinnon & Miller, 1987). For a couple of decades following the growth of Milan, what was known as "post-Milan systemic therapies" developed as an off-shoot of Milan. The idea behind post-Milan models was that therapists take on a more collaborative stance with clients and better understand the client context. Post-Milan therapies also recognized the role of the observer and second-order cybernetics. The terminology of post-Milan therapies served as a precursor to postmodern and poststructural perspectives of therapy. The Milan method planted seeds of thinking. Many concepts and interventions have laid a foundation for MFT theories that evolved since the time of early Milan thinkers.

References

Anslow, nee A. F. K. (2014). Systemic family therapy using the reflecting team: the experiences of adults with learning disabilities. *British Journal of Learning Disabilities, 42*(3), 236–243. doi: 10.1111/bld.12048

Barbetta, P. & Umberta, T. (2021). The Milan approach, history, and evolution. *Family Process, 60*(1), 4–16. doi: 10.1111/famp.12612

Breunlin, D. C. & Jacobsen, E. (2014). Putting the "family" back into family therapy. *Family Process, 53*(3), 462–475. doi: 10.1111/famp.12083

Campbell, D., Draper, R. & Huffington, C. (1989). *Second thoughts on the theory and practice of the Milan approach to family therapy*. London, UK: Karnac.

Carr, A., (1991). Milan systemic family therapy: a review of ten empirical investigations. *Journal of Family Therapy, 13*(3), 237–263.

Kaslow, F. W. (2010). A family therapy narrative. *The American Journal of Family Therapy, 38*, 50–62. doi: 10.1080/01926180903430030

MacKinnon, L. K. & Miller, D. (1987). The new epistemology and the Milan approach: feminist and sociopolitical considerations. *Journal of Marital and Family Therapy, 13*(2), 139–155. doi: 10.1111/j.1752-0606.1987.tb00692.x

Mitchell, P., Rhodes, P., Wallis, A. & Wilson, V. (2014). A comparison of two systemic family therapy reflecting team interventions. *Journal of Family Therapy, 36*(3), 237–254. doi: 10.1111/1467-6427.12018

Penn, P. (1982). Circular questioning. *Family Process, 21*(3), 267–280. https://doi.org/10.1111/j.1545-5300.1982.00267.x

Pinelopi, P. & Tseliou, E. (2015). Blame, responsibility and systemic neutrality: a discourse analysis methodology to the study of family therapy program talk. *Journal of Family Therapy, 38*(4), 467–490.

Rhodes, P. (2013). Post-Milan systemic therapy. In A. Rambo, C. West, A. Shooley & T. V. Boyd (Eds.) *Family therapy review: contrasting contemporary models* (pp. 136–140). New York, NY: Taylor & Francis.

Scheel, M. J. & Conoley, C. W. (1998). Circular questioning and neutrality: an investigation of the process relationship. *Contemporary Family Therapy, 20*(2), 221–235. doi: 10.1023/a:1023/a:1025033610756

Selvini Palazzoli, M., Boscolo, L., Cecchin, G. & Prata, G. (1974). The treatment of children through brief therapy of their parents. *Family Process, 13*, 429–442. https://doi.org/10.1111/j.1545-5300.1974.00429.x

Selvini Palazzoli, M., Boscolo, L., Cecchin, G. & Prata, G. (1980). Hypothesizing – circularity – neutrality: three guidelines for the conductor of the session. *Family Process, 19*, 3–12.

Selvini Palazzoli, M. (1989). *Family games: general models of psychotic processes in the family*. London, UK: Karnac Books.

Simon, R., (September/October, 1987). Good-bye paradox, help invariant prescription. *Psychotherapy Networker.*   www.psychotherapynetworker.org/magazine/article/954/good-bye-paradox-hello-invariant-prescription

Simpson, L. (1990). The comparative efficacy of Milan family therapy for disturbed children and their families. *Journal of Family Therapy, 13*, 267–284. https://doi.org/10.1046/j..1991.00427.x

Treacher, A. (1988). The Milan method – a preliminary critique. *Journal of Family Therapy, 10*, 1–8. http://dx.doi.org/10.1046/j..1988.00295.x

Willott, S., Hatton, T. & Oyebode, J. (2012). Reflecting team processes in family therapy: a search for research. *Journal of Family Therapy, 34*(2), 180–203.

9 Structural Family Therapy

Asha Sutton

Introduction

Structural Family Therapy is founded on the idea that each family operates according to established patterns of interactions. It is through these patterns of interactions that both overt and covert rules are played out and set the parameters for what is allowable within the family system. As a traditional model of family therapy, Structural Family Therapy de-emphasizes the role of the individual and instead focuses on multiple subsystems and restructuring the subsystems so that the hierarchy of the family as well as the boundaries, patterns, rules and general family functioning is healthy for all members of the system. The approach does not inherently seek to omit stress and conflict from occurring within the lives of members of the system, instead, Structural Family Therapy strives to help families effectively navigate how it is they manage life's inevitable stress and conflict.

Founder

Salvador Minuchin (1921–2017) is generally regarded as the founder of Structural Family Therapy. Born and raised in Argentina, Minuchin trained as a child psychologist. Throughout the 1960s, he worked with the likes of Nathan Ackerman and Jay Haley.

Minuchin's training with child survivors of the Holocaust and children from poverty-stricken areas helped to shape his ideas around the importance of examining families in their contexts.

In 1965, Minuchin became the director of **the Philadelphia Child Guidance Clinic**. During its inception, the clinic specialized in meeting the needs of low-income urban families. In the 1970s and 1980s, Minuchin focused his attention on training clinicians at the Philadelphia Child Guidance Clinic. He is responsible for training such clinicians as Harry Aponte, Jorge Colapinto and Michael Nichols. In 1981, Minuchin opened what is known today as The Minuchin Center for the Family in New York. He retired from The Minuchin Center in 1996.

Minuchin's (1974) *Families and family therapy* text is a seminal book in the field as it is the first to outline key Structural Family Therapy principles. Additional texts that helped to shape field's knowledge of Structural Family Therapy included *Family therapy techniques* (Minuchin & Fishman, 1981), *Families of the slums* (Minuchin, Montalvo, Buerney, Rosman & Schumer, 1967), *Family healing: tales of hope and renewal from family therapy* (Minuchin & Nichols, 1993), *Psychosomatic families: anorexia in context* (Minuchin,

DOI: 10.4324/9781003382621-12

Rosman & Baker, 1978), and Colapinto's (1991) chapter on Structural Family Therapy in the *Handbook of family therapy*.

Systemic foundation

On a fundamental level, Structural Family Therapy's focus on the whole rather than the individual parts underscores the systemic foundations of the model. With a focus on **wholeness**, the model seeks to generate **second-order change** in that there is an emphasis on fundamentally changing ineffective patterns of interaction among members of the system. While the individual is seen as an independent **subsystem**, structural family therapists are most interested in how individuals interact within and across subsystems (Minuchin, 1974). With a focus on **boundaries**, structural family therapists seek to understand what the implicit and explicit rules are as it pertains to who is considered a member of the system and the parameters by which members are expected to operate (Minuchin, 1974; Minuchin & Fishman, 1981). This helps to better understand how clearly defined the subsystems are within the family.

Example: three-generational households

In a three-generation household consisting of grandparents, parents and young children, a structural family therapist might seek to get a sense of the family's expectations around childcare-related matters. They are interested in learning more about explicit and implicit ways in which the family communicates about who is responsible for caring for the young children. Is the parental subsystem assuming their role as parents in that they take on the primary caretaking responsibilities such as decisions around the children's diet, bedtime, educational activities, etc.? If grandparents are actively engaged in child rearing efforts, do they heed to the parenting desires of the parental subsystem or do they make they own decisions around parenting regardless of the desires of the parental subsystem? Understanding how such boundaries are defined provides a great deal of information about what is permissible within and across subsystems.

Structural family therapists also seek to make **closed systems**, which are resistant to outsiders entering in, more open. It is in an **open system** that members of the system are able to seamlessly move in and out of the system without a threat to the stability of the system (Minuchin, 1974; Minuchin & Fishman, 1981). For example, in an open system, members in a couple subsystem are able to maintain friendships outside of the system and such friendships are not a threat to the intimacy that is uniquely shared within the couple subsystem. Similarly, in a family system in which a new child is born into, the new parents are able to make key parenting decisions yet are open to and non-threatened by the suggestions and recommendations of more experienced parents, such as grandparents or parents with older children.

Structural family therapists also strive to assess for and strike a balance when it comes to **relational complementarity**. Members of a system often assume distinct roles that help to balance the system (e.g., dominant/submissive; active/passive). Minuchin and Fishman (1981) identified the benefit of complementarity and emphasized the need for members of the system to find balance in their roles. Without such balance, members of the system become rigid to the point where the complementary nature of the roles becomes ineffective in navigating life stressors.

Example: relational complementarity – pursuer /distancer

Some couples experience what is commonly known as a pursuer/distancer dynamic. Typically, one member of the couple is the pursuer and the other is a distancer. This dynamic manifests itself in a variety of ways and interactions. In a healthy context, the pursuer helps the couple maintain necessary intimacy and closeness knowing that there will be times when the distancer sets necessary limits around such exchanges. When taken to an extreme, a pursuer might engage in aggressive pursuing behavior that is ultimately met by extreme distancing behavior by the distancer. Being stuck in the cycle of pursuing only to be met with distancing can create conflict in the couple system in that there is a lack of balance in both the efforts of the pursuer to be close and the acceptance of the limits set by the distancer.

The Structural Family Therapy model also focuses on family rules and how they are enforced (Minuchin & Fishman, 1981). Therapists evaluate **negative and positive feedback loops,** which are meant to either maintain or disrupt the homeostasis of the system. An example of this would be an adolescent seeking to have a discussion with their parents regarding extending their curfew. The willingness to engage in a discussion about the possibility of a curfew extension and the increased responsibility that comes with it, is indicative of a positive feedback loop. That is, the parents are cognizant that this is a change to their system; yet, they are open to the instability that might be a result of this change. If the adolescent is able to abide by the new curfew, the positive feedback will likely create a new homeostasis for the family system. If the adolescent is unable to abide by the new curfew, the result will most likely be a negative feedback loop in which the parents may decide to revoke the revised curfew and instead decide to stick with the original agreed upon curfew. By examining the ongoing positive and negative feedback, structural family therapists can get a sense of the stability of the system.

Philosophical underpinnings

Structural Family Therapy is open to a wide range of family configurations (Minuchin, 1984). Family configurations that are distinct from the traditional two-parent family structure should not be considered as non-normative, but rather should be viewed as a family structure that is experiencing a set of experiences unique and apart from what is known as the traditional two-parent structure. Despite these differences, the structural approach seeks to help all families through transitional periods.

The function of the **couple subsystem** is to operate separate from their **family-of-origin** (Minuchin, 1974; Minuchin & Fishman, 1981). Members of the couple subsystem are meant to support, accommodate and nurture the needs of one another. This should be the goal of the couple subsystem, whether they are married, cohabitating or dating. As couples acquire a sense of who they are within their partnerships, they are tasked with finding balance between staying connected to their family-of-origin and remaining open to new ideas and changing contexts that are sure to come as a result of merging one's life with someone outside of the family-of-origin.

The birth of children presents new challenges to the couple subsystem in that the parental subsystem emergences (Minuchin & Fishman, 1981). This is a new shift for the system, which requires adjustment. Often one of the greatest challenges for the **parental subsystem** is maintaining the spousal subsystem simultaneously. This can become quite the challenge due to the demands of caring for children, which is now placed on the parental subsystem. These demands seemingly consume the time and energy of the couple. The couple is tasked with finding balance between the demands of parenting and the continued nurturing needed in order to maintain the autonomy and closeness, which has ideally been established prior to the birth of children.

Ideally, the parental subsystem provides a safe environment where children learn the rules of the system and can practice how to be increasingly independent over time (Minuchin, 1974; Minuchin & Fishman, 1981). As children age, the family structure must adjust to each new developmental milestone. By encouraging an open family system, the parental subsystem passes along and models a respect for rules that promote clear boundaries and reciprocal relationships within the family system.

Structural family therapy also acknowledges **the role of siblings**. The sibling subsystem is a byproduct of the biological birth or non-biological addition of children to the family system. Once again, a secure and balanced couple subsystem helps to lay the foundation for a secure sibling subsystem. It is through the sibling subsystem that children first experience what it means to navigate interpersonal challenges in the context of a peer relationship (Minuchin, 1974; Minuchin & Fishman, 1981). Whether it be negotiating sharing of toys or communicating the need for individual space, the sibling subsystem allows children the context by which they are able to develop the necessary skills to effectively get their needs met among peers, yet garner support while navigating and negotiating the terrain that is the hierarchal structure of the family. When families are able to support its members, children grow into secure adults that are able to successfully get their needs met by navigating interpersonal peer conflict and negotiating hierarchical relationships, all while maintaining appropriate boundaries within and between subsystems.

The **acknowledgment of family development** is important to the work of a structural family therapist. Families are in a constant stage of change. Whether it be moving from single adults, to a cohabitating/married couple, to the birth of children, providing care for aging parents, divorce, remarriage or death, families may need support as they transition through such experiences. These often normative, life experiences require **restructuring of hierarchy and boundaries** in order to ensure that the needs of members are adequately addressed through the transitions (Minuchin & Fishman, 1981).

Boundaries are also seminal to the work of structural family therapists. Structural family therapists have identified three types of boundaries: clear, enmeshed and disengaged (Connell, 2010; Minuchin, 1974; Minuchin & Fishman, 1981). While boundaries are invisible, they are an important indicator for how subsystems interact with one another. It is ideal for subsystems to have clear boundaries within and between them. It is through clear boundaries that individuals are able to be their own person and contribute in relationships in an appropriate give and take manner. Families with enmeshed or diffused boundaries are overly engaged in the lives of members. In these families, members do not have sufficient space to grow and develop into their own selves and there is an over-reliance on the support and nurturance of families.

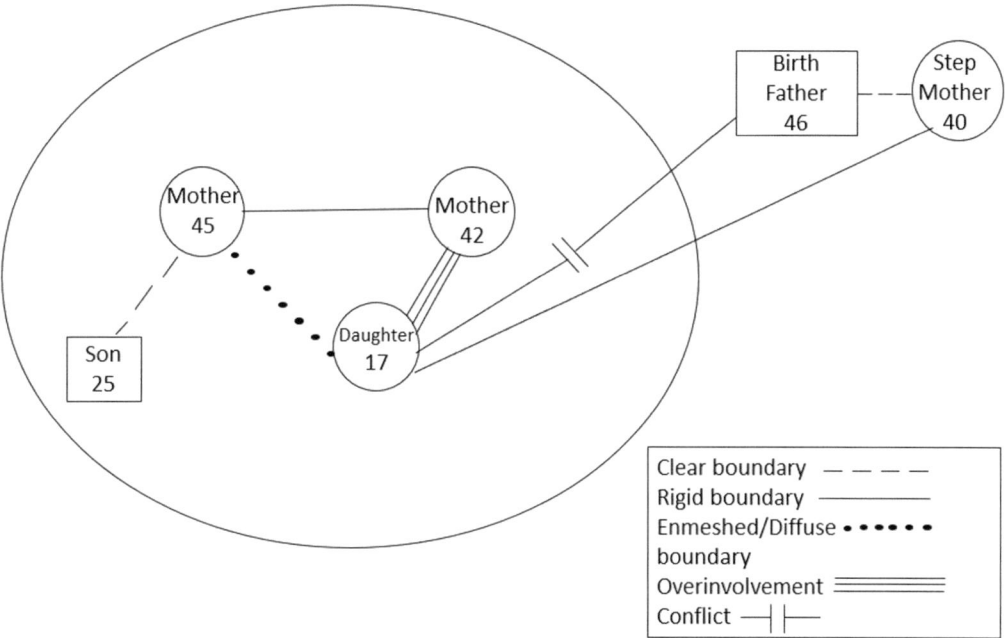

Figure 9.1 Structural Mapping.

Families that have rigid or disengaged boundaries tend to be disconnected from one another. They function autonomously and separately from one another with limited opportunities for connectedness. This leads to a lack of involvement in the lives of other family members and results in a slow response of the needs of family members.

Conceptualization of issues

Structural Family Therapy focuses on the extent to which subsystems operate in a clear fashion and respect the established hierarchy and boundaries across and within subsystems. The approach believes that when boundaries within and across subsystems are enmeshed or disengaged, the functioning of the system is unbalanced and thus not supporting members at an optimal level. In addition, when the hierarchy of the system is such that adults, parents or responsible caregivers are not the leaders of the family system, the system lacks the necessary leadership to guide younger members of the system (children) in a healthy developmentally appropriate manner. Problems are thought to be the result of a lack of balance in the system and an underutilization of inherent strengths that naturally occur within the family system (Minuchin, 1974; Minuchin & Fishman, 1981).

How change occurs

According to Minuchin (1974), **change occurs in three phases.** First, the therapist must join the family system. This is an important first step as it provides the space for therapist to enter the system and get a sense of how the family functions. While in many ways, the therapist takes on a position of leadership, joining the family requires that the therapist respect the current structure of the family, how it is organized and its rules for functioning. This might also be seen as accommodating to the system (Minuchin & Fishman, 1981). Entering the system in such a manner is required in order for the therapist to garner acceptance by the family.

The second phase of change consists of the therapist assessing the underlying structure of the family system. While assessment is an ongoing part of the therapeutic process, identifying the family's current structure and rules for operating is an important step in identifying areas of functioning that are ineffective at meeting the needs of members. Mapping the structure of the family is a technique that Minuchin used to help visualize the family structure and helps the therapist to develop hypotheses about the family's functioning (Minuchin, 1974; Minuchin & Fishman, 1981). This technique is very similar to Bowen's use of the genogram (Bowen, 1976). Through observation and interactions with the family,

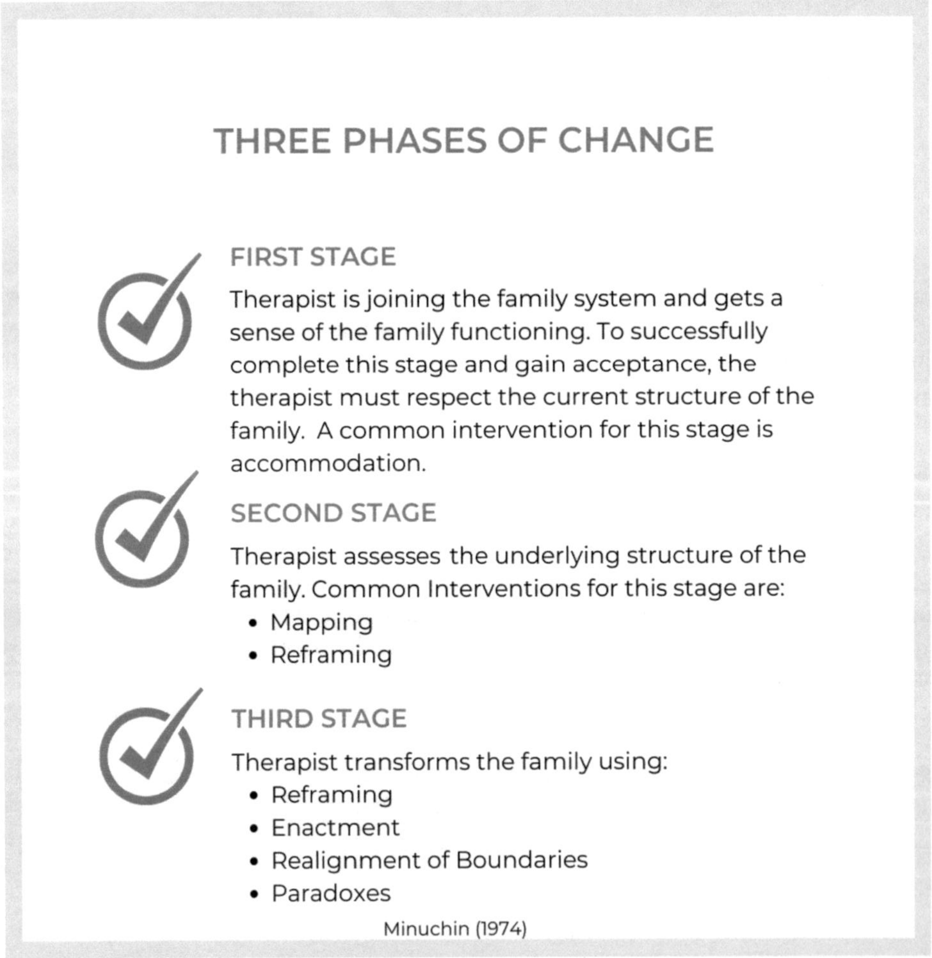

THREE PHASES OF CHANGE

FIRST STAGE

Therapist is joining the family system and gets a sense of the family functioning. To successfully complete this stage and gain acceptance, the therapist must respect the current structure of the family. A common intervention for this stage is accommodation.

SECOND STAGE

Therapist assesses the underlying structure of the family. Common Interventions for this stage are:
- Mapping
- Reframing

THIRD STAGE

Therapist transforms the family using:
- Reframing
- Enactment
- Realignment of Boundaries
- Paradoxes

Minuchin (1974)

Figure 9.2 Infographic: Phases of Change Minuchin.

the therapist maps out such aspects as boundaries and subsystems, as well as the quality of the familial relationships.

As members of the family describe problems, problems are reframed so that they are understood based on the family structure (Minuchin, 1974). For example, if the parents identify a problem with excessive sibling arguing, the therapist might reframe this problem as the children's conflict resolution skills are underdeveloped and the parents need support in modeling and establishing ground rules for supporting the children as they navigate peer conflict in a healthier manner. The hierarchy of the family might be assessed by identifying who answers questions first, who responds to questions that are meant for specific members of a subsystem or who is particularly quiet during the session. The idea is to get a sense of everyone's role in the family. Also, during the assessment phase, enactments are also used to help the therapist get a sense of how members of the system communicate as well as determining the extent that the expectations of the family are consistent with the development of members of the system.

Once the therapist gets a sense of the rules and roles in the family, the third and final stage of change consists of the therapist transforming the family system with the goal of realigning the system so that it is able to support the existing and future needs of its members. This is executed using such interventions as reframing, enactments, realigning boundaries, increasing intensity and use of paradoxes (Minuchin & Fishman, 1981).

Role of the client

As the therapist works to join with the family, one of the responsibilities of members of the family system is to be open and accommodating to the style of the therapist (Minuchin & Fishman, 1981). The partnership that is formed through joining requires mutual engagement between the therapist and family. Throughout the therapeutic process, the family must also remain receptive to expanding their perspective about how it is they make sense of their family interactions. Moreover, clients must accept the influence of the therapist as the therapist works to restructure the hierarchy of the family and realign boundaries.

Role of the therapist

A structural family therapist is meant to be an active participant in the therapeutic process. Active participation includes joining with the client, staging enactments, realigning the system and active listening in order to identify strengths of the family and challenge the family's assumptions about the meaning of their current interactions. The therapist is tasked with being a part of the family but also being an agent of change within the family. It is in this way that they are directive in facilitating change. Although structural therapists have expert knowledge on what they believe is a healthy structure for a family system (e.g., clear boundaries, sufficient parental hierarchy), they are still collaborative with the family as they allow the family members to define what aspects of their structure are working or not working for the family.

Interventions

Joining. The intervention of joining is seminal to the work of structural family therapists. Through joining, structural family therapists are able to become a part of the family system and ultimately help to realign the system. There are several key aspects of joining, which includes accommodating to the system and their ways for interacting, matching the language of the client and displaying empathy (Minuchin, 1974). An example of joining with a family who has school-aged children might include engaging in conversation about the children's school interest, discussing parenting-centered activities or relating to the challenges that come with parenting young children. The idea is for the therapist to be a member of the family system and not act as an outsider.

Reframing. Clients may enter treatment with a very clear way by which they communicate about and understand their problems. Reframing is a technique that helps to expand the manner in which clients understand their problems (Minuchin & Fishman, 1981). Specific to Structural Family Therapy, problems are reframed to be understood within the context of the larger family system. For example, an African American father and mother enter therapy with their 16-year-old son, citing complaints that his parents are too strict when it comes to curfew and hanging out with his friends. After conversations, in which the parents share their concern for the son's safety due to fear of being stopped by the police, a structural family therapist might reframe the parent's actions as a loving attempt to protect the son rather an attempt to be overly restrictive. This ultimately helps to expand the perspectives that behaviors are understood.

Enactments. Minuchin and Fishman (1981) outline the utility of enactments, both as a tool for assessment and as an intervention strategy. As a tool for assessment, the therapist might look for what is known as "spontaneous transactions", which naturally occur as the family discusses why they are seeking treatment. During the enactment, the therapist is able to observe instances where the boundaries are not clear and are ineffective at addressing the needs of the family. As a tool for intervention, the therapist might instruct a family to model how it is they discuss a challenging topic. This is also known as "eliciting transactions". The therapist is then able to interrupt the enactment and provide redirection as it relates to helping members of the system communicate in a clear manner respectful of the hierarchy and boundaries of the family system.

Throughout treatment, family members are able to practice new ways of interacting and receiving feedback from both the therapist and other members of the system. Enactments provide families with the opportunity to have successful interactions, which ultimately can lead to the development of hope that things can be different for the family and how they operate.

Realigning boundaries. In instances where the boundaries of a family are enmeshed or disengaged, there is a need to realign the boundaries so that they are clear (Minuchin, 1974; Minuchin & Fishman, 1981). Recall, clear boundaries ensure members of the system are able to operate independently of one another, yet share a connection that allows for reciprocity within the relationship. Among other techniques, realignment can occur verbally as well as physically. A therapist may decide to take the side of a lesser powered family member and give voice and validation to the experiences of the family member. This provides an opportunity to empower the member and shift how other members of the family view and interact with the member of the system. A therapist may also decide to shift the family's focus from the identified patient to another family member. This helps to break the family's pattern of shifting blame on one specific member of the system. Physically realigning boundaries consist of the therapist making adjustments to where clients sit in the room and even ignoring family members. This discourages coalitions, strengthens subsystems and delineates clear boundaries within the family system.

Increasing intensity and use of paradoxes. Through the use of paradoxes, therapists have the potential to increase the emotional intensity of clients (Minuchin & Fishman, 1981).

The clinician must be mindful of the appropriateness of increasing the emotional intensity in the room. Therapists can raise the emotional intensity by shifting their tone of voice, pace of speech, word choice (Minuchin & Fishman, 1981). When this occurs in conjunction with using paradoxes, a realignment of the family system may result. For example, if the mother of a wife is triangulated in the spousal subsystem to the point that the wife does not make decisions without consulting the mother, the therapist might highlight the need for separation and independence from the wife's mother. The therapist might ask the wife if she also consults her mother when it comes time for the couple to be intimate with one another. While the statement is paradoxically exaggerated to highlight the lack of hierarchy and clear boundaries, increasing the emotional intensity between the husband and wife can lead to unbalancing the system and shift the wife's enmeshment with her mother and help the couple to move closer to one another in regards to communicating more authentically about their relationship.

Identifying strengths. Since problems are thought to be the result of unacknowledged and underutilized inherent strengths of the family, structural family therapists focus on identifying the strengths of the family system. The assumption is made that, despite the challenges the family system has faced, somehow the family has managed to survive. Identifying the resources that have helped to sustain the family thus far helps to shift both the family's and the therapist's perspective from that of deficit- to strength-based while expanding the family's interpretation of how it is they function interpersonally (Minuchin & Fishman, 1981).

Termination of therapy

Structural family therapists maintain that families are able and capable of making changes in order to support all members of the family system. Treatment is terminated when the following goals are met:

- creation of effective hierarchal structures within the family system
- development of a spousal subsystem that is distinct from the parental subsystem
- establishment of the couple and parental subsystem at the top of the hierarchy
- clear boundaries are established between the role of the sibling subsystem and the role of the parental subsystem
- development of clear boundaries across members of the system, which includes a reduction in and/or elimination of disengaged or enmeshed boundaries

Therapy can be terminated when systems have been realigned so that the couple and/or parent subsystem has begun to consistently make decisions that are in the best interest of all members of the system. The support that adults provide one another, and children, are based on the development of members of the system and are communicated in a clear and consistent manner.

Key legal and ethical considerations

It is incumbent upon the therapist to ensure that they are practicing in a manner that is consistent with the current ethical standards outlined by one's professional code of ethics as well as state mandated reporting statutes. As structural family therapists assess the extent to which children are being adequately cared for by caretakers, it is important not to overlook possible evidence of child maltreatment. Evidence of this may also arise when observing excessive use of power and control from members at the top of the family hierarchy as well as observations of family boundaries that are excessively enmeshed or diffused boundaries. These attributes may be an indication of neglect and/or abuse. Clinicians should also remain mindful of possible maltreatment of elderly as well as individuals who are dependent on the care of others for daily functioning.

Another area that is important to be mindful of is the role that development plays in supporting members of the family system. A structural family therapist must not assume that chronological age establishes the hierarchy and rules of a family system. There may be situations where, as a result of a delay in development, it is necessary for a family system to operate in a "non-traditional" manner. For example, it might be appropriate for an older parent to assume more decision-making responsibilities for an adult son or daughter who has an identified developmental delay or handicap. Not assessing for these unique circumstances has potential negative consequences when it comes to attempting to rebalance the system based on traditional life stages.

Use with a diversity of clients

Structural family therapy can be used across a diverse population of clients as well as to address multiple presenting problems. This is the case, even though the approach most closely aligns with traditional models of therapy, which has leanings on very clear and distinct conceptualizations of how families should function. From a structural perspective, therapists work to understand the problems through the lens of the family. Taking an organized approach of first asking the leaders of the family (e.g., parents, caretakers, presenting adults), and then moving to understand the problem through the lens of children and other auxiliary members of the family, structural family therapists are open to learning from and understanding the problem from the family's perspective.

Particularly as it relates to the intervention of reframing and emphasizing a strengths-based perspective, structural family therapists believe that clients have the ability to identify solutions that work for them. The role of the therapist is to help the client identify these solutions in an organized fashion that consists of clear communication and flexible boundaries within and across subsystems. Structural family therapists are focused on identifying underutilized strengths in order to help the family interact and function beyond the current prescribed rules of the system. It is through this process that the structural approach can be used across a diverse range of populations. Studies have applied the structural approach to African American (Hall & Greene, 2003; Perry et al., 2013; Williams, Foye, & Lewis, 2016), Hispanic (Robbins et al., 2008; Santisteban & Mena, 2009;) and Asian families (Kim, 2003; Yang & Pearson, 2002), families in the foster care system (Lewis, 2011), families with an incarcerated parent (Tadros & Finney, 2018), same sex male couples (Greenan & Tunnell, 2003) and same sex parents (Coates & Sullivan, 2005).

Because structural family therapists employ a specific model of health for families, they need to be particularly sensitive to whether or not the model in its traditional form fits clients' cultural beliefs. As the expert in the therapy room, they should be sensitive to the power dynamic between therapist and client and consider how contexts of power and privilege influence families' problems and interactions (Fisher-Borne et al., 2014; Mosher, Hook, Davis, DeBlaere & Owe, 2017). It is key for structural therapists to reflect on their own beliefs about healthy family structure and how those personal beliefs may influence how they perceive and treat client families. Therapists should learn about what cultural values commonly organize family structure across diverse groups, but also need to be curious about each client family's unique belief system related to family roles, boundaries and expectations (Fisher-Borne et al., 2014; Mosher et al., 2017).

Research support

Structural Family Therapy has been used to address the needs of adolescents involved in gangs (McNeil, Herschberger & Nedela, 2013), intimacy and sexual desire in couples (Young, Negash & Long, 2009) and clients impacted by parental alienation syndrome (Gottlieb, 2013). The approach has been found to be effective with juvenile delinquents, families with a member with Anorexia Nervosa, families dealing with substance abuse and alcoholism, and low-income families (Aponte & Van Deusen, 1981; Minucuhin et al., 1978). Structural Family Therapy has also been found to be effective in addressing adolescent substance use (Sim, 2007), pornography addiction (Ford, Durtschi & Franklin, 2012) and to treat clients diagnosed with intermittent explosive disorder (Fisher, 2017). There have also been adaptions of the approach for treatment of bipolar disorder (Miklowitz, 2012) and application within public schools (Gerrard, 2008), colleges (Parcover, Mettrick, Parcover & Griffin-Smith, 2009) and in programs that facilitate partnerships between schools, families and the community (Messina, Kolbert, Hyatt-Burkhart & Crothers, 2015).

One critique of the research on Structural Family Therapy is that much of it is based on case studies. Weaver et al. (2013) conducted a pilot study on the effects of Structural Family Therapy on child and maternal symptomatology using more rigorous experimental methods. They found that mothers who participated in Structural Family Therapy experienced improvement in depression and anxiety symptoms and they reported improvements in their children's symptoms. However, children's ratings of their own symptoms showed no significant change after treatment.

Structural family therapy has also given birth to the empirically validated models of ecosystemic Structural Family Therapy (Lindblad-Goldberg, Dore & Stern, 1998), multisystemic therapy (Henggeler, Schoenwald, Borduin, Rowland & Cunningham, 1998), multidimensional family therapy (Liddle, 2002), brief strategic therapy (e.g., Szapocznik & Williams, 2000) and functional family therapy (Sexton, 2011). These models are at least in part built on Structural Family Therapy, as described with brief strategic therapy in the previous chapter.

There continues to be a need to research the effectiveness of Structural Family Therapy. Parker and Molteni (2017) have found that, while systemic treatments offer theoretical support for treatment of families impacted by autism, the research has yet to confirm the empirical support for their longitudinal effectiveness for treatment of autism spectrum disorder.

Self-of-the-therapist considerations/reflections specific to the approach

When applying the structural approach, it is important to consistently be mindful of the manner in which a therapist understands and positions themselves in the approach. More specifically, therapists need to consider to what extent they believe systems should operate in the outlined manner of the approach. Reflecting upon their own experiences, structural family therapists should take an inventory as to the extent to which their own family-of-origin did or did not operate as outlined by the Structural Family Therapy approach and what impact this may have had on the growth and development of the clinician. It is through this assessment that clinicians can evaluate the benefits of the approach and the extent to which the approach may or may not adequately support clients.

References

Aponte, H. & Van Deusen, J. (1981). Structural family therapy. In A. S. Gurman & D. P. Kniskern (Eds.), *Handbook of family therapy* (pp. 310–360). New York, NY: Brunner/Mazel.

Bowen, M. (1976). Theory in the practice of psychotherapy. In P. J. Guerin (Ed.), *Family therapy: theory and practice* (pp. 42–90). New York, NY: Gardner Press.

Coates, J. & Sullivan, R. (2005). Achieving competent family practice with same-sex parents: some promising directions. *Journal of GLBT Family Studies, 1*(2), 89–113. doi:10.1300/J461v01n02_06

Colapinto, J. (1991). Structural family therapy. In A. S. Gurman & D. P. Kniskern (Eds.), *Handbook of family therapy* (Vol. 2, pp. 417–443). New York, NY: Brunner/Mazel.

Connell, C. (2010). Multicultural perspectives and considerations within structural family therapy: the premises of structure, subsystems and boundaries. *Rivier Academic Journal, 6*(2), 1–6.

Fisher, U. (2017). Use of structural family therapy with an individual client diagnosed with intermittent explosive disorder: a case study. *Journal of Family Psychotherapy, 28*(2), 150–169.

Fisher-Borne, M., Montana Cain, J. & Martin, S. L. (2014). From mastery to accountability: cultural humility as an alternative to cultural competence. *Social Work Education, 34*(2), 165–181.

Ford, J. J., Durtschi, J. A. & Franklin, D. L. (2012). Structural family therapy with a couple battling pornography addiction. *The American Journal of Family Therapy, 40*, 336–348. doi:10.1080/01926187.2012.685003

Gerrard, B. (2008). School-based family counseling: overview, trends, and recommendations for future research. *International Journal for School-Based Family Counseling, 1*(1), 1–30. doi:10.1177/01430343

Gottlieb, L. (2013). *Strengths-based nursing care: health and healing for person and family.* New York, NY: Springer Publishing.

Greenan, D. E. & Tunnell, G. (2003). *Couple therapy with gay men.* New York, NY: Guilford.

Hall, R. L. & Greene, B. (2003). Contemporary African American families. In L. Silverstein & T. Goodrich (Eds.), *Feminist family therapy: empowerment in social context* (pp. 107–120). Washington, DC: American Psychological Association.

Henggeler, S. W., Schoenwald, S. K., Borduin, C. M., Rowland, M. D. & Cunningham, P. B. (1998). *Multisystemic treatment of antisocial behavior in children and adolescents.* New York, NY: Guilford.

Kim, J. M. (2003). Structural family therapy and its implications for the Asian American family. *The Family Journal, 11*(4), 388–392. doi:10.1177/1066480703255387

Lewis, C. (2011). Providing therapy to children and families in foster care: a systemic-relational approach. *Family Process, 50*(4), 436–452. doi:10.1111/j.1545-5300.2011.01370.x

Liddle, H. A. (2002). *Multidimensional family therapy for adolescent cannabis users* (Cannabis Youth Treatment Series, Vol. 5; DHHS Publication No. 02-3660). Rockville, MD: Center for Substance Abuse Treatment, SAMHSA.

Lindblad-Goldberg, M., Dore, M. & Stern, L. (1998). *Creating competence from chaos.* New York, NY: Norton.

McNeil, S., Herschberger, J. & Nedela, M. (2013). Low-income families with potential adolescent gang involvement: a structural community family therapy integration model. *The American Journal of Family Therapy, 41*, 110–120. doi:10.1080/ 01926187.2011.649110

Messina, K. C., Kolbert, J. B., Hyatt-Burkhart, D. & Crothers, L. M. (2015). The role of mental health counselors in promoting school family collaboration within the tiered school-wide positive behavioral intervention and support (SWPBIS) model. *The Family Journal, 23*(1), 277–285. doi:10.1177/1066480715574471

Miklowitz, D. J. (2012). Family treatment for bi-polar disorder and substance abuse in late adolescence. *Journal of Clinical Psychology, 68*(5), 502–513. doi:10.1002/jclp.21855

Minuchin, S. (1974). *Families and family therapy*. Cambridge, MA: Harvard University Press.

Minuchin, S. (1984). *Family kaleidoscope*. Cambridge, MA: Harvard University Press.

Minuchin, S. & Fishman, H. C. (1981). *Family therapy techniques*. Cambridge, MA: Harvard University Press.

Minuchin, S. & Nichols, M. P. (1993). *Family healing: tales of hope and renewal from family therapy*. New York, NY: Free Press.

Minuchin, S., Montalvo, B., Buerney, B. G., Rosman, B. & Schumer, F. (1967). *Families of the slums*. New York, NY: Basic Books.

Minuchin, S., Rosman, B. & Baker, L. (1978). *Psychosomatic families: anorexia in context*. Cambridge, MA: Harvard University Press.

Mosher, D. K., Hook, J. N., Davis, D. E., DeBlaere, C. & Owen, J. (2017). Cultural humility: a therapeutic framework of engaging diverse clients. *Practice Innovations*, 2(4), 221–233.

Parcover, J. A., Mettrick, J., Parcover, C. A. D. & Griffin-Smith, P. (2009). University and college counselors as athletic team consultants: using a structural family therapy model. *Journal of College Counseling, 12*, 149–161. doi:10.1002/j.2161-1882.2009.tb00112.x

Parker, M. L. & Molteni, J. (2017). Structural family therapy and autism spectrum disorder: bridging the disciplinary divide. *The American Journal of Family Therapy, 45*(3), 135–148. doi: 10.1080/01926187.2017.130365

Perry, A. R., Robinson, M. A., Moore, S. E. Alexander, R., Lemelle, A. J. Reed, W. & Taylor, S. (2013). Post-prison community reentry and African American males; implications for family therapy and health. In. K. M. Lindahl, H. R. Bregman & N. M. Malik (Eds.), *Handbook of African American health*. New York, NY: Springer.

Robbins, M. S., Szapocznik, J., Dillon, F. R., Turner, C. W., Mitriani, V. B. & Feaster, D. J. (2008). The efficacy of structural ecosystems theory with drug-abusing/dependent African American and Hispanic American adolescents. *Journal of Family Psychology, 22*(1), 51–61. doi:10.1037/0893-3200.22.1.51

Santisteban, D. A. & Mena, M. P. (2009). Culturally informed and flexible family-based treatment for adolescents: a tailored and integrative treatment for Hispanic youth. *Family Process, 48*(2), 253–268. doi:10.1111/j.1545-5300.2009.01280.x

Sexton, T. L. (2011). *Functional family therapy in clinical practice: an evidence-based treatment model for working with troubled adolescents*. New York, NY: Routledge.

Sim, T. (2007). Structural family therapy in adolescent drug abuse: a Hong Kong Chinese family. *Clinical Case Studies, 6*(1). 79–99. doi: 10.1177/1534650105275989

Szapocznik, J. & Williams, R. A. (2000). Brief strategic family therapy: twenty-five years of interplay among theory, research and practice in adolescent behavior problems and drug abuse. *Clinical Child and Family Psychology Review, 3*(2), 117–134.

Tadros, E. & Finney, N. (2018). Structural family with incarcerated families: a clinical case study. *The Family Journal*, 26(2), 253–261.

Weaver, S. J., Lubomski, L. H., Wilson, R. F., Pfoh, E. R., Martinez, K. A. & Dy, S. M. (2013). Promoting a culture of safety as a patient safety strategy: a systemic review. *Annals of Internal Medicine, 5*(158), 369–374.

Williams, N. D., Foye, A. & Lewis, F. (2016). Applying structural family therapy in the changing context of the modern African American single mother. *Journal of Feminist Family Therapy* 28(1), 30–47.

Yang, L. & Pearson, V. J. (2002). Understanding families in their own context: schizophrenia and structural family therapy in Beijing. *Journal of Family Therapy, 24*(3), 233–257. doi:10.1111/1467-6427.00214

Young, T. L., Negash, S. M. & Long, R. M. (2009). Enhancing sexual desire and intimacy using the metaphor of the problem child: utilizing structural-strategic family therapy. *Journal of Sex and Marital Therapy, 35*, 402–417. doi:10.1080/00926230903065971

10 Strategic Family Therapy

Emily Schmittel

Introduction

Strategic Family Therapy is one of the first marriage and family therapy (MFT) models to be directly informed by systemic concepts (Watzlawick, Beavin, & Jackson, 1967). Focused on treating family dynamics, strategic therapists are committed to brief interventions that are targeted specifically on the client-identified presenting problem (Madanes, 1991). Due to its use of non-linear, paradoxical directives, many have questioned if strategic therapy is an ethical approach. Although these ethical concerns have been largely attributed to misunderstandings about the model, this led to a reduction in research focused on studying the original formulations of strategic therapy. However, adaptations of the model (e.g., Brief Strategic Therapy), have been rigorously studied and found to be efficacious. Based on the important historical contributions of this model to the systemic practice of MFT and the ongoing emphasis in the field for evidence-based models, it is essential that MFT trainees have a solid foundation in strategic therapy.

History of strategic family therapies

Mental Research Institute

Strategic therapy was directly informed by the work of anthropologist Gregory Bateson and his research team, who studied dynamics of families with a member who has Schizophrenia (Watzlawick, Weakland & Fisch, 1974). They were particularly focused on applying concepts of cybernetics to family systems and better understanding double-bind communication patterns. Several members of Bateson's research team, specifically Richard Fisch and Don Jackson, went on to form the Mental Research Institute (MRI) in Palo Alto, CA. Eventually joined by John Weakland and Paul Watzlawick, the MRI group studied both problem formation and resolution from a systemic perspective, and developed early concepts that led to multiple iterations of strategic therapy. In addition to Bateson, the MRI group was influenced by the strategies of Milton Erikson (Madanes, 1991). This led to their focus on finding the briefest solutions to problems through unusual, paradoxical interventions to create second-order change (Watzlawick et al., 1974).

In the late 1960s, Jay Haley left the MRI group to create his own strategic model that expanded on the MRI group's concepts and integrated structural considerations when assessing and treating the problem. Haley co-developed his approach with his wife, Cloé Madanes. Haley's addition of structural concepts grew out of his close work with structural family

DOI: 10.4324/9781003382621-13

therapy founder Salvador Minuchin (Haley, 1987; Madanes, 1991). The organization of the therapy process and focus on hierarchy in conceptualizing and treating problems are the hallmark differences between the original MRI group's approach and that of Haley and Madanes.

Systemic foundations

At the heart of strategic assessment and intervention practices is systems theory (Watzlawick et al., 1974). Based on this theory, strategic therapists assess **circular patterns of interaction** that maintain the problem and what types of solutions have been attempted that also allow the problem to continue. Through a systemic lens, strategic therapists determine what type of directive to apply to the system to elicit the needed type of change. Some of the core systemic concepts that inform this model include homeostasis, circular causality, complementarity and first- vs. second-order change.

Homeostasis

Homeostasis refers to a system's tendency to stay the same and resist change.

Strategic therapists assume that, when a family has identified one person in the family as a problem, this serves a function of maintaining homeostasis. If a family is stable through labeling one person as the problem, the system will resist any efforts by the therapist to change (Haley, 1987). However, if the system is in crisis, or destabilized, they may be more likely to change, inducing interventions from the therapist as they are seeking to return to a homeostatic, or stabilized, state. Strategic therapists truly believe that families want their problems to reduce and are unaware of how they contribute to the maintenance of the problem; clients are not viewed as consciously or intentionally using a family member to maintain homeostasis.

Circular causality

Using the concept of homeostasis, strategic therapists view problems as a sequence of interactions that occur between family members, as opposed to a problem that exists within one person's behavior or cognition isolated from context (Haley, 1987). Strategic founders emphasized that it is unproductive to get stuck in seeking an answer to whose behavior came first in a circular interaction because this information is not helpful to problem resolution and an answer may not clearly exist (Watzlawick et al., 1974). Even if there is a formal, individual diagnosis, strategic therapists look at how circular patterns seek to reduce or exacerbate the symptoms related to the diagnosis.

Complementarity

Complementarity refers to homeostatic, circular patterns in which family members mutually engage. This is a common phenomenon in families, and is not always dysfunctional. In this type of dynamic, in order for a family member to hold a role, another family member has to hold the opposite of that role (Watzlawick et al., 1967). Some examples of complementary patterns that are problematic include:

- weak-strong
- good-bad

- pursuer-distancer
- logical-emotional
- overfunctioner-underfunctioner

Often one of these roles is viewed as preferred, while the other is viewed negatively with desire for the other person to change. From a systemic perspective, in order for one person to abandon their role, the other partner must abandon their role as well (Watzlawick et al., 1967). For example, for one partner to stop pursuing, the other partner must stop distancing. This dynamic can shift when second-order changes are applied.

First- and second-order change

Strategic therapies are concerned with what types of changes are attempted within systems that can help maintain or resolve the system's current functioning (Watzlawick et al., 1974). First order changes are typically logical, linear changes that allow a system to continue to function without any changes to its structure (e.g., rules, roles, patterns). When families experience a problem, they often can identify that a change is needed; however, typically their efforts to change a problem are first-order changes. While, at times, first-order change in therapy is sufficient, typically first-order changes allow the problem to continue or make the problem worse because the current roles, rules and overall pattern of interaction is allowed to continue.

Second-order changes are those that alter the structure of the system (Watzlawick et al., 1974). Predominantly, strategic therapists seek to create second-order changes to achieve a true resolution of clients' presenting problems. Keep this point in mind as you consider strategic interventions, which often seem unusual to the beginning therapist because second-order changes can require radical and illogical interventions to truly disrupt a current pattern of functioning. While it's a natural tendency to assume that logical, linear interventions make sense, systemic principles demonstrate that logical approaches allow the core problem to continue to exist because the system can continue functioning in the same manner.

To illustrate this example, I like to think about when I was in a long-distance relationship with my partner while we were both in graduate school in different states. When I would miss him, I would call and text him more. During that time, he was quite busy and not available to have a lot of contact throughout the day due to the demands of his education. I became miserable as I was pursuing more closeness and feeling rejected each time I reached out with no response. I kept applying, what at the time, felt like a logical solution. If I want more contact, I need to reach out more, so I continued doing so. At the height of my distress, I decided I was going to stop reaching out. I was certain this was the end of the relationship and I was done trying to work on it. To my surprise, our relationship and my general happiness almost immediately improved. I was no longer stressing over him not responding to me and he picked up more of the responsibility of calling me. As a new MFT graduate student, a light bulb went off. In this moment, I applied a second-order of change in my relationship, which disrupted our homeostasis, that wasn't working. My logic told me that making this change was me accepting the relationship was over, which in fact was not what happened at all as we remain together 14 years later as I write this story.

MRI brief family therapy: conceptualization and assessment of problems

Based on their systemic orientation, strategic therapists will assess the interactional sequence that occurs related to homeostasis and the problem (Watzlawick et al., 1974). This involves tracking the cycle in which the family moves from homeostasis, escalates to conflict, expresses a symptom and then self-corrects back to homeostasis. Strategic therapists are focused on disrupting this cycle as it occurs in the present, rather than assessing detailed history about the problem, which is considered to take a lot of time without contributing much to problem resolution.

Assessing communication

There are several core principles the MRI group considered in assessing communication in families. Most importantly, they emphasized that all behaviors are communication; **we cannot not communicate** (Watzlawick et al., 1967). Imagine if one of your family members gave you the silent treatment. Even if they aren't saying anything, they are still communicating a message that they are hurt or angry.

Communication also involves multiple levels of messages that occur simultaneously. For example, we might communicate one message with our words, and another message at the same time with our body language. This same family member might say "I'm fine" when you ask them what's wrong, but their frown and crossed arms communicate that they are not fine. Problems in relationships often occur when there is a lack of congruence between multiple levels of communication.

One particular type of incongruent communication that strategic therapists assess for is a **double-bind** (Bateson, Jackson, Haley & Weakland, 1956). This type of communication sends two messages simultaneously that are in direct contradiction to one another. A common example of this is when someone tells their partner to "be spontaneous". They are sending a command to their partner to follow their instructions, however, if their partner follows their instructions, then they are not being spontaneous as they are just doing what they are told.

Problem formation

The MRI group assessed problems as resulting from the solutions that families apply to their problems. There are three types of solutions that MRI therapists looked for that are maintaining the problematic interactional sequence: 1) Needed action is not taken; 2) Action is taken to change the unchangeable; and 3) Action is taken at the wrong level (Watzlawick et al., 1974).

When action is needed but not taken. This first type of problem formation is when families deny that a problem exists, when one in fact does exist (Watzlawick et al., 1974). Families regularly engage in this type of denial to maintain their appearance in a social context. Watzlawick provides the following quote to illustrate this concept: "*They are playing a game.* They are playing at not playing a game. If I show them, I see they are, I shall break the rules and they will punish me. I must play the game of not seeing that I play the game" (Laing, 1970, p. 1, as cited in Watzlawick et al., 1974, p. 43).

Imagine a family with parents that highly value sports. They are athletic and both played sports throughout high school and college. As they raise their children, they enroll them in multiple sports and emphasize this is an important part of their development. They put a lot of pressure on their children to practice and demonstrate high performance in each sport they participate in. When a game doesn't go well, the parents are visibly angry and disappointed, and lecture the children on what they did wrong that should be corrected. Each time a new sport begins, the parents ask the children if they are excited to start, to which the children don't dare express any true feelings. Rather, they agree they are excited and don't bring up their anxiety about beginning the sport. In this system, the "game" they are playing at is based on the rigid family rules, that we love sports and the only option is for us to excel at them. There is no space to acknowledge dislike or dissatisfaction with these activities. Additionally, there is no space to acknowledge they are faking their enjoyment of sports or just playing as a way to follow the family rules.

When action is taken to change something that is unchangeable. Issues arise in families when a member believes that a solution exists for a problem and tries to apply the solution to something that cannot be solved (Watzlawick et al., 1974). This occurs when we expect that experiences should always be positive without challenges or suffering. This is especially the case through family life cycle transitions such as getting married, having children or retiring. Cultural messages tell us that these accomplishments should be wholly positive, so we may be disappointed when they come with discomfort, and then seek solutions for this suffering that is normal and may not be solvable. A good example of this is with the transition to parenthood. For first time parents, having a new baby is an exciting, emotional event often marked by high highs and low lows. On top of the lack of sleep and round the clock care that infants need, parents in this phase of life are also often still building their careers and working toward financial stability. Some new parents may find it surprising that the first weeks of having a baby are not as joyful as they expected. This can lead to negative views of self, such as, "I must not be a good parent because I don't love this experience" or feeling angry at their partner for not enjoying these early weeks. This can lead to increase in symptoms of sadness, negative self-talk and partner conflict. Whereas accepting that this is a difficult stage, during which it's normal to feel some sadness or lack of enjoyment, could allow the partners to validate one another's experience and bond through experiencing these challenges together.

Change is attempted at the wrong level. The next circumstance under which problems form is when a family member places another in a paradox through trying to illicit change at the wrong level (Watzlawick et al., 1974). This could be when someone applies a first-order solution to a problem that needs second-order change.

A classic example of this is when a parent tells a child to be more responsible and independent or a partner more spontaneous. If the child follows these directions, they are then being more dependent, and a partner following instructions to be spontaneous is thus being less spontaneous by doing what he is told.

Again, keep in mind that insight about problems such as this is not viewed as helpful (Watzlawick et al., 1974). Another example that Watzlawick points out is when a family member wants someone else to do something because "they want to, not because I told them to". Then, if the person does as they are told, they are still in trouble because their desire to perform an action (which cannot be forced) did not arise. Another example of change at the wrong level is when a couple is stuck in a pursue-withdraw pattern. Imagine a husband would like to connect more with his wife, who he notices has pulled away emotionally. As he pursues her for increased connection, she distances herself further. The more he experiences her distancing herself, the more he pursues her, pushing her further away. Here, his solution of pursuing not only does not fix the original problem, but in fact it makes it worse.

MRI brief family therapy: problem resolution strategies

In this approach, you will find that therapists are not concerned with understanding why an intervention works, but rather whether or not the intervention is successful at resolving the problem (Watzlawick et al., 1974). This model believes that understanding the cause of a problem doesn't help with creating the solution, and in fact efforts to achieve this understanding can distract time and energy away from applying the accurate solution. When families are stuck in a repetitive problem, two questions are asked: "How does this undesirable situation persist?" and "What is required to change it?" (1974, p. 4). Related to these questions, there are four steps of the change process utilized by the MRI group (1974, p. 108):

Problems and goals are very clearly defined in this approach. This has the purpose of keeping therapy highly targeted on the problem, thus making it a briefer therapy process than other models. Once the first three steps of treatment are complete, the therapist will use several different techniques for the fourth step to create change, including: reframing, behavioral prescriptions (more-of-the-same and less-of-the-same) and restraining (Watzlawick et al., 1974). Many of the interventions from the MRI group are paradoxical due to the belief that straightforward interventions are likely to only create first-order changes, which would allow problems (and current homeostasis) to continue.

Therapeutic double-binds

Most interventions in this approach are considered therapeutic double-binds, which is a category of interventions in which the therapist seeks to undo double-bind communication patterns that occur between family members. As double-bind communication creates a no-win circumstance for families, therapeutic double-binds are intended to create a no-lose outcome circumstance for families (Watzlawick et al., 1967; Goldenberg & Goldenberg, 2004). Typically, therapeutic double-binds send the message to the client not to change. If the person follows the therapist's instructions, then the client learns that they have some degree of control over the symptom, which helps them to see they have control to solve the problem. If the client resists the therapist's instructions, they've then established control over the problem and solved the problem (1967).

Reframing. One technique for eliciting second-order change is reframing. This is a technique that seeks to assign new meaning to the problem so that it is no longer viewed as a problem. This is a useful strategy for changing someone's perspective on an unchangeable problem, which can then change the rules by which the person follows in relation to the problem (Watzlawick et al.,1974). This works when the problem isn't the problem, but rather the perspective of the problem. Reframes need to fit the client's world view, which is why it is important for the therapist to adequately join with and get to know the client.

Prescribing more-of-the-same. A common therapeutic double-bind is prescribing the symptom. The therapist could encourage families to "practice" the symptom or to keep doing what they are doing because they aren't ready for change. They might also encourage families to do the symptom even more intensely than the symptom occurs. For example, if a family is coming in for parent-child conflict that occurs several times a week, the therapist might assign the family to have fights daily (Watzlawick et al., 1974).

Restraining. Clients often worry that therapy either isn't working or isn't working quickly enough. To combat this unhelpful anxiety, MRI therapists often instructed their clients to not change too quickly (Watzlawick et al., 1974). This helped to address any client fears of not changing fast enough. Additionally, this technique can have the effect of clients wanting to prove their therapist wrong, in which they change more quickly.

Consider a couple who have felt disconnected and begin to experience improvements. They are working hard to spend more time together and are having more emotionally connected conversations. An MRI therapist might tell them in the next session, you are changing really quickly, you might benefit from going slower. If they then experience regression or a slow-down in change, it is in line with what the therapist prescribed, but if they resist this instruction and change more quickly, it is also a success.

Prescribing less-of-the-same. At times, MRI therapists prescribe clients to do the opposite of what they are doing that is not working. After assessing what solution is applied that is failing to solve the problem, or worsening the problem, they will devise an instruction for the client to do the opposite or less of the same reaction (Watzlawick et al., 1974). Watzlawick provides the case example of a young couple whose parents are overinvolved by staying in the couple's home for long periods of time, insisting on paying for various expenses and completing chores around the home despite protests for them to stop from the couple. The more the couple protests, the more conflict arises and the parents continue their behavior. A less-of-the-same prescription given by Watzlawick and colleagues was for the couple to protest the parents' behavior less and to act more dependent by expecting parents to take care of these tasks. This led the parents to determine that the couple was becoming much too dependent on them and that it was time for them to no longer be using their support.

Haley and Madanes: conceptualization and assessment of presenting problems

Much like in the MRI approach, Haley and Madanes' strategic model conceptualizes the problem as a specific behavior that is believed to be one part of a larger sequence of interactions between family members that repeatedly occurs.

Madanes (1991) further emphasizes that therapists using this approach seek to identify a unique "strategy for each specific presenting problem" (p. 19) for each client as opposed to applying a similar model across cases. To ensure therapy is brief, the therapist does not veer off the issues that the client identifies as the problem (Haley, 1987; Madanes, 1991). Symptoms are viewed as voluntary behaviors that clients can change (Haley, 1963), often resulting from family members' attempts to control how to define their relationship. As a result, the therapist works to help the family members redefine their relationship in new ways so that the symptom is no longer needed (Goldenberg & Goldenberg, 2004).

Family structure and power

As previously noted, Haley and Madanes integrated concepts on family structure into their model, so an assessment of the problem would also consider family life cycle stages, hierarchies, cross-generational coalitions and boundary problems (Haley, 1987). This informs a model for health in which parents should have more power than children and that cross-generational coalitions are problematic. For example, parents should have a united front, as opposed to one parent uniting with a child against the other parent (Madanes, 1991). Madanes further emphasized that there should be equity in the marital subsystem.

Madanes identified several different dimensions for understanding the problem from a systemic perspective (Madanes, 1991). Any number of the following dimensions could be utilized in a case conceptualization:

- involuntary vs. voluntary
- helplessness vs. power
- metaphorical vs. literal
- hierarchy vs. power
- hostility vs. love

Clients view the problems they have that bring them to therapy as involuntary, which ultimately leads to helplessness and hopelessness. In order to empower clients, strategic therapists seek to shift clients to viewing their problems as voluntarily maintained (Madanes, 1991). Strategic therapists also assess how symptoms give clients power. For example, the overfunctioner in a couple system, while often the most frustrated, also maintains a high degree of power as the "good partner".

Imagine a couple in which one partner tends to take care of most of the childcare, cooking meals and other daily household chores. When they won't be available for these tasks, they plan so that they are easy for the underfunctioning partner such as through setting up extra help, cooking meals ahead or creating a schedule for the parent to follow. Consider how this also gives them a great deal of control over what happens in the household, as well as how and when tasks are completed. They also maintain a position of the "good" partner, who should be appreciated and revered, while the other partner holds the position of the "bad" partner who is lazy, incompetent and undeserving of appreciation.

Madanes also points out that symptoms can be viewed as a metaphor of another problem in the system. A child's anger toward his sibling might be symbolic of discontent in another subsystem.

Symptoms also can develop due to a need for more hierarchy in the family system, or out of need for there to be less power of one subsystem. For example, a child might rebel as a way of communicating they would like more autonomy in a rigid, authoritarian household. Finally, a family member's behavior could be motivated by love or hostility (Madanes, 1991). An example would be a parent yelling at their child due to love and desire for their child's success.

Haley and Madanes: problem resolution strategies

You'll recall from previous sections that strategic therapists are mostly focused on second-order change and do not use insight-oriented interventions. Not only do they believe insight-focused interventions are unhelpful and time-consuming, but they also believe that clients already have insight about their problems and, if that were enough to create change, they wouldn't be in therapy (Haley, 1987; Madanes, 1991).

Consequently, strategic therapists take responsibility for the change process by assuming an active role in which they clearly structure sessions and issue directives. Throughout this section, consider how Haley's approach is more structured than the MRI group.

Role of the therapist

In this model, therapists hold a position of power in the therapeutic context as the expert on the therapeutic process. Consequently, the therapist is expected to directly address and resolve whatever problem is identified by the client (Haley, 1987, p. 2). While there is a clear structure to therapy, directives are designed to fit each family's unique needs. Because attempts to control one another are viewed as part of the reason symptoms develop, this model emphasizes the importance of the therapist having a hierarchical position in which they maintain control over the treatment process (Haley, 1963).

Haley (1987, p. 4) acknowledged that with a social perspective on presenting problems, therapists at times may intervene at other levels beyond the family system, including the community or political context. When interacting with clients' systems, he recommends that therapists be sensitive to their ability to contribute to the persistence of problems through these interactions (1987, p. 3). He emphasized it was important for therapists to be mindful of how their language and collaboration with other providers could affect the client. For example, he criticized the use of individual-focused, diagnostic language, which he believed supported homeostasis of the problem.

Additionally, he was aware that therapists are at risk for creating coalitions or conflict with other professionals involved in the case, which could further maintain the problem (Haley, 1987).

Despite the hierarchical role strategic therapists take, at times the therapist will take a one-down stance of hopelessness. This directly relates to the concept of complementarity, which hypothesizes that, if one person assumes a position of hopelessness, the other assumes an opposite position of hopefulness (Watzlawick et al., 1967; Watzlawick et al., 1974). Strategic therapists also use this stance, to demonstrate they respect the system and its rules (Segal, 1991).

Stages of treatment

Haley (1987) laid out a specific structure for the initial assessment phase of therapy, which occurs in the first session. While members of the MRI group did not see it as necessary to have all family members present, Haley (1987) urged that all people involved in or affected by the problem be present at the first meeting. Typically, this includes the whole family system, but for other types of issues could also include people from other systems, such as the school system when a child is having school-related problems. While strategic therapists begin collecting information and planning therapy with the first phone call, there are five stages to the first interview with a client family:

1. social stage
2. problem stage
3. interaction stage
4. goal-setting stage
5. task-setting stage

Social stage. The social stage is when therapists begin the therapeutic relationship. Key tasks include interacting with each family member in a way that ensures that they feel their perspective is valued (Haley, 1987). The therapist should not move on to discussing the problem with anyone until they have addressed each person in a social manner to help them feel more comfortable in the room.

Although therapists redirect clients away from the problem during this stage, the therapist is already beginning their assessment. Some areas of observation include clients' level of interest in being at the session and mood (Haley, 1987). Strategic therapists work to match the mood of the client, whether it is happiness, anger or desperation. How family members interact with one another in this stage is also of interest. Therapists will observe for coalitions or conflicts within and between parental subsystems, sibling subsystems or parent-child subsystems. Any subtle information about dynamics is noted, such as where family members sit. Similarly, the therapist also considers how family members interact with the therapist. This gives information about the attitude toward therapy and expectations for the process. Although the therapist makes these early observations, clinical impressions should not be reviewed with the family and they should be held onto lightly as they will likely change throughout the treatment process.

Problem stage. After the therapist has socially interacted with each member and ensured that the family is as comfortable as possible, the therapist shifts the conversation to discussing the presenting problem (Haley, 1987). To open this dialogue, the strategic therapist shares what they already know about the case and why the entire family was invited to the session. Specifically, the therapist emphasizes that they want to get everyone's perspective on the problem. This is followed by a general open-ended question to the family to stimulate the discussion about the problem. Some examples of how to open this conversation include:

- "What is your problem?"
- "What is it you want from me?"
- "What changes do you want?"
- "Why are you here?" (1987, pp. 19–20)

Strategic therapists are considerate about who they ask about the problem first (Haley, 1987), as this can influence the therapeutic relationship and engagement in the therapy process. In the quote below, Haley gives an example on how therapists' bias can influence what they ask and to whom they direct questions.

A therapist who considers children to be victims of parents may tend to side with children in the way she inquires about their problem. Such a therapist may ask the problem child what the problem is, implying that she thinks the child is probably misunderstood (1987, p. 20).

To avoid biases, therapists are encouraged to consider the following points when identifying how to interact with the family in this initial interview (Haley, 1987):

- Who is concerned about the problem, and who is in therapy reluctantly?
- What is the hierarchy of the family?
- Who will be most responsible for bringing the family back in?
- Who is most and least involved in the problem?

Considering the above points, the therapist should start by asking questions to the person who is the least part of the problem, as opposed to the identified patient, and be highly respectful and considerate to those with more power. Therapists avoid starting with the identified patient to ensure that they are not further shaming or blaming this family member. It is critical that therapists set aside their own perspective on who should have power in the family system and assess whichever person seems to be in control of the family system, even if this is a child or adolescent (Haley, 1987).

Therapist role in the problem stage. How the therapist listens to the family discuss the problem is also vital at this stage. Some recommendations include (Haley, 1987):

- Accept family members' explanations without interpretation
- Do not provide any advice
- Gather facts and opinions only; do not elicit emotions
- Ensure the therapist demonstrates a disposition in which they are interested in being helpful as they stay focused on the presenting problem
- Ensure each family member has a chance to speak with minimal interruptions from other family members
- Match the family's speed for discussing problems
- Maintain control and structure of the session

Patterns to observe. While therapists are concerned with some content of the problem conversation, they are most interested in the process of the conversation, including the dynamics that the family displays as they discuss the problem. There are several types of patterns that strategic therapists look for to understand the systemic nature of the problem.

- Incongruence between a client's affect and what they are saying
- How often a client has previously discussed the problem
- Who is blamed for the problem?
- Each family members' reaction to other family members' descriptions of the problem
- How descriptions of the problem relate to the quality of relationships within related subsystems. For example, how a parent describes a child's behavioral problem might also provide information about the spousal subsystem (Haley, 1987)

Interaction stage. After observing the family discuss their opinions about the problem and engaging each family member in the discussion, the therapist shifts therapy to the interaction stage. If the interaction stage starts before the problem stage is done, it is essential that the therapist return to the problem stage, otherwise clients won't all feel heard and may be more likely to get stuck in conflict in the interaction stage (Haley, 1987). The goal of this stage is to talk to each other, as opposed to the therapist, about the presenting issue. Even after being given the instructions to talk to one another about the problem, clients will fall back into talking to the therapist. It's the therapist's role to be active in redirecting clients back to discussing the problem with one another.

Another goal is to involve all family members in the conversation, so if two family members are only in the conversation, but another family member is present, the therapist works to bring the third client into the conversation. This will elicit the family's typical dynamics around the problem that they aren't able to articulate to the therapist (Haley, 1987). The therapist will also, in this stage, ask the client to display their symptoms directly in the room.

At the end of this stage, the therapist needs to have a clear explanation from each family member about the desired changes they'd like to see occur through therapy (Haley, 1987). Problems and therapy goals need to be defined in a measurable way. This helps with client engagement and cooperation, as well as helps everyone determine if the goal has been met. Unlike many other family therapy approaches, in strategic therapy, the target of therapy stays on the person with the presenting problem, as opposed to encouraging the family to identify other issues with other family members.

Goal-setting stage. After the interaction stage is complete, the therapist and clients identify the specific problem they are targeting in therapy along with clear, measurable goals. This ensures that therapy has an explicit focus and that everyone can identify if and when change is occurring (Haley, 1987).

Task-setting stage. After goals have been identified, the therapist concludes the meeting with specific instructions for the assignment they will carry out after session (Haley, 1967). Directives, which will be discussed in the next section, are the main intervention strategy of this approach. It's recommended that directives are given with some type of explanation that makes the recommendation appear sensible, especially when the directive is paradoxical (Goldenberg & Goldenberg, 2004).

Directives

Haley (1987) points out that directives have several different functions. In addition to the core purpose of creating behavioral change, directives provide meaning to the therapist role. Clients need to see therapists as having an important role in the change process, both during and outside of sessions. Directives help to bring the therapy process (and the therapist) into the rest of the client's week between sessions.

Additionally, directives assist therapists in an ongoing assessment about clients and presenting problems throughout treatment. Even if clients don't do a directive, the therapist learns something (Haley, 1987). Therapists can issue directives to be followed in or after sessions (Madanes, 1991). How a directive is given is critical in this approach.

Directives should be carefully tailored to each client, clear and specific (Haley, 1987). Clients might not follow through with instructions that are ambiguous. It is also important that directives are not merely suggestions. Directions should be given imperatively. If clients are asked if they would like to follow through with instructions, clients will get the impression that it is an optional instruction and be less likely to follow through.

Strategic directives involve each family member in some way (Haley, 1987). This reinforces that therapy is focused on changing the family as a whole, as opposed to just focusing on one person. To ensure everyone understands their role, after giving the task, the therapist should follow up and have each family member review their responsibility to make sure they understand what is being asked of them.

How the therapist follows up on the task in the following session is also essential to therapeutic process. The therapist always checks in to determine if clients have fully or partially completed the directive (Haley, 1987). While the therapist always praises a family for following through with the task, there are a couple of different ways they can respond to a lack of follow through. Haley (1987) recommends the therapist either respond "nicely" or harshly to the failed task. The "nice" approach involves the therapist apologizing for not fully understanding what the clients needed by saying something like, "I must have misunderstood you or your situation to ask that of you – otherwise, you would have done it." (1987, p. 71). In the harsher approach, the therapist directly states that the family failed and did not take advantage of a chance to change.

Haley (1987) points out that, if the therapist tells the family it was ok, they did not complete the task, it diminishes the therapist role as essential to achieving client goals.

Directives are generally classified into two categories: straightforward and indirect (Haley, 1987). Therapists can use straightforward directives when they have enough power in the family system to have family members follow through with their instructions, and when clients have some degree of control over the problem. Indirect directives are used when the therapist does not have this level of power, and the client perceives themselves as having very little control over the problem.

Straightforward directives. There are two ways to give this type of directive (Haley, 1987). The therapist can ask a person to stop a behavior. Haley (1987) considers this approach to be the hardest to receive client follow-through, and only likely to be successful if the therapist is dramatic in their request. Rather than telling someone to stop their behavior, the therapist can direct them to do something else instead. Directives to do something different can be done in two ways. They can be provided either as good advice or focused on changing a series of behaviors in the family. Haley (1987) offers some practical recommendations for motivating a family to follow straightforward directives:

- Intensify the desperate nature of the situation or that each of the family's attempts to solve the problem has failed.
- Recommend small changes that are additive to any changes that have been successful.
- Direct small changes during session.
- Frame any tasks as directly related to client goals.

In this model, it is assumed that clients generally have already heard good advice on the problem and don't have an issue with knowing what they should do. Clients are believed to know what they are supposed to do but are unable to follow through with it. Due to this perspective, strategic therapists tend to focus more on changing series of family patterns through the use of paradoxical directives (Haley, 1987).

Paradoxical directives. Paradoxical tasks simultaneously tell clients to change and not to change (Haley, 1987). Paradoxical directives are considered effective because they disrupt the family's current homeostasis. It's also believed that, although clients genuinely desire change, they are also likely to be resistant to linear directives to make changes. As a result, the therapist will give directives with the expectation that the client will not follow what is being asked, but make the changes needed to resolve the presenting problem (Madanes, 1991). If a more linear directive is used, it might only create first-order, rather than second-order change, which would allow the problem to maintain (Haley, 1987). Two types of paradoxical directives are used in the strategic approach proposed by Haley (Goldenberg & Goldenberg, 2004; Wachtel & Wachtel, 1986): prescriptive directives and descriptive directives. Prescriptive directives are those that give the instruction for a client to do something, often more or less of a behavior. Descriptive directives are those that describe the problem in a different way, such as a reframe.

Haley (1987, p. 81) provides the following steps for implementing a paradoxical intervention:

1. Create a therapeutic alliance with the client.
2. Develop a clear definition of the problem.
3. Set clear goals.
4. Provide a plan to address goals, and at times a rationale for the plan.
5. "Disqualify the current authority on the problem" (1987, p. 81).
6. Give the specific directive.
7. Observe the client's changes or lack of changes in response to the directive.
8. Acknowledge the client as the person who was successful if change has occurred, rather than the therapist taking credit for change.

Redefine, prescribe, restrain. Paradoxical techniques developed by the MRI group are used in this model, including the use of reframing, prescribing the symptom and restraining (Goldenberg & Goldenberg, 2004; Weeks & L'Abate, 1982). These interventions can be used independently, or in a series (Papp, 1983):

Reframe → Prescribe → Restrain

Through these steps, the therapist works to shift the meaning of the symptom through a reframe, then prescribes a paradoxical task which clients follow (or don't follow) in order to create behavioral change in relation to the symptom. Then to maintain those changes the therapist offers a restraining intervention, such as telling the client not to change too quickly (Papp, 1983).

Ordeals. An ordeal is an intervention in which the therapist assigns a task that would be more of a problem to engage in than the presenting problem. Every time the symptom occurs, clients are assigned to also follow through with an ordeal. Assigning an ordeal can also be useful, in which the therapist makes it more difficult for the clients to carry out the problem than the solution. The ordeal not only has the purpose of making it more difficult to engage in the symptom, but it also creates a second-order shift in a system, as it requires a change in the usual sequence of interactions (Haley, 1984). For example, if a parent and child have to go out for ice cream every time they fight, it is going to be cumbersome for both of them if it occurs often enough. Additionally, this task will disrupt the usual sequence of events with a potentially positive activity that might create opportunities for strengthening their relationship.

Pretend techniques. Madanes (1991) offered a softer paradoxical approach through the use of pretend techniques. Rather than simply instruct clients to increase a symptom, she would ask them to "pretend" to have the symptom or to pretend to have achieved the goal of therapy. Madanes believed this approach was more useful than asking clients to have the symptom, since it provided opportunities for families to be more creative and flexible to explore old and new patterns that can occur related to the symptom.

Developmental considerations

Strategic therapy, like many other systemic approaches, consider the role of the family life cycle in the presentation of problems (Haley, 1973; Madanes, 1991; Szykula & Morris, 1986). Problems are most likely to occur when a family is transitioning from one stage to another, such as the transition from a family with children to a family with adolescents. They may experience difficulties re-aligning hierarchies, boundaries or family rules in response to biopsychosocial changes that come with the change in age.

When children are referred for therapy, it's recommended that therapists start by working with the parental subsystem (Szykula & Morris, 1986). First, therapists target any "problem-perpetuating solution-attempts" (1986, p. 174) that parents are stuck using. To address this, therapists provide directives for the parent to try with their children outside of therapy.

Therapists need to make some adaptations to their approach when young children are part of the family system and present in therapy (Haley, 1987). Therapist should create a context in which children are able to communicate through play. As a result, the therapist will need to be prepared to have toys and drawing utensils to facilitate age-appropriate opportunities for expression. This also provides a context in which the therapist can observe other family members' abilities to interact and include young children in the family.

Considerations for ethical and culturally sensitive practice

Since its formation, therapists have debated the ethical nature of strategic therapy (Solovey & Duncan, 1992). A common reaction to this approach is that it requires the therapist to take on an excessive position of power in which they are using manipulative tactics to get clients to change. As a result, critics have questioned whether strategic therapists violate clients' ability to provide informed consent to the methods used, if therapists are abusing their power in the therapy relationship and if strategic therapists are respecting clients' autonomy to make their own decisions. While Haley has addressed these ethical concerns (1987), Solovey and Duncan (1992) provide a clear defense of the ethical nature of strategic approaches. There are several components of the AAMFT code of ethics (American Association for Marriage and Family Therapy [AAMFT], 2015) that therapists consider when determining the ethical application of strategic therapy. The following sections will indicate how strategic therapy addresses these ethical standards to the same extent as our other MFT models.

Clients provide informed consent to treatment and abuse of the therapeutic relationship (AAMFT, 2015)

According to the AAMFT code of ethics (2015), clients need to be able to provide informed consent to treatment. This involves them having a clear understanding of what therapy entails and the impact of this on their lives. This allows them to autonomously decide if they would like to participate in this process. In accordance with this standard, therapists should not purposefully deceive their clients or engage in treatment processes that their clients haven't knowingly consented to (Solovey & Duncan, 1992). Doing so would also be an example of a therapist abusing their power. As a result, Haley points out that strategic therapists do not lie or deceive their clients. While unusual tasks or questions are posed to provoke second-order change, Haley (1987) suggests that therapists should only use interventions that they honestly and authentically believe.

Despite the point that clients knowingly consent to treatment, therapists of all models need to acknowledge that they often conduct interventions (small or large) in sessions that occur without the client's direct awareness. For example, a therapist's subtle body language or facial expressions can influence clients' thoughts, behaviors and emotions without the client having a direct awareness of this impact. Therefore, strategic therapists argue that they are particularly ethical for their honesty about their awareness that at times they implement interventions without the client overtly knowing (Solovey & Duncan, 1992; Haley, 1987). Despite these points, as with any model, strategic therapists should consider that there are power differentials inherent in the therapist-client relationship; these power differences can also be influenced by client-therapist differences in race, class, ethnicity, sexual orientation and/or gender (Fisher-Borne, Cain & Martin, 2015; Mosher, Hook, Captari, Davis, DeBlaere & Owen, 2017).

Client autonomy in decision making (AAMFT, 2015)

It's been argued that the strategic therapist's lack of sharing hypotheses and interpretations about clients' behaviors allows them autonomy to make their own decisions about changing those behaviors (Haley, 1987). Because the therapist doesn't impose their interpretations onto the client, space is created for co-construction of therapy (Solovey & Duncan, 1992). Solovey and Duncan note that interventions, such as a reframe, help to shift meanings and beliefs of clients to create opportunities for clients to have self-agency to solve their own problems.

Benefit of the therapeutic relationship (AAMFT, 2015)

Strategic therapy was designed with the intention of ensuring that the client-identified problem is addressed as briefly as possible. This prevents long-term treatment that only minimally addresses client issues requiring a high amount of time and financial resources from the client (Haley, 1987). From this perspective, once the problem is resolved, therapy should end, rather than searching for additional problems.

Non-discrimination (AAMFT, 2015)

Strategic therapy is inherently flexible for application to diverse groups as it has few universal beliefs about what is healthy for a family. Since families identify the problem and their preferred outcomes, therapists are less likely to impose their own cultural beliefs (Haley, 1987). However, strategic therapists still need to consider applying cultural competence and cultural humility when working with families (Fisher-Borne et al., 2015; Mosher et al., 2017). To promote competence, they need to be curious about their clients' background and gather information to ensure interventions are culturally relevant. In order to maintain cultural humility, strategic therapists need to engage in self-reflection about personal biases and the privilege they may bring into the therapy room (Fisher-Borne et al., 2015; Mosher et al., 2017). Strategic therapists need to be aware that dominant cultural norms can reinforce discrimination and marginalization of minority groups, which can influence symptom development (Fisher-Borne et al., 2015). They should explore what cultural norms and values are important to the client and relevant to the presenting problem and consider how value differences might affect the therapeutic relationship. Because ruptures in the alliance can occur when therapists misunderstand a client's cultural context, strategic therapists should be sensitive to repairing the alliance if and when this occurs (Mosher et al., 2017). The following section is an example of a case study in which the therapist demonstrates how she adapted strategic therapy to fit the clients' needs.

Adaptation example

In a case study, a therapist adapted strategic therapy to treat a heterosexual couple who identified that their presenting problem was related to the male partner's cross-dressing (Gallo, 2016). The main adaptation to this approach included an affirmative stance toward cross-dressing based on the premise that, "providing counseling to a person who identifies as a cross-dresser requires counselors to be accepting, without personal judgment, of a client's cross-dressing behavior and own unique means of personality and sexual expression" (2016, p. 78). This involves recognizing cross-dressing as a psychologically healthy desire and as a means for expressing one's feminine side. As a result, it's recommended that therapy includes finding ways to fully integrate cross-dressing into one's life and identity, as efforts to reduce this behavior are likely to not only be ineffective, but also harmful. A strategic lens gave the therapist flexibility to integrate cross-dressing into the client's identity and system, as opposed to viewing cross-dressing as part of a disease. Through reframes, the therapist and couple determined that the main problems were the wife's loss of power and the husband's shame regarding his authentic desires to cross-dress. Because the husband was more open to changing, the therapist gave him straightforward directives such as telling his wife every time he cross-dressed to reduce the secrecy around this behavior. Another intervention in this case that was more paradoxical was the use of an ordeal, in which the couple was instructed to have the husband cross-dress for an entire weekend without changing their planned schedule. Because this would have been more difficult than the current presenting problem, the couple avoided the ordeal and increased their acceptance of the husband's current patterns of cross-dressing (Gallo, 2016).

Research support

Research on early formulations of strategic therapy has been limited to studies that were conducted over 20 years ago with small samples sizes (e.g., Gallo, 2016; Szkula & Morris, 1986;). The limited research on strategic therapy results from the difficulty of manualizing this approach to study with larger samples. One exception to this involves a moderately-sized comparison study of 49 families, in which Strategic Family Therapy was found to be just as effective as behavioral family therapy in treating children with behavioral problems and depression symptoms (Steinberg, Sayger, & Szykula, 1997). It should also be noted, however, that concerns over the model's ethical nature led to a reduction of scholarly research on the model overall, as the field shifted to other approaches (Gardner, Burr & Wiedower, 2006).

Case studies have been used throughout the Strategic Family Therapy literature, such as the article previously discussed of a couple where the presenting problem was related to the male partner's cross-dressing (Gallo, 2016). In another case study, strategic couple's therapy was used to treat one partner's Anorexia Nervosa symptoms (Murray, 2014). While there are limitations to a single-case study, the positive results presented in this article warrant further exploration of how strategic therapy can be used to effectively treat Anorexia Nervosa and other disorders. In this study, the therapist identified ways in which the husband's Anorexia Nervosa both empowered and disempowered both partners. For example, the wife was empowered through being the "healthy" partner, who could blame and shame the husband by bringing up his symptoms in arguments. However, the husband remained empowered by using his symptoms to restrict activities such as eating out together. One example of an intervention prescribed was for the husband to report everything he ate to his wife to exaggerate the power dynamic. Another case example was provided in the literature illustrating the results of when therapists working in a juvenile justice system were trained in strategic therapy. Therapists and clients impacted by this training largely reported high rates of success with multistressed clients presenting with complex needs (Bobrow & Ray, 2004).

Brief Strategic Family Therapy

Although extensive quantitative research has not been conducted on the original versions of strategic therapy laid out by the MRI group or Haley and Madanes, we can't ignore the large base of evidence that has been accumulated on Brief Strategic Therapy (BSFT), which combines strategic and structural concepts. BSFT consists of three core components: system, structure and strategy. During assessment and treatment, the family is conceptualized as a whole containing interdependent parts. So, an adolescent substance abuse or behavior problem is viewed as part of a larger repetitive cycle of family interactions in which family members provoke one another's responses. Since the problem is part of this sequence of interactions, in order to solve the problem, the systemic dynamic has to change (Szapocznik & Williams, 2000). As a result, interventions are planned, targeted to the specific problem and present-focused. Reframing is a commonly used technique, along with efforts to re-align boundaries and hierarchy within the parent-child subsystem (Robbins & Szapocznik, 2000).

Most studies on BSFT have been conducted with Latino youth treating substance abuse and behavioral problems (Szapocznik & Williams, 2000). Through this research, BSFT has contributed key recommendations for culturally competent practice with this population. Findings show that interventions are most effective when therapists consider how parent-adolescent relationships are influenced by cultural differences between parents who immigrated to the U.S. and their first-generation children. Promotion of biculturalism, where both Latino and American values are honored, has helped families better reach their goals. This model also considers how cultural values might inform expectations for therapy. For example, Cuban families were found to prefer a therapist who was "active, directive, and present-oriented" (2000, p. 119), which helped to determine that a strategic approach would be an appropriate fit.

While BSFT was initially developed through pilot studies, clinical trials have been conducted on comparing BSFT to individual (Szapocznik et al., 1989) and group interventions (Santisteban et al., 2003). One study demonstrated that while both BSFT and individual psychodynamic therapy were effective in decreasing adolescent symptoms in comparison to a control group, those in the BSFT group had better family-related outcomes at a one-year follow-up (Szapocznik et al., 1989). In another clinical trial, adolescents with conduct disorder and socialized aggression were randomly assigned to either BSFT or a group therapy intervention. Adolescents in the BSFT treatment group had a significant reduction in symptoms post-treatment, while those in the group therapy intervention did not.

Case example

Paris and Corrine are a couple who have been living together for two years. Paris initiated therapy due to being "fed up" with her partner's lack of contributions around the house and in the relationship. In the first phone call, the therapist learned that Paris works as an attorney for a major law firm, while Corrine recently started an MBA program after she had difficulty finding work with her BA. Paris reported that she is the primary financial provider for the family and she tends to organize tasks around the household (e.g., laundry, pet care, meal-planning). Paris reported that she thinks that Corrine is "depressed". Paris states that she tries to be understanding, but ultimately isn't sure how much more she can take of "doing everything by myself". She reports they are living like roommates, sometimes sleeping in separate bedrooms after they fight. Early on the therapist identifies that Paris has created a double-bind for Corrine, with the directive "I want you to be more responsible".

The therapist shares in the first session her understanding of the problem from an initial phone call and that the main goal of the first session is just to learn more about both of their perspectives on the problem and to start coming up with some solutions.

Maintaining a business-like approach, the therapist first asks Paris, what changes are you hoping to see happen from this process? The therapist starts with Paris because she initiated therapy and may be the most invested. This can help to ensure the couple continues coming in. The therapist then asks Corrine next what she hopes to get out of the process. Asking Corrine second can also help prevent it from seeming like the therapist is blaming her for the problem. Corrine responds that she's not exactly sure, she does not know if this is something that can be fixed. Paris is clearly unhappy with her, but she thinks she is really doing her best. It seems like it's never enough, no matter what she does. She would like for Paris to give her some credit, to notice that she does what she can and for that to be enough for her. She also would like for them to communicate better when they fight, they never really resolve their fights and she hates it when Paris sleeps in the other room after a fight. She wants Paris to be excited to be with her again, rather than disgusted by her. It seems hopeless that they can get back to where they used to be. The therapist then gathers information about why it's important for them to attend therapy and how long the problem has been occurring and how the cycle of interaction occurs.

In the early stages of the intake, the therapist gathers facts, avoids feelings and advice-giving:

- It sounds like it was a hard time for you both, how did things change for you, Corinne, when you couldn't find work?
- When do these fights about being responsible occur the most?
- Paris, you come home from work and Corrine is relaxing, and then these fights start. What do you do, Paris, when this battle starts? When you want her to take this initiative to be responsible?
- What do you do at those times, Corinne, when she tells you to be more responsible?
- What do you do, Paris, when she avoids or half-way does these tasks?
- What do you when she pulls away, Corinne?

To instill confidence in the therapist and the process, the therapist communicates that these challenges you have been facing are quite common with couples when they go through a lot of difficult changes like they have with school and work. She lets them know that she thinks that she can help them with this.

Next the couple is directed to discuss the problem between each other. This helps the couple practice directly talking about the problem. Additionally, the therapist can observe their patterns of interactions when they talk about the problem to help inform goals and the task that will be assigned for outside the session.

After the therapist hears each client's perspective and directly observes their interactions, she moves into setting goals. She recommends that the therapy goals include Corrine taking on more responsibilities at home and spending more positive time together. Once she confirms that the couple agrees to the goals, she moves forward with setting the tasks for outside of session.

To help achieve your goals this week, I have some homework that I'd like you to both complete if you are willing. Paris, the first part of your homework this week is **not** to make a to-do list for Corrine. Corrine, your homework is to make up your own to-do list. Your to-do list can have as few or as many things on it as you like. You know best what your schedule is and what is reasonable for you to complete. I know that you are busy getting ready for school to start and volunteering, so don't put too much on your list. Since you are also really busy, it's ok if you just do these tasks part of the way, don't worry about doing it perfectly, because that will likely be too much for you to have to take on. I want this to be successful, so make sure not to overdo any of these tasks. Corrine, the other part of your homework is that you cannot share your list with Paris. If she tries to ask you what's on your list or what you did on the list that day, just remind her gently that it is not her concern. It's whatever you want it to be, based on your abilities and schedule. I'm more worried that you will put too much on this list, so just make sure not to do that.

Paris, your homework is to imagine that you are an investigative journalist this week and you are writing an article on how bad a partner Corrine is. You are looking for all the big or small ways in which Corrine is a bad partner. There might be evidence that she is a good partner, but that's not relevant to the article you are writing. Next session, bring your journalist notes for this bad partner article so that we can keep talking about how bad a partner Corrine is.

Both tasks assigned present a therapeutic double-bind. It would result in a success whether the couple follows the therapist's instructions or not. How the clients follow through also provides additional information about them and the problem that the therapist can use in designing future interventions.

Summary

Strategic therapy holds an important place in our history as MFTs. Therapists who practice other models within the MFT still utilize many concepts originally developed by this approach, especially the practical applications of systems theory. If you are just learning about this approach, you may find that they have some concerns about the ethical nature of this model and its evidence base.

We encourage you to further address these questions by exploring the voices on both sides of this argument that are present in the literature. Ultimately, you will have to decide what you believe about problem formation and resolution to determine if strategic therapy is the right fit for you.

References

American Association for Marriage and Family Therapy. (2015). AAMFT code of ethics. Retrieved from www.aamft.org/iMIS15/AAMFT/Content/Legal_Ethics/Code_of_Ethics.aspx

Bateson, G., Jackson, D. D., Haley, J. & Weakland, J. (1956). Toward a theory of schizophrenia. *Behavioral Science, 1*, 251–307.

Bobrow, E. & Ray, W. A. (2004). Strategic family therapy in the trenches. *Journal of Systemic Therapies, 23*(4), 28–38.

Fisher-Borne, M., Cain, J. M. & Martin, S. L. (2015). From mastery to accountability: cultural humility as an alternative to cultural competence. *Social Work Education, 34*(2), 165–181.

Gallo, M. (2016). A case study of cross-dressing: using a strategic therapy lens in couple's counseling. *The Family Journal, 24*(1), 77–84.

Gardner, B., Burr, B. & Wiedower, S. (2006). Reconceptualizing strategic family therapy: insights from a dynamic systems perspective. *Contemporary Family Therapy: An International Journal, 28*(3), 339–352.

Goldenberg, I. & Goldenberg, H. (2004). *Family therapy: an overview.* Pacific Grove, CA: Brooks/Cole-Thomson Learning.

Haley, J. (1963). *Strategies of psychotherapy.* New York, NY: Grune & Stratton.

Haley, J. (1973). Strategic therapy when a child is presented as the problem. *Journal of the American Academy of Child Psychiatry, 12*(4), 641–659.

Haley, J. (1984). *Ordeal therapy.* San Francisco, CA: Jossey-Bass.

Haley, J. (1987). *Problem solving therapy* (2nd ed.). San Francisco, CA: Jossey-Bass Publishers, Inc.Laing, R. D. (1970). *Knots.* New York, NY: Pantheon Books.

Madanes, C. (1991). *Strategic family therapy.* San Francisco, CA: Jossey-Bass Inc.

Mosher, D. K., Hook, J. N., Captari, L. E., Davis, D. E., DeBlaere, C. & Owen, J. (2017). Cultural humility: a therapeutic framework for engaging diverse clients. *Practice Innovations, 2*(4), 221–233.

Murray, S. (2014). A case of strategic couples therapy in adult anorexia nervosa: the importance of symptoms in context. *Contemporary Family Therapy: An International Journal, 36*(3), 392–397.

Papp, P. (1983). *The process of change.* New York, NY: The Guilford Press.

Robbins, M. S. & Szapocznik, J. (2000). Brief strategic family therapy. *Juvenile Justice Bulletin.* Washington DC: Office of Juvenile Justice and Delinquency Prevention. Retrieved May 16, 2011, from www.ncjrs.gov/html/ojjdp/jjbul2000_04_3/contents.html

Santisteban, D. A., Coatsworth, J. D., Perez-Vidal, A., Kurtines, W. M., Schwartz, S. J., LaPerriere, A. & Szapocznik, J. (2003). Efficacy of brief strategic family therapy in modifying Hispanic adolescent behavior problems and substance use. *Journal of Family Psychology, 17*(1), 121–133.

Segal, L. (1991). Brief therapy: the MRI approach. In A.S. Gurman & D.P. Knishern (Eds.), *Handbook of family therapy* (pp. 171–199). New York, NY: Brunner/Mazel.

Solovey, A. D. & Duncan, B. L. (1992). Ethics and strategic therapy: a proposed ethical direction. *Journal of Marital and Family Therapy, 18*(1), 53–61.

Steinberg, E. B., Sayger, T. V. & Szykula, S. A. (1997). The effects of strategic and behavioral family therapies on child behavior and depression. *Contemporary Family Therapy: An International Journal, 19*(4), 537.

Szapocznik, J., Rio, A. T., Murray, E., Cohen, R., Scopetta, M. A., Rivas-Vasquez, A., Hervis, O. E. & Posada, V. (1989). Structural family versus psychodynamic child therapy for problematic Hispanic boys. *Journal of Consulting and Clinical Psychology, 57*, 571–578.

Szapocznik, J. & Williams, R. A. (2000). Brief strategic family therapy: twenty-five years of interplay among theory, research and practice in adolescent behavior problems and drug abuse. *Clinical Child and Family Psychology Review, 3*(2), 117–134.

Szykula, S. A. & Morris, S. B. (1986). Strategic therapy with children: single-subject case-study demonstrations. *Psychotherapy: Theory, Research, Practice, Training, 23*(1), 174–180.

Wachtel, E. F. & Wachtel, P. L. (1986). *Family dynamics in individual psychotherapy: a guide to clinical strategies.* New York, NY: Guilford Press.

Watzlawick, P., Beavin, J. B. & Jackson, D. D. (1967). *Pragmatics of human communication: a study of interactional patterns, pathologies, and paradoxes.* New York, NY: W.W. Norton & Company, Inc.

Watzlawick, P., Weakland, J. H. & Fisch, R. (1974). *Change: principles of problem formation and problem resolution.* New York, NY: W.W. Norton & Company, Inc.

Weeks, G. R. & L'Abate, L. (1982). *Paradoxical psychotherapy: theory and technique.* New York, NY: Brunner/ Mazel.

11 Experiential Family Therapy

Amanda Veldorale-Griffin

Introduction

Experiential therapy primarily refers to two approaches developed in the early history of family therapy by Virginia Satir (Human Growth Model) and Carl Whitaker (Symbolic-Experiential Therapy). However, other models have been developed from these original approaches such as Emotionally-Focused Couples Therapy (EFT) (Johnson, 2004) and Internal Family Systems (Schwartz, 1995). Here is a brief list of these approaches:

1. *The Satir Growth Model*: This model was developed by Virginia Satir and emphasizes using therapist warmth and a supportive stance to help family members connect with one another and change maladaptive patterns of communication.
2. *Symbolic-Experiential Therapy*: This model was developed by Carl Whitaker and emphasizes the meanings that family members assign to their interactions with one another. He utilized both warmth, humor and confrontation to unbalance the system and encourage change.
3. *Emotionally-Focused Therapy (EFT)*: This model was developed by Sue Johnson and incorporates attachment theory into an experiential framework for helping couples. It has been researched extensively and is considered at the forefront of evidence-based approaches to couples therapy (Johnson, 2004). This model will be addressed in a later chapter of this text.
4. *Internal Family Systems*: This model was developed by Richard Schwartz and applies systems thinking to a person's internal workings. The therapist works in the moment to resolve relationships between a client's internal parts, or the relationships between family members' internal parts (Schwartz, 1995).

Across all models of experiential therapy, there is a focus on emotions and using warmth, empathy and self to promote a strong therapeutic alliance, which serves as the main driver of change. Interventions typically seek to access and heighten in-the-moment experience, which is believed to be most likely to create second-order change.

Founders

There are two people who shaped experiential family therapy at its inception – Carl Whitaker and Virginia Satir. Carl Whitaker originally trained as an obstetrician/gynecologist but decided to seek additional training in psychiatry in order to better understand his

DOI: 10.4324/9781003382621-14

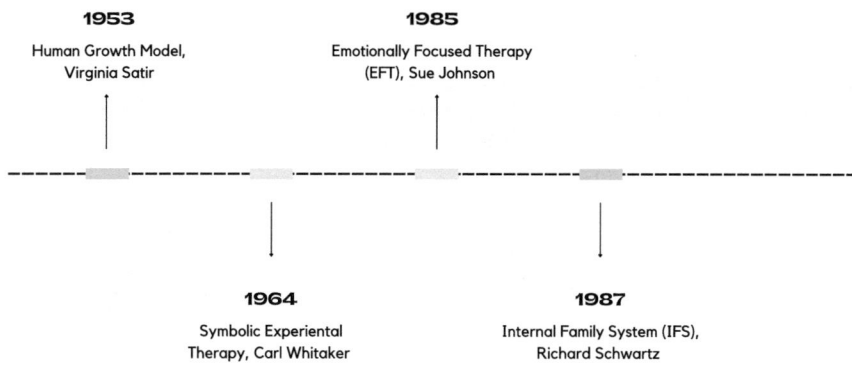

EXPERIENTIAL THERAPY TIMELINE

1953
Human Growth Model,
Virginia Satir

1985
Emotionally Focused Therapy
(EFT), Sue Johnson

1964
Symbolic Experiential
Therapy, Carl Whitaker

1987
Internal Family System (IFS),
Richard Schwartz

Experiental Therapy Model

Figure 11.1 Infographic: Experiential Family Therapy Timeline.

patients. After this experience, his subsequent positions were focused on psychiatry practice, including chair of the psychiatry department at Emory University (Whitaker, 1989). While working with patients suffering from Schizophrenia, he noticed a reemergence of symptoms when families were reunified with their families, which led him to wonder about the impact of family systems on individual symptomology (Whitaker & Keith, 1981). After resigning from Emory University in 1955, Whitaker founded (along with many of the faculty from Emory University) the Atlanta Psychiatric Clinic, where he turned his attention to the research and practice of what would become experiential psychotherapy (Napier & Whitaker, 1978). Napier and Whitaker were critical of theory and challenged therapists to focus more on being their authentic selves in therapy rather than spending too much time theorizing about what was happening in session.

Virginia Satir was a social worker who began in private practice in 1951. She was also part of the early days of the Mental Research Institute (MRI), where she served as the first director of training until 1966. Her therapeutic model emphasized enhancing familial communication and nurturing individual growth. She used a variety of techniques, including family sculpting, role-play and coaching to create new, in-the-moment experiences for families. She also made extensive use of warmth, empathy and self-of-the-therapist to facilitate change (Satir, 1972; Satir & Baldwin, 1983). Her change process model and nurturing approach served to help shape Experiential Family Therapy (Jencius, 2017; Nicholas & Schwartz, 2006).

Theoretical and philosophical underpinnings

Systemic foundation

Experiential therapy is rooted in systems theory and adds that family interactions are regulated by emotions and emotional expression (Satir, 1991; Napier & Whitaker, 1978). Experiential therapy is based on many of the systemic concepts that have been reviewed in this text, including wholism, interdependence of subsystems, circular causality, homeostasis, first- vs. second-order change and context. As a result of this systemic perspective, experiential therapists try to stay focused on the process of interactions over the content of conversations (Napier & Whitaker, 1978).

Wholism, interdependence of subsystems and circular causality

Wholism refers to the belief that behavior is only understood when viewed within the context of the system. No one part of the system can be understood without looking at the whole sum of its parts and interactions between parts. Related to wholism, experiential therapists believe that parts of a system are interdependent and that problems arise due to interactions between parts of the system. No one individual constructs and maintains the family rules, patterns of interaction or dysfunction.

Through a systemic perspective, the symptom or identified patient is believed to serve some function within the family, therefore cannot be treated in isolation from the system. For example, a child's acting out at school may serve to pull his parents' attention away from their own conflict to focus on the child.

Experiential therapists also are interested in family structure, including family roles, rules and hierarchy (Napier & Whitaker, 1978). According to Carl Whitaker, problems occur within the family when they become inflexible in the roles, rituals and routines they have put in place in an attempt to avoid the conflict and messiness that is inherent to all family systems (Napier & Whitaker, 1978). When families become uneasy with the uncertainty and conflict they are faced with, they seek out other ways of trying to make their interactions more manageable and predictable. Over time, the patterns of interactions that family members engage in can become part of (or seen as part of) their personalities. That is, rather than viewing different communication stances or roles as reactions to family interactions, they become viewed as something inherent to the person.

For example, Mary is the good kid and John is the bad kid. When this happens, people shut down about their experiences and hide their genuine feelings. Satir highlights five common family roles – martyr, victim or helpless one, rescuer, good child/parent and bad child/parent – that individuals within the system may adopt. These roles both serve to maintain one another and the family dynamics and can also become viewed as unchanging personality traits rather than a natural product of the current interactions within the system (Satir, 1998).

Experiential therapists categorize families as open systems or closed systems. Families are considered closed when family members are required to all think and behave the same, rather than be allowed to engage in authentic self-expression, which is allowed in an open system (Satir, 1988). Satir (1988) highlights that, when a person is rigidly required to suppress their own thoughts and feelings, individual development is hampered, leading to disturbances in mood and behavior.

Homeostasis

Systems are believed to seek homeostasis. Symbolic-Experiential Family Therapy posits that people create rules and interact in patterned ways in order to adhere to their system's expectations of behavior (Satir, 1988). In this model, therapists want to know about the homeostatic sequences of events that occur and may use circular questioning to gather this information.

One homeostatic pattern that experiential therapists often try to address is a transgenerational pattern of emotional avoidance (Napier & Whitaker, 1978). An effort to maintain homeostasis can lead people to repress their emotions and deny their own experiences or that of their children. Whitaker noted that parents deny or relabel children's experiences, which serves to dissociate them from their own world. He also noted that families may achieve their sense of serenity (homeostasis) through the preservation of family myths (Satir, 1988), which help create the rules that maintain the family's interactional patterns.

Satir deeply believed in a system's tendency to maintain status quo and resist change. As a result, she developed a stage model of change that clients progress through in order to disrupt homeostasis and achieve second-order change. A key aspect of this is that families learn to tolerate some degree of chaos, which forces the system to reorganize (Satir, Banmen, Gerber & Gomori, 1991). Experiential therapists also recognize that homeostatic family systems have positive and negative feedback mechanisms, with positive feedback moving the system away from its stable homeostasis, and negative feedback returning the system to homeostasis (Napier & Whitaker, 1978). While experiential therapists work with in-the-moment interactions, they recognize that patterns often originate from transgenerational experiences and patterns.

First- vs. second-order change

Second- vs. first-order change

Second-order change is believed to occur through heightening emotional intensity and increasing family members' ability to tolerate discomfort to achieve a new homeostasis. This new homeostasis is preferably characterized by increased vulnerability, emotional expression and authenticity. Additionally, the hope is that family members achieve a balance between connectedness and individuality (Napier & Whitaker, 1978).

Context and chronology

Experiential therapists recognize that family systems exist within larger systems and along a time continuum. They realize that economic, cultural and political contexts will trickle down and influence family dynamics (Napier & Whitaker, 1978). Satir's growth model also highlights the importance of family chronology, that is the key events in a family's or individual's life (Satir, 1983; Satir, 1988; Satir et al., 1991). These events, which include births, deaths, marriages, divorces, moves, wars, natural disasters, etc., provide the context with which the therapist can view and understand the family.

Humanism

Experiential family therapy finds its roots in the humanistic tradition of Carl Rogers (Satir et al., 1991). Rogers proposed three essential traits for therapists: (a) congruence or genuineness; (b) accurate empathy; and (c) unconditional positive regard (Rogers, 1951). Congruence refers to the idea that the therapist is authentic and true to themselves during their sessions, rather than putting on a therapeutic "face". In other words, the therapist's internal experience and outward reactions are congruent. This helps therapists to build trust with their clients and provide them with a model of authentic expression that does not deny or minimize their experience or emotions.

Accurate empathy refers to the therapist's ability to understand their clients' experiences at a deep level and convey that understanding to their clients. This helps clients to feel truly heard and validated. Unconditional positive regard refers to the idea that the therapist views their clients as whole people who are worthy of respect just the way they are. It encompasses the notion that therapists do not judge their clients and help ensure that clients feel cared for in the therapeutic relationship and have the emotional safety to share their experiences. It is important to note that this does not mean that the therapist will always approve of or condone their clients' actions, but that, even when they don't, they accept their client as a person who is doing their best in that given moment. In this way, they are able to validate their client's experience in the moment without labeling it as right or wrong, normal or abnormal; it just is what it is (Satir, 1983). These ideas form the basis of the warm, empathic approach, strong use of self and focus on the therapeutic alliance that are key components of Experiential Family Therapy.

Main assumptions and conceptualization of issues

Underlying all models are some inherent assumptions. The most basic of these models to the experiential therapies is the idea that change occurs by opening people up to new experiences. It is from this fundamental assumption that the model gets its name – Experiential Family Therapy. By helping clients get in touch with their emotions and be deeply involved in their experience, the experiential therapist can help them address their problems.

The Symbolic-Experiential approach founded by Carl Whitaker emphasized **freedom** and **personal responsibility**. One underlying assumption of this model is that people have the power to choose what actions they take. Thus, the experiential therapist looks for clients to take ownership of their future and "write their own destiny" (Neill & Kniskern, 1983). Moreover, according to this model, psychopathology is not inherently negative. Rather, the experiential therapist believes that people are able to grow through the pain they experience, and that anxiety can act as the catalyst to move people out of their homeostasis and into needed change.

Virginia Satir's growth model emphasizes the importance of **self-worth** and what Satir refers to as **congruence,** or the ability to authentically express one's self. Her model is based on four key assumptions, which are derived from humanistic and systems perspectives (Satir et al., 1991).

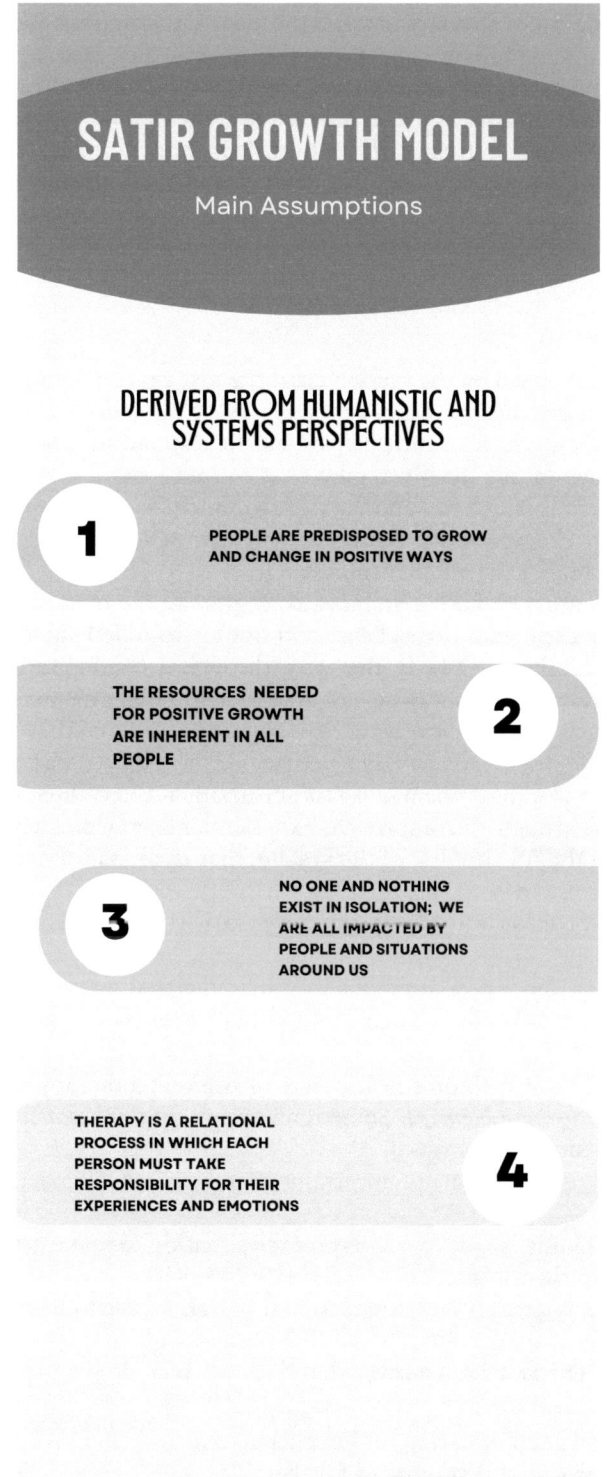

Figure 11.2 Infographic: Satir Growth Model Main Assumptions.

From these basic assumptions, one can begin to see how Experiential Family Therapists come to conceptualize issues. Primary to this is the idea that symptoms are not the "problem", but rather what distracts families from the real problems they face, such as illness, death, marriage, divorce and birth. Whitaker viewed these as the primary struggles families faced and saw symptoms as signs of people trying to wrestle with these issues without becoming "social robots" (Whitaker & Ryan, 1989). Both Satir and Whitaker viewed problems as arising when family members are not able to be authentic with one another about their experiences and emotions, instead relying on prescribed roles and rituals, while shutting down true intimacy and validation (Satir, 1988; Napier & Whitaker, 1978).

How change occurs

Experiential therapy is based on the fundamental premise that changing experience changes affect. That is, when families have new experiences of one another, it changes how they feel about one another, which in turn helps them to respond in new ways. One way this change occurs is when family members take risks to move either closer to or farther from other family members (Napier & Whitaker, 1978). In order to help promote this change, Experiential Family Therapists use the power of their self, including their personalities, gender and age, to create existential encounters.

These encounters must be both genuine and reciprocal; the therapist must be willing to engage fully and honestly with their clients and not try to hide behind their "professional role" (Napier & Whitaker, 1978). In this way, through a combination of warm support and provocation, experiential therapists are able to help family members lower their walls and connect with each other in new ways. It is important to note that Experiential Family Therapists are not focused on changing people. Rather, they assist family members in discovering their own feelings, opening up to one another about them, and join with them in their confusion. Through this approach, experiential therapists help families to create their own change in the functioning of the system, that is, second-order change. This focus also helps the therapist to confront their own anxiety about creating change and allows them to set that aside in order to be in the moment with their clients and help them feel truly understood.

Virginia Satir took the above approach and hypothesized a specific six-stage model of change for creating second-order change (Satir et al., 1991). The stages include:

1. *Late status quo:* This is the homeostatic state or beginning therapy state.
2. *Introduction of a foreign element:* Something occurs that unbalances the system (e.g., a crisis or a therapeutic intervention).
3. *Chaos:* The family enters a state of uncertainty and heightened anxiety. They try to regain the status quo.
4. *Integration:* The family is able to reinterpret the situation to make new meaning of it and incorporate it into their lives.
5. *Practice:* The family creates new interactional patterns based on the integration of the foreign element.
6. *New status quo:* The new homeostasis that does not include symptomology.

She used warmth and genuine caring for her clients to help them move through these stages and create a new status quo that worked for them.

Roles of the therapist and client

The experiential therapist is a collaborator and coach in the process of therapy. They take on the role of the expert in therapy, but not on the client's experiences or their life. This dynamic creates a situation where the therapist alternately leads their clients or follows them, bringing them along when necessary and allowing them to direct the change and take charge of creating new experiences at other times. The primary responsibility of the experiential family therapist is for building and maintaining the therapeutic alliance, as well as modeling a congruent (or authentic) way of being.

In addition to this key responsibility, Carl Whitaker highlighted two important "battles" that occur within the process of therapy, and which he saw as part of the therapist's role (Whitaker & Bumberry, 1988). The first of these is the **battle for structure**. This occurs before therapy even begins and has to do with who will be involved in therapy, when and how. The therapist in this type of therapy is in charge of providing the structure of the therapy process. They take on a position of power, or leader role where they are "in charge". Napier and Whitaker highlight that this is important as it requires a powerful presence to challenge the family's homeostatic patterns that, while not working, feel familiar. Taking on this role allows the family to establish trust that the therapist can do what is needed to create change. Part of learning whether or not therapists can provide this structure also involves the family testing it.

Whitaker posited that, in an effort to maintain their homeostasis, families make an effort to control their participation in therapy. He believed that progress could only be made by involving the whole system and he would set clear boundaries about who he would need to have in session in order to work with the family.

The second battle is the **battle for initiative** (Whitaker & Bumberry, 1988). This, Whitaker proposed, occurs when families reject the responsibility for change. At this point, it is the therapist's role to place the work of change back in the hands of the family (Jencius, 2017). While the Experiential Family Therapist will coach, encourage and assist clients in making change, ultimately it is the clients who will do the emotional work of change. They will be the ones to take the emotional risks that will allow them to experience their lives in new ways and connect with their family members through more open and honest communication.

Co-therapy

Carl Whitaker was a proponent of using co-therapy, in which two therapists guide the therapy process. While one benefit of this was for training new clinicians, the primary purpose is to provide a pseudo-parent experience for clients. Some experiential therapists argue that co-therapists should be mixed gender, however Whitaker didn't think this was necessary (Napier & Whitaker, 1978). The co-therapy relationship gives therapists the flexibility to move in and out of coalitions with various family members, model healthy family interactions with one another and maintain a balanced perspective on the family system.

Interventions

Although Experiential Family Therapy is not a technique-driven approach, there are a number of interventions that Experiential Family Therapists can use to help families have new, in-the-room experiences of one another. A few of these interventions are described in more depth below. As you review these methods, consider the here-and-now nature of these approaches, in contrast to other models' methods that might focus either on the past or future. Most interventions in experiential therapy are directed toward unbalancing homeostasis, usually through intensifying emotional experience, as it presents itself in the moment in therapy (Napier & Whitaker, 1978; Satir et al., 1991).

Use of self

As previously mentioned, the experiential therapist's use of self is one of the key elements of this therapeutic model. The use of self includes being congruent in their internal and external experiences and may also include self-disclosure, when appropriate. This form of honest communication provides a model for clients and also serves to form the basis of a safe therapeutic relationship where clients can take risks in their communication without fear of judgment or negative consequences (Satir, 1988; Satir et al., 1991).

Reflection

Reflection is one of the key ways in which therapists demonstrate their accurate empathy (Vogt, 2014). The therapist may mirror the client's communication by repeating all or part of something a client has expressed or they may highlight some emotion underlying what a client has just expressed. This can help clients to become of aware of and acknowledge hidden emotions. It also helps the therapist to join with their client and create a strong therapeutic alliance.

Validation

When the therapist validates a client's experience or emotional response, they are giving the message that that experience is valid and that it is not wrong to feel a particular way. Like with reflection, this intervention helps create emotional safety and strengthen the therapeutic alliance. It is especially important to help clients gain comfort with emotions that they have not previously been aware or expressed (Vogt, 2014).

Family sculpting

In this intervention, popularized by Virginia Satir, family members are asked to pretend as though their other family members are clay and arrange them (both in tableau and in action). This serves as a visual portrayal of each person's take on the family system and their place within it (Satir, 1988; Satir et al., 1991). It can also be used as a way of reenacting important moments from the past.

Conjoint family drawing

In this technique, family members are asked to draw a picture of their family. The family does this together and the pictures they create can highlight differences in viewpoints between family members and help them to acknowledge roles or emotions in the family that they had not previously considered (Bing, 1970).

Role-playing

This technique is designed to help bring experiences to life in the here-and-now and can be used with both past and future experiences (Satir, 1983; Satir, 1988).

Parents may be asked to take on the role of the child or the therapist may introduce the Gestalt "empty chair technique" to help family members bring someone "into the room". In this way, the family member can get practice expressing their emotions and playing out patterns of interaction that remove them from any rigid roles.

Case example

A single mother, Anna (36), and two daughters, Patricia (16) and Catalina (12), present for therapy. They are originally from Puerto Rico and have been living in the mainland U.S. for three years. The mother reports that the daughters are disrespectful and don't listen to her. The older daughter states that she has to do everything around the house because her mom is working all the time and that her sister doesn't have to do anything because she's "the baby". The 12-year-old reports that her sister yells at her all the time and bosses her around.

Questions:

1. How might you assess the family dynamics in this case?
2. What interventions could you use to help the family create a better homeostasis?
3. How would your approach be different as a symbolic-experiential therapist versus a therapist using Satir's Human Process Growth Validation Model?

Example intervention approach

Following an initial assessment phase during which the therapist gathers a detailed family history and understanding of the presenting problem, the therapist engages the family in a family sculpt. The therapist explains to the family that they are going to do an activity that is a bit different and that it might feel strange at first, but that is okay. The therapist instructs Ann, Patricia and Catalina to all stand up. They are told that they will be taking turns sculpting the family how they see everyone. The therapist instructs the mom to go first and to place the girls however she wants to demonstrate their family dynamic. The therapist explains that she can adjust how close they are, if someone is turned away, has raised hands, is down on their knees, etc. Anna places both girls far apart with raised fits facing each other and herself on her knees between them. The therapist comments on what she sees and asks clarifying questions to Anna and inquires how Patricia and Catalina feel in these positions. Anna reveals that she feels she is in a constant state of battle with her girls. Catalina and Patricia both report feeling that things are different and express excitement to do their own sculpts. Patricia goes next. She places Catalina and Anna very close to each other, with Anna almost cradling Catalina. She places herself in the other corner of the room. Again, the therapist engages in a debriefing process and Patricia is able to express that she feels cut off from the family and like her mom only cares about Catalina. Finally, Catalina has a turn and places her mom off to one corner of the room. She puts herself near Patricia with her sister pointing at her. Through the debriefing with the therapist, Catalina is able to express that she feels like her mom doesn't want to be around them and so she is left with her sister bossing her around. The therapist inquires how each of them is feeling in the moment during the intervention and offers validation of their experiences.

Termination of therapy

Therapy ends when the clients decide that it is appropriate to do so (Napier & Whitaker, 1978) and, ideally, they have entered into a new status quo (Satir et al., 1991). It is considered "successful" when the family members' emotional barriers have been broken down and they are communicating openly without engaging in mystification or holding on to family myths. When this occurs, families will no longer cling to their previously rigid family roles, but instead will be able to relate to one another as individuals with their own unique feelings and experiences. They will engage with each other more honestly and openly, and they will be able to validate the emotions and experiences of other members of the family. Napier and Whitaker (1978) suggest there are a few signs it is time to terminate therapy, including when the atmosphere becomes more casual, less professional and there is a lack of focus to the sessions.

Key legal and ethical considerations

Chief among the potential ethical considerations in the practice of Experiential Family Therapy are concerns regarding engaging in "psychotherapy of the absurd". This was a concept introduced by Carl Whitaker, in which he would behave in unconventional, and even outlandish ways to perturb the system. One obvious example of the potentially problematic nature of this was related by Keith and Whitaker (1982). They discuss a therapist responding to a female adolescent's complaint of being bored by sitting on her lap and stating that he would "take the blame" if she got an erection. While most therapists would never consider anything so bizarre, there is still an inherent risk in being openly confrontational and provocative with clients. Thus, therapists must be cautious not to push clients too far past their limits, use methods that are not age appropriate or open them up to too intense emotions. This is particularly important for clients who have a trauma history. Increasing emotional intensity beyond a client's limits has the potential to trigger trauma symptoms in an unhelpful way (Briere, 2002). They also need to be sensitive to the effects of encouraging clients to be vulnerable with family members who may exploit that vulnerability after a session (Johnson, 2004).

Therapists must also be careful in their use of touch as part of the therapeutic process. While providing a supportive hand on a shoulder or hug to a client can be a powerful connecting moment, it also has the potential to be seen as overly invasive or inappropriate by some clients. Again, this is particularly relevant to clients with a trauma history, who could be triggered by physical touch. One way therapists can combat this is by asking permission from clients before touching them. This allows clients to also practice setting boundaries.

Use with a diversity of clients

The research on the use of experiential therapies with diverse clients is quite limited, making it difficult to draw any definitive conclusions on the topic. Hollist, Miller, Falceto and Fernandes (2007) suggest that the fundamental assumptions of EFT make it well-suited to treat the depression frequently associated with marital discord among Latinas. However, no specific research has been conducted to confirm this hypothesis. Because it is a client-centered therapy model that emphasizes the importance of a strong therapeutic relationship and self-of-the therapist work, Experiential Family Therapy is well-suited for giving clients a voice and allowing an open discussion of issues of race, discrimination, stigma, etc. that may be affecting clients. Therapists need to ensure that in their building of the therapeutic relationship they explore cultural values that are uniquely relevant for each client and are aware if any ruptures occur to misunderstandings about culture. Additionally, experiential therapists need to add a critical lens that assesses how social inequities may be influencing presenting issues (Fisher-Borne, Montana Cain & Martin, 2014; Hook, Davis, Owen & DeBlaere, 2017). Empirical and conceptual articles suggest that it is particularly important that issues of racial socialization and racism be overtly addressed in therapy (e.g., Brown, 2008; Laszloffy & Hardy, 2000). Because of this, it is vital for experiential therapists to engage in ongoing self-of-the-therapist working, exploring their own values and beliefs, and examining why they think, feel and respond in the ways they do. It can be helpful to engage supervisors or professional colleagues in dialogue around these issues to help highlight hidden biases or other factors the therapist may not be aware of. As experiential therapists engage in their self-of-the-therapist work to enhance their authenticity in therapy, they also need to reflect on their own cultural values that may influence the therapy process as well as how aspects of their identity bring privilege and power into the therapist-client relationship (Fisher-Borne et al., 2014 Hook et al., 2017). For example, experiential therapists have a clear model of health that promotes emotional expression and intensity. This may need some shifting if a client is from a culture that values inhibition of emotions (McGoldrick, Giordano & Garcia-Preto, 2005).

The systemic nature of the model is also likely to be beneficial in working with diverse populations, as familial support can serve as an important protective factor (Brown, 2008). Finally, the warmth of the experiential model may make it a positive model for working with Latino families (Bean, Perry and Beddell, 2001). However, Experiential Family Therapy may be less suited for working with certain populations, such as Arab families. Specifically, research suggests that therapy for these clients may be more effective if it is directive in nature and employs more passive communication patterns (Al-Krenawi & Graham, 2000).

Self-of-the-therapist reflection questions:

1. What are your beliefs about expressing emotions?
2. What emotions are you most comfortable with?
3. What emotions are uncomfortable for you to sit with?
4. What was your role in your family of origin?
5. What aspects of your identity are most important to you? Why?

Research support

Little research has been conducted on the effectiveness of Symbolic-Experiential Family Therapy or Satir's Growth Model, making it difficult to speak to the empirical effectiveness of the models. It is difficult to empirically validate because these models are uniquely applied based on each client's unique presentation and in-the-moment needs in therapy. While some may critique this nature of the models, experiential therapists argue that this in-the-moment tailoring to the client is the essence of what creates change.

Although little testing of the model has occurred, a great deal of research has been conducted on the importance of the therapeutic alliance and therapist contributions to that relationship, which is an essential component of Experiential Family Therapy. Studies in this vein have found that the therapeutic alliance is an important predictor of positive treatment outcome, and that this remains true even when potential confounding variables are controlled for (Del Re, Fluckiger, Horvath, Symonds & Wampold, 2012). Moreover, it has been shown that a therapist is a vital agent of change in the therapeutic process (Blow, Sprenkle & Davis, 2007) and their personality, specifically their agreeableness, has an indirect effect (via the therapeutic alliance) on the decrease in depressive symptoms among clients (Kushner, Quilty, Uliaszek, McBride & Bagby, 2016). These results suggest that the self-of-the-therapist and their ability to create a strong relationship with their clients is an important factor in predicting successful treatment.

Additionally, multiple studies have assessed the utility of experiential methods, specifically activities that provoke in-the-moment experiences in order to facilitate change. In one study, Pos, Paolone, Smith and Warwar (2017) found that emotional arousal in session indirectly predicts positive therapy outcomes. Auszra, Greenberg and Herrmann (2013) found that activating and processing emotion predicts reduction in depression symptoms. One recent case study was published on the usefulness of treating adjustment disorder with Symbolic-Experiential Family Therapy (Bauman & Belous, 2016).

One of the best studied off-shoots of experiential therapy is Emotionally-Focused Couple's Therapy (EFCT). The research on this particular model suggests that EFT is effective in creating long-term change in couples' relationship satisfaction and helps them to improve their attachment security and reduce marital discord (see James, 1991; Johnson & Greenberg, 1985; Soleimani et al., 2014; Wiebe et al., 2017; Wiebe, Johnson, Moser, Dalgleish & Tasca, 2017). This model will be reviewed in more detail in Chapter 13.

Internal family systems (IFS) is another experiential therapy that has emerging evidence demonstrating it can be used to treat a variety of presenting issues (Haddock, Weiler, Trump & Henry, 2017). In a pilot study with 37 female college students, IFS was found to be as effective in treating depression as cognitive behavioral therapy. Several case studies on IFS have also been published, showing its utility in treating various presenting issues and populations, including trauma (Sweezy, 2011), children (Wark, Thomas & Peterson, 2001) and couples integrating a feminist perspective (Prouty & Protinsky, 2002). While IFS includes unique aspects beyond the approaches of Whitaker and Satir, this research lends support to models that emphasize an in-the-moment focus on emotional experiences of clients.

References

Al-Krenawi, A. & Graham, J.R. (2000). Culturally sensitive social work practice with Arab clients in mental health settings. *Health and Social Work, 25,* 9–22.

Auszra, L., Greenberg, L. S. & Herrmann, I. (2013). Client emotional productivity – optimal client in-session emotional processing in experiential therapy. *Psychotherapy Research, 23*(6), 732–746.

Bauman, M. L. & Belous, C. K. (2016). Using symbolic-experiential family therapy to treat adjustment disorder: a case study. *American Journal of Family Therapy, 44*(5), 285–300.

Bean, R. A., Perry, B. J. & Beddell, T. M. (2001). Developing culturally competent marriage and family therapists: guidelines for working with Hispanic families. *Journal of Marital and Family Therapy, 27*(1), 43–54.

Bing, E. (1970). The conjoint family drawing. *Family Process, 9,* 173–193.

Blow, A. J., Sprenkle, D. H. & Davis, S. D. (2007). Is who delivers the treatment more important than the treatment itself? The role of the therapist in common factors. *Journal of Marital and Family Therapy, 33,* 298–317.

Briere, J. (2002). Treating adult survivors of severe childhood abuse and neglect: further development of an integrative model. In J. E. B. Myers, L. Berliner, J. Briere, C. T. Hendrix, T. Reid & C. Jenny (Eds.), *The APSAC handbook on child maltreatment,* (2nd ed., pp. 175–202). Newbury Park, CA: Sage Publications.

Brown, D. L. (2008). African American resiliency: examining racial socialization and social support as protective factors. *Journal of Black Psychology, 34*(1), 32–48.

Del Re, A. C., Fluckiger, C., Horvath, A. O., Symonds, D. & Wampold, B. E. (2012). Therapist effects in the therapeutic alliance-outcome relationship: a restricted- maximum likelihood meta-analysis. *Clinical Psychology Review, 32*, 642–649.

Fisher-Borne, M., Montana Cain, J. & Martin, S. L. (2014). From mastery to accountability: cultural humility as an alternative to cultural competence. *Social Work Education*, 34(2), 165–181.

Haddock, S. A., Weiler, L. M., Trump, L. J. & Henry, K. L. (2017). The efficacy of internal family systems therapy in the treatment of depression among female college students: a pilot study. *Journal of Marital and Family Therapy*, 43(1), 131–144.

Hollist, C. S., Miller, R., Falceto, O. G. & Fernandes, C. L. C. (2007). Marital satisfaction and depression: a replication of the marital discord model in a Latino sample. *Family Process, 46*(4), 485–498.

Hook, J. N., Davis, D., Owen, J. & DeBlaere, C. (2017). *Cultural humility: engaging diverse identities in therapy*. Washington, DC: APA.

James, P.S. (1991). Effects of a communication training component added to an emotionally focused couples therapy. *Journal of Marital and Family Therapy*, 17, 263–275.

Jencius, M. (2017). Experiential family therapy. In J. Carlson & S. B. Dermer (Eds.), *The SAGE encyclopedia of marriage, family, and couples counseling*. Thousand Oaks, CA: SAGE Publications, Inc.

Johnson, S. (2004). Integration in EFT: a reply to Simon. *The Family Journal*, 14(1), 8–12.

Johnson, S. M. & Greenberg, L. S. (1985). Differential effects of experiential and problem-solving interventions in resolving marital conflict. *Journal of Consulting and Clinical Psychology, 53*, 175–184.

Keith, D. V. and Whitaker, C. A. (1982). Experiential-symbolic family therapy. In A. M. Horne & M. M. Ohlsen (Eds.), *Family counseling and therapy*. Itasca, IL: Peacock.

Kushner, S. C., Quilty, L. C., Uliaszek, A. A., McBride, C. & Bagby, R. M. (2016). Therapeutic alliance mediates the association between personality and treatment outcome in patients with major depressive disorder. *Journal of Affective Disorders, 201*, 137–144.

Laszloffy, T. A. & Hardy, K. V. (2000). Uncommon strategies for a common problem: addressing racism in family therapy. *Family Process, 39*(1), 35–50.

McGoldrick, M., Giordano, J. & Garcia-Preto, N. (2005). *Ethnicity and family therapy* (3rd ed.). New York, NY: The Guilford Press.

Napier, A. & Whitaker, C. A. (1978). *The family crucible*. New York, NY: Harper & Raw.

Neill, J. R. & Kniskern, D. P. (Eds.). (1983). *From psyche to system: the evolving therapy of Carl Whitaker*. New York, NY: Guilford Press.

Nichols, M. P. & Schwartz, R. C. (2006). *Family therapy concepts and methods* (7th ed.). Boston, MA: Pearson Education, Inc.

Pos, A. E., Paolone, D. A., Smith, C. E. & Warwar, S. H. (2017). How does client expressed emotional arousal relate to outcome in experiential therapy for depression? *Person-Centered and Experiential Psychotherapies*, 16(2), 173–190.

Prouty, A. M. & Protinsky, H. O. (2002). Feminist-informed internal family systems therapy with couples. *Journal of Couple & Relationship Therapy*, 1(3), 21–36.

Rogers, C. R. (1951). *Client-centered therapy*. Boston, MA: Houghton Mifflin.

Salin, L. (1983). Review of from psyche to system: the evolving therapy of Carl Whitaker by J. R. Neil & D. P. Kniskern (Eds). American Journal of Orthopsychiatry, 53(4), 764–747.

Satir, V. M. (1972). *Peoplemaking*. Palo Alto, CA: Science and Behavior Books.

Satir, V. M. (1988) *The new peoplemaking*. Palo Alto, CA: Science and Behavior Books.

Satir, V. M. (1983). *Conjoint family therapy* (3rd ed.). Palo Alto, CA: Science and Behavior Books.

Satir, V. (1991). *The Satir Model*. Palo Alto, CA: Science and Behavior Books.

Satir, V. (1998). *Conjoint Family Therapy*. Palo Alto, CA: Science and Behavior Books.

Satir, V. M. & Baldwin, M. (1983). *Satir step by step: a guide to creating change in families*. Palo Alto, CA: Science and Behavior Books.

Satir V., Banmen, J., Gerber, J. & Gomori, M. (1991). *The Satir model: family therapy and beyond*. Palo Alto, CA: Science and Behavior Books.

Schwartz, R. C. (1995). *Internal family systems therapy*. New York, NY: The Guilford Press.

Soleimani, A. A., Najafi, M., Ahmadi, K., Javidi, N., Kamkar, E. H. & Mahboubi, M. (2014). The effectiveness of emotionally focused couples therapy on sexual satisfaction and marital adjustment of infertile couples with marital conflict. *International Journal of Fertility and Sterility, 9*(3), 393–402.

Sweezy, M. (2011). The teenager's confession: regulating shame in internal family systems therapy. *American Journal of Psychotherapy, 65*(2), 179–188.

Vogt, R. (2014). Therapist's core competencies in utilizing emotionally focused therapy [PDF document]. Retrieved from http://surl.li/ijwmp

Wark, L., Thomas, M. & Peterson, S. (2001). Internal family systems therapy for children in family therapy. *Journal of Marital and Family Therapy, 27*(2), 189–200.

Whitaker, C. (1989). *Midnight musings of a family therapist*. New York, NY: W. W. Norton.

Whitaker, C. A. & Bumberry, W. M. (1988). *Dancing with the family*. New York, NY: Brunner/ Mazel.

Whitaker, C. A. & Keith, D. V. (1981). Symbolic-experiential family therapy. In A. S. Gurman and D. P. Kniskern (Eds.), *Handbook of family therapy*. New York, NY: Brunner/Mazel.

Whitaker, C. A. & Ryan, M. O. (1989). *Midnight musings of a family therapist*. New York, NY: Norton.

Wiebe, S. A., Johnson, S. M., Lafontaine, M., Moser, M. B., Dalgleish, T. L & Tasca, G. A. (2017). Two-year follow up outcomes of emotionally focused couples therapy: an investigation of relationship satisfaction and attachment trajectories. *Journal of Marital and Family Therapy, 43*(2), 227–244.

Wiebe, S. A., Johnson, S. M., Moser, M. B., Dalgleish, T. L & Tasca, G. A. (2017). Predicting follow up outcomes in emotionally focused couples therapy: the role of change in trust, relationship-specific attachment, and emotional engagement. *Journal of Marital and Family Therapy, 43*(2), 213–226.

12 Bowen Family Systems Theory

Michael Knerr

Introduction

One of the major theoretical approaches used by marriage and family therapists (MFTs) to help us understand how people relate comes from Bowen Family Systems Theory (Bowen, 1978; Friedman, 1991). Bowen Theory was developed through Dr. Murray Bowen's study of whole family units and his theory evolved over the course of many years. Since its development, Bowen Theory has become prominent in the field of family therapy and continues to be used clinically and tested through ongoing research (Miller, Anderson & Keala, 2004).

Bowen Theory is a broad theory based on an understanding of evolutionary processes and biological systems. Bowen Theory posits **eight interlocking concepts** that are used to help explain the operations and dysfunctions of families, the development of symptoms and suggest possible treatment interventions (Bowen, 1978; Friedman 1991; Kerr & Bowen, 1988). Since the theory is based in an evolutionary, systemic worldview, it also extends beyond immediate nuclear family processes and seeks to explain the transmission of behaviors across extended generations and into general society. In this sense, Bowen Theory is quite broad, seeking to help explain the development of relationship processes across generations.

Bowen's **major concepts** are *differentiation, emotional systems, multigenerational transmission, emotional triangles, nuclear family, family projection process, sibling position and societal regression* (Friedman, 1991; Kerr, 1988; Kerr & Bowen, 1988). Even without having yet provided specific definitions of these concepts, it is clear from their scope that Bowen Theory is a universal approach to explaining all types of human behaviors from individual actions to larger societal choices. Each of these eight concepts and how they fit together to try and explain human interactions will be discussed in this chapter. Once the concepts are clear, we can move onto the applications of the theory in a family therapy context. The second half of the chapter will focus on how Bowen Family Systems Theory can be applied in the therapy room.

Founders

Murray Bowen's Family Systems Theory was developed over a long period of time beginning with Bowen's early work as a psychiatrist at the Menninger clinic in the 1940s (Bowen, 1978; Friedman, 1991; Kerr & Bowen, 1988). This was the beginning for Bowen of being able to look at the family as a unit and the start of thinking about how the whole unit operates and the implications for individual patient symptoms. Bowen eventually moved

DOI: 10.4324/9781003382621-15

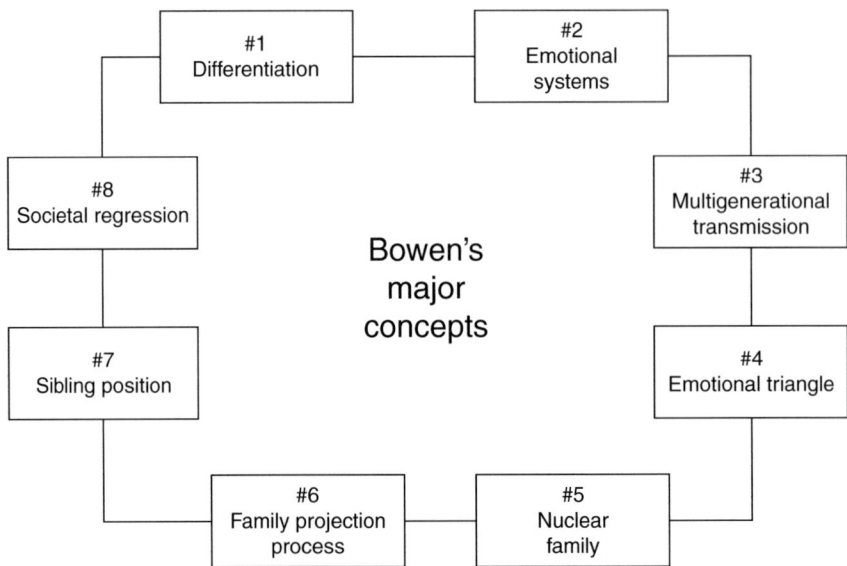

Figure 12.1 Bowen's Major Concepts.

to working at the National Institute of Mental Health in the mid-1950s and then onto Georgetown University in the early 1960s. Throughout these moves, Dr. Bowen continued to explore ideas of the family as a unit and understand their operations as a system, similar to other biological systems he had studied in medical school. Dr. Bowen remained at Georgetown University where his theoretical writings about family functioning developed into what we now call **Bowen Family Systems Theory** (Bowen, 1978; Kerr & Bowen, 1988; Friedman, 1991). In 1966, the original outlines of the theory were published using six major concepts. Later in the 1970s, two additional concepts were added to the model after further reflection and study. Along the way, a number of other people have become key contributors to understanding and applying Bowen Theory. For a full understanding of the theory and its application, students can also look at the writings of **Michael Kerr (1988)**, **Peter Titelman (2003)**, **Philip Guerin** (Guerin, Fogarty, Fay & Kautto, 1996) **and David Schnarch (1991)**, to name a few.

Systemic foundation

The application of a systems theory approach to human behavior was a new and interesting way to think about human behaviors in the 1940s and 1950s. Though trained in the psychoanalytic tradition of Freud, Bowen took his thinking in two distinctly different directions (Bowen, 1978; Friedman, 1991; Kerr & Bowen, 1988)

First, Bowen began to move the focus from the study of individuals to **the study of the relationship system**, suggesting that "dysfunctional" or symptomatic behaviors in individuals did not reside solely within the person. Rather than seeing mental health problems as "organic" and caused by something inside the person, Bowen began to look at the relational system as a factor in symptom development. This opened up new places to intervene – changing the relationship system/pattern – to provide symptom relief (Bowen, 1978; Friedman, 1991; Kerr & Bowen, 1988).

Second, Bowen looked at humans as part of the **natural system of evolution**, rather than as something unique from all other species. In this sense, Bowen saw the development of relational systems as "natural", a part of evolution and thus applicable to all human relationships. Understanding these relationship processes is then no different to understanding the process of cell biology. In theory, one could then study the processes of human relationships and discover "how people operate" much the same way we can study cell biology and explain how cells operate. Bowen extends the idea that the human body is a biological system (many parts that make up a whole) to understanding that humans interacting with other humans is a relational system. Understanding the operations of a relationship system also provides insight into what happens when these relational systems do not work, again in similar fashion to what happens when cells within a body function improperly (Bowen, 1978; Friedman, 1991; Kerr & Bowen, 1988).

In practice, this means that Bowen Family Systems Theory is much more interested in studying the family relationship system and understanding how that system operates than it is in examining individual symptomatic behaviors. Bowen's theoretical concepts seek **to outline the general characteristics that all relational systems have in common**.

Once these are understood, one can see where the system is not operating well and the symptomatic outcomes that result. In applying the theory to treatment, this provides the MFT with ideas about where to make changes in the system to help all members of that system function at their best (Bowen, 1978; Friedman 1991; Kerr & Bowen, 1988;).

Philosophical underpinnings

As is probably apparent by now, Bowen Family Systems Theory works from a **modernist philosophical approach** to human behavior. This means that Bowen's theory is **seeking to explain all human behavior** and makes assumptions that apply, no matter the culture, geography, history or values of the people group. Bowen Theory seeks to describe universal truths that explain how humans interact. For Bowen, these truths are not philosophical, but biological/evolutionary in their nature (Bowen, 1978; Friedman 1991; Kerr & Bowen, 1988). Bowen Theory is trying to find ways to describe relational interactions the same way another scientist is seeking to explain or describe other concepts in the physical universe. For example, a theory develops about how light behaves, and this guides research until measures can be developed to test the theory, which then brings revisions to our understanding of light. Bowen Theory makes similar assumptions about how humans interact and is seeking to find the basic ground rules of those interactions in much the same way, though admittedly finding reliable measures of human interactions is perhaps a more difficult process. Still, Bowen Theory believes these relationship interactions are discoverable because the theory **assumes they are not something someone developed or constructed, but are in fact rooted in our basic evolutionary biology**. In this sense, Bowen Theory takes a modernist philosophical approach to the problem of human behaviors in that it is seeking to understand the universal truths that guide all types of human interactions.

Main concepts

Bowen Family Systems Theory is comprised of eight major interlocking concepts. It is important to understand each concept individually – how it is defined, examples and applications – as well as how all eight concepts work together to provide an overall explanation of family functioning (Bowen, 1978; Friedman 1991; Kerr & Bowen, 1988).The following section will provide definitions of the major concepts and then some discussion of how they each work together to explain family outcomes.

Differentiation of self

While all the concepts are significant and interconnected in Bowen theory, the most central concept to the whole theory is that of differentiation (Friedman, 1991). **Differentiation is a multifaceted concept that deals with a person's ability to manage their need for both intimate connection with others and personal autonomy.** In order to manage the anxiety of this dilemma, the well differentiated person needs to be able to distinguish internally their feelings from their thoughts. This ability allows the person to avoid intense emotional reactivity and instead make thoughtful relationship choices even under stress (Bowen, 1978; Friedman, 1991). A well differentiated person is able to strike a balance so that their relationships are marked by true intimacy and emotional connection, while at the same time allowing maintenance of one's own personal identity. The inability to manage the competing needs for both closeness and distance, seen often as either volatile emotional reactivity or significant emotional cutoff, is often a key problem area for people entering therapy. According to Friedman (1991), **differentiation refers, "more to a process than to a goal that can ever be achieved"** (p. 141). In this sense, the process of becoming more differentiated can be likened to the development of maturity.

It is helpful to many people just learning about differentiation to **think of it as a two-part construct.** Bowen used the idea of differentiation to help explain the evolution of the human brain and what makes humans different from animals. Bowen suggests that the key difference in the development of the human brain is the ability to make rational choices, to reflect and select one's behavior. This is in contrast to instinctive or automatic responses/reactions seen in nature. Bowen Theory suggests that the human brain has evolved to the point where conscious choosing is possible, but that we have not left behind the automated part of the brain either.

Thus, a key way to think about differentiation is the ability of people – especially under stress – **to manage their automatic/emotional reactions well enough to use higher level thinking and instead make choices about their interactions with others.** A person with a "higher" level of differentiation would thus be better at making thoughtful choices and not falling prey to their more automated reactions.

The second aspect of differentiation in Bowen Theory is focused on how people relate to each other. If the first half of the definition is primarily internal – managing one's reactions and choices – **the second half is external, managing one's relationship connections.** It can be helpful to think of differentiation in these two parts, but for Bowen Theory the two parts are always connected, thus differentiation is a single construct (Bowen, 1978; Friedman, 1991; Kerr & Bowen, 1988)

In terms of relating to others, Bowen suggests all people face the issue of differentiating themselves from other people – what defines me; me and you; you – while also staying connected to others in a genuine way. Too much connection with others and the person loses themselves. Too much emphasis on becoming a unique self and a person loses connections with others. The problem is that both are good goals, but they tend to run counter to each other. The result of this tension is a basic level of chronic anxiety present in all relationships.

A well differentiated person is one who can maintain genuinely deep connections with others and at the same time stand up for their own unique selves. Trying to do this is difficult which is why, once again, it is something Bowen emphasizes is a lifelong process rather than a goal one achieves.

Differentiation is used in Bowen Theory to help explain a number of facets of how family systems operate. One of the ways differentiation is used is to help explain why similar families can respond to the same kinds of crisis events in such different ways (Bowen, 1978; Friedman, 1991; Kerr & Bowen, 1988). While each family system is unique, Bowen was curious about why there is such a wide range of family outcomes when faced with similar crises – job loss, death, chronic illness, etc. Bowen suggests one explanation for why some families are able to overcome such stressors and even grow through them and others are not is because of the differentiation levels of the adults in the family system. Better differentiated members are thought to be more resilient in the face of crisis, able to make better choices and attend to the relational needs of all, thus making a better outcome possible.

One final implication of the differentiation construct is also a basic assumption of Bowen Theory. That assumption is that all of life comes with some **level of chronic anxiety** (Bowen, 1978; Friedman, 1991; Kerr & Bowen, 1988). According to Bowen Theory, one can learn to manage anxiety, but there is no time at which some level of chronic anxiety is not present – it is simply a fact of being a human being in relationships with others. Chronic anxiety is a natural outcome of the competing forces of seeking a truly defined self and a deeply connected relationship. Trying to do both forces all people into a state of some anxiety as they must consistently make choices in one direction or the other and face the risks of those decisions. For Bowen, this is simply a natural consequence of our evolutionary process and the challenge that all people must now face (Bowen, 1978; Friedman, 1991; Kerr & Bowen, 1988). This chronic anxiety is then something that all family systems have to figure out how to manage, which leads to the next concept – the nuclear family emotional process.

Nuclear family emotional process

For Bowen, what defines a family is the emotional process they use. Much more than the structure – single parent vs. two parents for example – Bowen is concerned with how the family operates. Their emotional process includes how the family (as individuals and a unit) thinks, feels, behaves and responds to one another. **This family emotional process is what makes each family distinct – what makes us "us".** It is part of what people are referring to when they say things like, "We're the kind of family that…" Such statements tell us something about that family's emotional process. The emotional process of the family is how they manage all of the chronic anxieties built into life as well as the particular, unique challenges they may face. For Bowen, this process is identifiable; one can see the patterns of interactions as well as the places where these patterns create their own problems/symptoms. If the adults in the system are better differentiated, then perhaps the family emotional process is one where people pull together and see crisis moments as times of adventure and challenge. On the other hand, the family emotional process may be less resilient with additional challenges causing people to cutoff or become symptomatic in response to crisis moments. For the MFT, assessing the family emotional process is a key element in understanding the family system and what has led them to seek therapy, even if they come to therapy with a clearly identified patient.

Triangles

Bowen Theory says that all families make use of triangles in their relationships as a means of keeping stability in the family. Often, this is not a problem for the family as the third party is able to temporarily provide relief from developing tensions between a family dyad. Bowen suggests that in general a dyad is not particularly stable as a relational unit unless things are generally calm (Bowen, 1978; Friedman, 1991; Kerr & Bowen, 1988) under increased duress, a third party is "triangled into" the relationship as a means of reducing the tension. This can be functional for maintaining the relationship, but it can also **become problematic when the triangled person falls into a fixed pattern of behavior.** This is related to the issue of differentiation in the sense that the triangled party may help the dyad to manage their chronic anxiety and allow for growth to occur, or they may begin to impede that growth process by allowing the parties to avoid the relationship anxieties and thus avoid becoming better differentiated. For the MFT, it is important to be able to identify the relationship triangles, assess their function and determine when a relationship needs to be de- triangled through therapist interventions.

   Problematic triangles show up in several ways within the family emotional process. Tracking the family emotional process tends to reveal where relationship triangles exist and following those triangles often leads to understanding the development of symptomatic behaviors. **In Bowen Theory, the most common locations for the development of symptoms are in three areas** – marital conflicts; dysfunction in one adult partner; or impairment to one or more children (Bowen, 1978; Friedman, 1991; Kerr & Bowen, 1988;). Bowen Theory suggests that these areas of symptom development are directly related to the theory concepts – differentiation levels, family emotional processes and triangles. For the MFT, this means that the Bowen assessment process is a systemic exploration of these concepts as the primary explainers of the family presenting problem. The next two concepts tell us something about how families develop their emotional family process in the first place. The final three concepts then highlight some other means by which the family emotional process can become dysfunctional.

Sibling position

This concept is based on the work of Toman (1993), who examined the impact of sibling position on child development. Bowen Theory suggests **that, based on one's sibling position, the experience of the family emotional process may differ.**

   Though all of the children are raised within the same nuclear family emotional process, how each child experiences that process can be shaped in part by their place in the system. Some sibling positions seem to be more likely than others to become the object of family projections or to be the child who is triangled into parental conflicts. Bowen thus suggests that, in order to fully understand the family emotional process, sibling position is something that should be noted in the development of the genogram.

Multigenerational transmission process

This concept is the idea that the family emotional process is passed down from one generation to the next. Thus, in examining client problems, it is useful for the MFT to create a multigenerational genogram to help explore how the family emotional process has developed over time (Bowen, 1978; Friedman, 1991; Kerr & Bowen, 1988). Families may change in either direction – as adults become more or less differentiated, their emotional

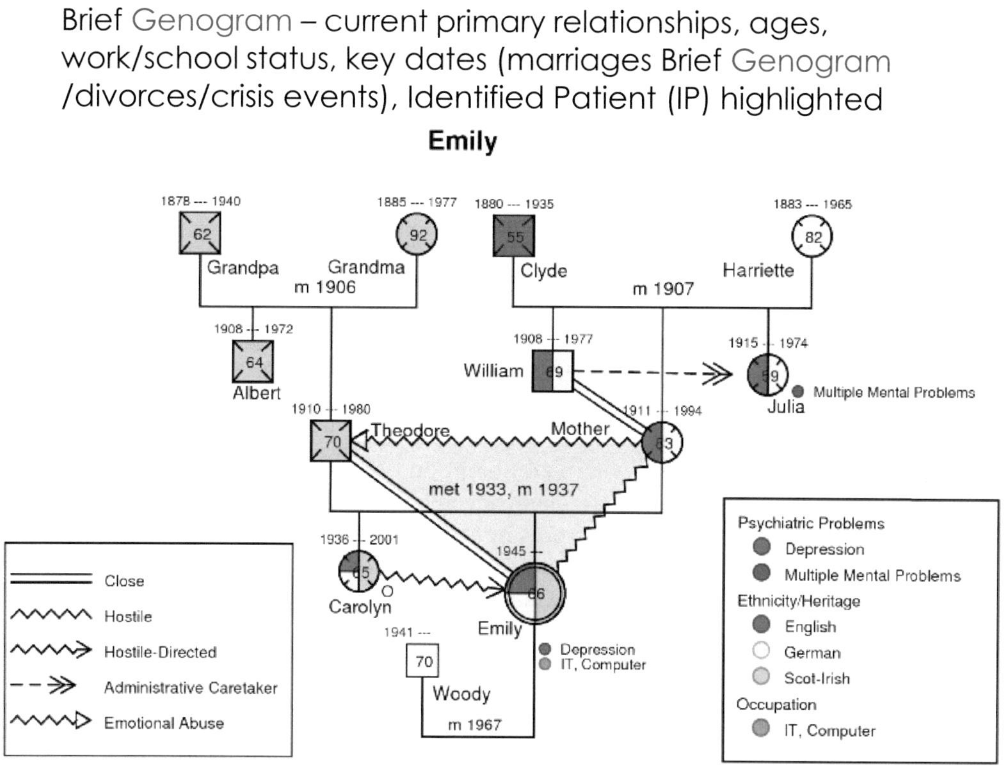

Brief Genogram – current primary relationships, ages, work/school status, key dates (marriages Brief Genogram /divorces/crisis events), Identified Patient (IP) highlighted

Emily

Figure 12.2 Brief Genogram.

processes also change. However, it is possible to see the patterns across generations and this can be helpful to clients in understanding why change can be so difficult to achieve. The transmission process is a natural phenomenon. **People simply absorb their family emotional process, and then they carry that same approach to relationships into the next generation.**

Family projection process

This concept is the idea that parents project onto their children their own anxieties and lack of differentiation. Often this occurs by triangulating a child into unresolved conflicts between spouses. No matter how hard we try, all parents do this to some degree to their children. Remember, differentiation is a lifelong developmental process, so we all have "junk" we pass onto our children. In worst case scenarios, this junk is projected onto the child – that is, **rather than the adult owning their own problems/anxieties, the child is seen as the sources of the problem.** The problem is "projected", meaning the child is seen as having the problem the parent has but needs to avoid solving. For example, the parent and eventually the whole family might "project" their own inability to manage anger onto the child by repeatedly claiming that this particular child is the one with an "anger problem" and needs to get help. This process of projecting one's own lack of differentiation onto their child can have a range of impacts from mild to severe on the child's development and own differentiation level (Bowen, 1978; Friedman, 1991; Kerr & Bowen, 1988). For the MFT, this means that one needs to assess the impact of this family projection process on individual clients in order to help them move to a higher level of differentiation.

Emotional cutoff

In response to a difficult family emotional process, some people employ emotional cutoff as a mechanism to survive. This is sometimes done geographically when the child moves far away and stops communicating with the rest of the family. However, one can also live right next door to one's parents and be emotionally cutoff. Emotional cutoff is about the person's relationship to the family emotional process (Bowen, 1978; Friedman, 1991; Kerr & Bowen, 1988). The person who is emotionally cutoff has been unable to resolve their emotional attachments in their family of origin. They are generally poorly differentiated and have to manage their distress with a combination of emotional and physical distance. In order to resolve an emotional cutoff, clients need help to see how to differentiate within their family of origin. Simply sending clients home and telling them it is important to have relationships with their family would likely cause more distress and be unhelpful. At the same time, **maintaining the emotional cutoff tends to stunt one's growth in relationships, so this is a key problem area to help clients resolve.**

Societal emotional process

The final concept in Bowen Theory may seem less applicable to specific therapy sessions, but it is in fact a vital component of the theory and its application. Since Bowen Theory seeks to explain all human relationship interactions, it is easily extended beyond the nuclear family system. In fact, the theory virtually demands that we consider larger societal contexts since all human relationships face the same systemic patterns. Likewise, larger social systems – schools, churches, hospitals, political groups, social movements – all have an ongoing impact on the nuclear family system since each of these is also a relational system. It becomes a false dichotomy to claim that the family system operates in one way, but the political system is different; or that one can be part of the family system and not part of the larger political/social system. Since all systems are interconnected by relationship patterns, we are all impacted whether we admit it or not. Thus, for Bowen Theory, part of understanding the nuclear family emotional process is rooted in understanding the larger societal emotional process (Bowen, 1978; Friedman, 1991; Kerr & Bowen, 1988)

In addition, just as a nuclear family emotional system sometimes faces a crisis and their response to that crisis shapes/and is shaped by their differentiation levels and previous history, the same is true of society in general. The societal-level emotional process can change in response to crisis events – natural disasters, terror events and political changes – both in good and bad ways. **Bowen Theory suggests that, with well differentiated leadership in place, society as a whole can develop improved emotional processes that allow all people to grow.** Likewise, with poorly differentiated leadership a society in crisis can see citizens regress and become less differentiated in their interaction patterns. As therapists, we must take these factors into account in the therapy process, otherwise we are simply affirming the larger status quo.

Case example

As you read this case vignette, consider Bowen's eight concepts. How can you use them to assess the couple described below? Jack and Jill come to you seeking to do couples therapy. Jack is 50, the CEO of his own law firm. Jill is 47, she met Jack when they were in law school together and they have been married for 18 years. Jill manages the household and their two children – Millie who is 16 and Max who is 13. Both children attend an exclusive private school and are expected to achieve academically and athletically, just like their parents did at their ages. Jill has been pushing Jack to come to couples therapy together for the past year or so, stating she feels like things are getting "out of control" and she is "afraid for their marriage". Jack is busy and has been putting it off for some time but agreed to come after there was some family drama two weeks ago. In his own words, Jack says he "Lost it" with their daughter and the two of them ended up screaming at each other in the driveway outside the family's vacation home. As for the marriage, Jill says things seemed to "get worse" during the year of Covid lockdown, with the kids attending virtual school from home while Jack was working 90+ hours a week from the office. She says she tries to talk to Jack, but, when she does, she gets upset, cries or pleads with him and he just "sits there and says almost nothing". Jack counters that he "can't figure out what makes her so upset" because they "have everything". He provides them all with plenty of money, a nice house, a vacation home at the lake, private schools, so he just doesn't see what there is to complain about. At least until his daughter screamed at him. He is concerned she has an anger management problem and thinks Jill should have done something more about it before it came to this.

What Bowen concepts did you spot in their story? This is the start of therapy, so for now these are simply things to note and explore later in treatment: nothing is definitive yet, but these are some starting points.

Nuclear family emotional process – It sounds like the couple are in a cycle where "the more she is upset, cries, pleads with him", the "more he shrugs, is confused, dismisses her concerns or avoids her" and the more this happens...

Differentiation levels – These seem to be low, as both partners "react" to the other and genuine connection and response seems limited, which explains the repeating cycle between them. Despite being able to see the cycle, neither one seems to be able to break it, instead automatically repeating the same patterns without being able to think of alternatives.

Triangles – Perhaps between mom, dad and the daughter? Mom and dad avoid solving their repeating cycle – even if the conflict is perhaps unseen by children. To manage the tension of unresolved conflict as a couple, the focus turns to their daughter with dad "demanding she do better" and Mom "hovering and helping with every challenge", thus leaving the daughter as the "problem child".

Societal emotional process – Covid disrupted a year of school/life routines, forcing the whole system to adapt to virtual school, limited social relationships and dramatic increases in time spent together in the home. The anxiety over "what will happen next" and the tension within the school community with competing protests about what should be done are felt by everyone in the home.

As therapy begins, creating a genogram with this couple would help the Bowen therapist explore these concepts. It also opens up space to investigate the impact of **sibling position,** possible **emotional cutoffs,** how the current family emotional process may represent "**multi-generational transmission**" and whether or not the family is currently using a **projection process** toward their daughter.

Conceptualization of issues

Bowen Theory makes the assumptions that all people are part of relational systems and that these systems have developed as part of the natural evolutionary process in the world. The eight concepts we just discussed form the framework for understanding how issues and symptoms develop within families and individuals. Thus, in contrast to the medical model that sought to find problems, especially mental illness symptoms, within the individual, Bowen Theory locates problems primarily within the relational system. In addition, rather than seeking a cause and a cure, Bowen Theory focuses on the system process and individual growth (Bowen, 1978; Friedman, 1991; Kerr & Bowen, 1988). In terms of problem conceptualization, this means that Bowen Theory uses the systemic lens and assumes that the process of change is lifelong. This does not mean that therapy must be a lifelong process, but it does mean that the Bowen therapist wants clients to understand they will need to keep working on their issues long past the end of the therapy relationship.

Like other systemic approaches to therapy, Bowen theory wants to assess and intervene in the family system to create changes. When starting with a new client and their presenting problem, the Bowen therapist wants to understand the particular problem/symptoms in the context of the larger relational system. In other words, how is a particular individual's report of depression an outcome of the relational system they live in day to day? In order to assess this relational system, the Bowen therapist would use the eight concepts listed above to understand how the client's system operates and how that is connected to their current struggle.

How change occurs

In Bowen Theory and therapy, change occurs as people understand their relational system and begin to change how they operate within that system. Practically speaking, this means helping each person in the system become more highly differentiated in their interactions. While the presenting problem may not focus on the family of origin, understanding one's family emotional process is a key to assessing the clients' current functioning. In terms of creating change, the Bowen therapist first seeks to help the client assess their own relational functioning, then begins the process of helping clients interrupt and change their old automatic behaviors and replace them with more thoughtful and intentional choices (Bowen, 1978; Friedman, 1991; Kerr & Bowen, 1988). Ideally, this is done together with multiple family members so that everyone can see and participate in the ways the system is changing. In simple terms, Bowen Theory sees change as a combination of insight and action based on what one learns about themselves and their family emotional processes.

Role of the therapist

The Bowen therapist's role is proactive as they often take on the position of **leader** or **coach.** The start of therapy often focuses on the use of a genogram to help clients explore their own family emotional process. In this stage, the Bowen therapist takes on a leadership stance as they need to help clients begin to see their presenting problem as something systemic (Bowen, 1978; Friedman, 1991; Kerr & Bowen, 1988) It is important for the therapist <u>to be clear as to the purpose of creating a genogram</u>, otherwise clients may reject the exercise as "not helping them solve their problem". Clients rarely come to therapy and think about their issues systemically, thus the Bowen therapist often needs to lead them to view their issues differently. If done well, clients often experience relief just knowing there is a new way to think about the problem and this sets the table for interventions.

Constructing a genogram

One of the best ways to do this with clients is by drawing the genogram on a whiteboard or flip chart so clients can see it as it takes shape and add comments and details as you construct it together. There are some standard symbols and formatting, but, for Bowen therapists, genograms happen in two parts. Part one is collecting basic factual data about the client, their family system, and one or two generations back. This includes names, ages, dates of major events – marriages, divorces, deaths – as well as other useful facts like jobs, education, geographical locations. Part two is about exploring family patterns (looking for hints regarding Bowen's eight concepts) and this might involve discussing with clients various patterns of behaviors, roles, health or mental health concerns, how various family members connect or distance themselves, accept or reject change. The genogram can then be used through the therapy sessions as a means of referring back to how the clients' system operated in the past and how they might like to see it change in the present.

Once the therapist has helped the client to see their problem differently – as an outcome of their system – this opens up new avenues for change and the Bowen therapist can begin to help clients think about how they want to change their interaction patterns within the system. These changes typically challenge clients to work at some aspect of becoming more highly differentiated and the various ways we can predict the system will resist their attempts and fight for homeostasis. In this stage, the therapist often becomes more of a coach, helping clients to consider their options, to create experiments and to grow from their attempts to interact with their relationship system in more thoughtful and mature ways.

Role of the client

As clients begin to see their problems within the context of their relational systems – both the family of origin and their current relational systems – **they are able to take this insight and design steps to change.** Clients often come to therapy feeling stuck, like they have already tried everything they can think of to change. The shift to seeing problems systemically and through the lens of Bowen Theory concepts can be refreshing and build hope. It also becomes a place of challenge for clients as they can see their role in the maintenance of the system. For clients, this often means shifting their focus from "what others do to them" to "how they react or respond" to the overall system. The client is asked to embrace the process of change and examine which skills they lack or need to develop further. For example, some clients have a well-defined sense of self, but struggle to make genuinely intimate connections. They may therefore "look mature", but, in the Bowen system, they still are not very highly differentiated. This client may need to work on different things than the client who is well connected but seems to have lost their sense of self. Bowen Theory seeks to help clients see where they are stuck, how their current family emotional process maintains that stuckness and develop their own steps to grow up.

Interventions

While Bowen Theory provides the MFT with a broad understanding of how humans interact and relational systems develop and get stuck, it is much less concerned with providing the therapist with specific interventions. A common complaint regarding the Bowen model is that, while it explains human behavior and problems, there are no specific steps for what to do with that explanation. For many people, this is a problem with Bowen Theory, but other therapists find the model refreshing for just this reason.

Bowen Theory leaves open many different possibilities for intervention strategies, making it ideal for therapists who want room for their own creativity in the therapy room. Bowen Theory marks out **large goals** for the therapist in terms of working with clients – increase differentiation levels, detriangle problematic relationships, resolve emotional cutoffs – but it is much less specific about how to do this. The "how to" of therapy is left open to the therapists' imagination to devise interventions for use within the overall framework of the theory.

Perhaps the only clear intervention specifically associated with Bowen Theory is the **use of the genogram** (Bowen, 1978; Friedman, 1991; Kerr & Bowen, 1988). Developing a genogram with a client is considered an essential part of understanding the client's family emotional process. The genogram makes clear how the system operates and points to areas for change. At the same time, creation of the genogram helps clients begin the process of seeing their presenting problem systemically and not as simply a problem within an identi-fied patient.

The genogram allows the therapist to do two things simultaneously – to assess the family functioning as the genogram is drawn and to begin hypothesizing with the client connections between the system and the problem (Bowen, 1978; Friedman, 1991; Kerr & Bowen, 1988). Thus, the genogram is both a tool for assessment and a means of intervention itself. In order to make the genogram something more than a simple family tree, we need to think about what we are assessing as the genogram is constructed. It is helpful to gather all the facts – ages, dates of marriages, children, education levels, mental health history, etc. – and there are many possible facts to gather. However, in Bowen Theory, we are especially interested in understanding the emotional family process. As we assemble the genogram, we are looking for how the family operates by using the eight Bowen concepts – where are the emotional triangles, what has been handed down through generations, how does sibling position change the family experiences, how well differentiated are people and how can you tell? Even as the client is reporting facts, the Bowen therapist is thinking about these concepts and how they fit together for this client and explain their family system. Understanding the system then helps the therapist to see how the client's symptoms/crisis/problem fits in the system. How is their issue a result of how their system operates? How is it a result of how multiple generations of systems have operated? As the genogram is constructed, it can be helpful to both ask clients for their observations and to make some observations of your own regarding the system and how it connects to their presenting problem. The Bowen therapist can then take on a coaching stance as they begin to suggest possible changes in the way one interacts with their relational system. Often these come in the form of small experiments designed to help the client see what they can learn about themselves and their system when they do something outside of their usual, automatic patterns.

Using the genogram to create interventions

One way to move from creating the genogram to create change is to ask the clients to explore the "unwritten rules" of their family system. This can be done in sessions, or as a homework assignment for clients to work on between sessions and bring back. This simple exercise gets the family to start thinking about their system (nuclear family emotional processes) both past and present.

Here are some basic steps you could use:

1. Have clients imagine their family system when they were between the ages of 8–18.
2. Explain the idea of "unwritten rules" – things everyone knows and follows in the family, but that are probably not explicitly stated. For example, an explicit rule might have been "Curfew is at midnight, if you come home late you will be grounded for a week". An "unwritten rule" might be something like this, "If you need $20, get it from mom's purse when she is not looking because she always has cash and she will never notice." This is something all the kids "know", even though no one ever told them directly this is the rule.
3. Give clients some categories to consider where these unwritten rules might occur. For example, there are likely unwritten rules regarding money, academics, gender roles, conflict resolution, mood expression, social life, health and diet. There are many possibilities you could select.
4. Have clients think about these unwritten rules, jot down a few notes about them indi vidually, then take some time to compare lists and discuss similarities and differences.

If the genogram is a key intervention in assessing the system, a second important intervention in Bowen Theory is the person of the therapist (Bowen, 1978; Friedman, 1991; Kerr & Bowen, 1988). Bowen Theory suggests that the key to helping clients lies in the therapist themselves. In a sense, the therapist entering the family system is the "intervention". By making contact with the therapist, the family is introducing something new into their system and the interactions with the therapist provide them the opportunity to grow and become better differentiated. However, this is based on the assumption that the therapist themselves has the ability to stay non-reactive and maintain their own self in the face of distressed/conflicted clients. Thus, an important intervention offered by the Bowen therapist is the therapist themselves. By remaining non-anxious in the face of crisis and helping the clients see their system more clearly, the Bowen therapist provides clients a chance to change their system. This also means that the Bowen therapist needs to be someone who does their own work.

Differentiation is a lifelong process, not something one achieves; and so the Bowen therapist needs to commit to their own process of "doing their own work" to continue to grow in their own levels of differentiation, knowing that they will never reach an end point (Bowen, 1978; Friedman, 1991; Kerr & Bowen, 1988). Termination of therapy

Termination of therapy in the Bowen Family Systems Model is a joint decision between client and therapist. Since the theory promotes a lifelong growth process rather than a definite "cure", deciding when to discontinue treatment is open ended. Ideally, the Bowen therapist has developed good rapport and a coaching stance with clients who have taken ownership of their own growth processes. In such a case, making a mutual determination for termination is done as clients report on progress and goal achievement. Sometimes, clients choose to maintain therapy but on a less regular basis, using a quarterly or annual checkup process to make sure they continue in the direction of greater health. There is no specified number of sessions required for Bowen therapy, though it tends to see therapy as a longer-term process than some other MFT models.

Research support

Bowen Theory is a large theory with many complex constructs and thus it can be difficult to develop treatment outcome studies using the model. Since there are not many clearly defined treatment stages of interventions, it can also be difficult to measure how the therapist is applying the theory and compare its effectiveness to other treatment models. This means that research often focuses on parts of the Bowen model rather than the therapy model as a whole.

Miller, Anderson and Keala (2004) reviewed Bowen studies that were examining basic research conducted to test various propositions of Bowen Theory. While there are no clinical outcome tests examining the effectiveness of Bowen Theory as a treatment model, the authors suggest the review of basic research is useful in building confidence in the value of Bowen Theory. The authors review studies that provide empirical support for hypothesized relationships between differentiation, chronic anxiety, marital satisfaction and distress.

Sabatelli and Bartle-Haring (2003) tested a model that explored the relationship between married couples' family of origin experiences and their current levels of marital adjustment. There is also research that has explored the effect of differentiation on adolescent behaviors, including such issues as risk-taking behavior, problem severity when entering therapy and test anxiety (Knauth, Skowron & Escobar, 2006; Peleg-Popko, 2002).

Skowron (2000) undertook a study to examine the role of differentiation in marital satisfaction. Using a sample of 39 couples who completed the DSI and the Dyadic Adjustment Scale, Skowron reported that a substantial amount of the variance in marital adjustment (74% in husbands and 61% in wives) can be accounted for by the couple's level of differentiation. She reports that couples who were less reactive, emotionally cutoff or fused with others also reported higher levels of marital satisfaction. More specifically, she found that emotional cutoff was predictive of marital upset and that the husband's level of cutoff was significant in predicting satisfaction or dissatisfaction (Skowron, 2000).

Bowen Theory's broad approach to the understanding of human relationships allows its application to be made in a variety of clinical circumstances. For example, some clinicians have used Bowen Theory as a basis for the development of sex therapy treatments (Schnarch, 1991). Others have used Bowen Theory as a basis for exploring the impact of one's family of origin on current family processes (Klever, 2004). Bowen Theory has sparked research and further theorizing regarding emotional cutoff, working with relationship triangles and applications to larger social systems (Guerin, Fogarty, Fay & Kautto, 1996; Titelman, 2003).

Research seems supportive of the various Bowen Theory concepts as they connect to client problems and interventions. Bowen Theory has been used with couples, individuals, families and other relational systems such as management teams or church boards. The theoretical concepts appear to have values, but since the application of the model is less structured, it has been difficult to measure overall effectiveness of Bowen Theory as a treatment model.

Key legal and ethical considerations

One key area for reflection on the ethics of Bowen Theory is in the area of gender and power. Some feminist family therapy approaches were highly critical of Bowen Theory, claiming the basic concept of differentiation empowered a masculine approach to life (Hare-Mustin, 1978). This claim was based on the idea that Bowen Theory valued thinking over feeling, thus reflecting the dominant position of male socialization. In response to feminist critique of Bowen Theory, Silverstein (2005) notes the critique regarding intellectual and emotional systems and potential male bias but suggests that these critiques miss the larger points made by Bowen regarding emotional systems. Instead, she points out that more problematic is the fact that Bowen Theory does not address gender roles or the impact of power dynamics on relationship interaction patterns (Silverstein, 2005). Gender socialization can have an impact on relationships because it becomes a factor in one's emotional reactivity. To deal with these issues, Silverstein suggests that, in the same way that Bowen wants to account for the impact of sibling position, one should also consider gender role socialization. One's gender position has an impact on the kinds of automatic emotional responses utilized. Put another way, gender impacts one's position in the family and in Bowen Theory part of becoming well differentiated is the ability to take a solid self-defined position in one's family.

Another issue for the Bowen therapist to consider as a potential area for ethical risk is working with clients who have become emotionally cutoff from their family system.

Within Bowen Theory, it is generally seen as unhealthy to be emotionally cutoff from one's family. However, there are times when such a cutoff is both necessary and reasonable. For example, asking family members to re-establish relationships with abuse perpetrators in the family system may be putting the client in harm's way. It can be tempting for new therapists to push clients to resolve emotional cutoffs because they see it as important in the theory. However, clients still need to maintain their own sense of autonomy in therapy. The Bowen therapist may take on a role of coach, but client feedback is important and should not be overlooked. The Bowen therapist needs to attend to their own self-of-the-therapist issues should they find themselves trying to compel clients to do something.

Self-of-the-therapist

Bowen Theory requires the therapist to be self-reflective and to continue pursuit of their own growth in differentiation throughout their lifetime. The Bowen therapist has never "arrived" but is always seeking growth opportunities because the therapist's ability to be differentiated in the therapy room is a key to helping families change (Bowen, 1978; Friedman, 1991; Kerr & Bowen, 1988). For most people, this means the Bowen therapist will need to develop their own personal genogram, explore their own family of origin emotional system and be willing to continue to work at being well differentiated within one's own family of origin and in their current relationships. This likely means the Bowen therapist will need to be in therapy themselves, perhaps not all of the time, but regularly throughout life as they change and grow.

Use with a diversity of clients

Bowen Theory attempts to describe all human relational processes from a universal standpoint. Thus, the Bowen therapist is attentive to particular differences in culture and values but would still maintain that the family emotional processes are similar in how they operate. While some cultures may value or define a "genuine relationship connection" differently, Bowen Theory assumes that all people are seeking this within the constructs of their particular culture. Bowen Theory is seen as applicable with any client, no matter how different they may be from the therapist. It is the therapists' job to understand and bridge these differences – to be well differentiated in the therapy room – and then to help clients develop the relational system that works for them.

As a model in which the therapist takes an expert stance, the therapist needs to be aware of their own cultural values and be mindful that they are not imposing beliefs about family systems that are not relevant to clients' cultural contexts (Fisher-Borne et al. 2015). For example, differentiation may look different for a person from an individualistic culture versus a collectivist culture (e.g., Sauerheber, Nims & Carter, 2014).

An example – Bowen Therapy considerations with Muslim families

Sauerheber, Nims and Carter (2014) provide recommendations for adapting Bowen's theory for Muslim couples that align with standards of cultural competency and humility. First, they highlight that Muslim families experience discrimination in the U.S., which can lead to symptoms and warrant the need for additional connection and support from one's family of origin. Additionally, family therapists should be aware of Islamic values related to marriage and family roles and expectations, especially since there are many misconceptions about Islam in western societies. They provide one example of how therapists might adapt their assessment based on cultural knowledge, highlighting that the common exploration of a couple's friendship and dating history may not be as relevant to some Muslim couples. In many traditional families, a decision to marry originates more from family support than friendship or dating, which is not always allowed. Commonly, marital expectations align with traditional gender roles with women caring for household responsibilities, and men being the primary breadwinner. However, it is emphasized that therapists remain curious about cultural values, rather than assuming commonly held beliefs or practices will fit for a Muslim family as there is great diversity in adherence to cultural practices across families. When implementing a genogram, therapists need to explore relationships with any family members residing in the family's country of origin. They should inquire about how living in different countries affects relationships as well as potential differences in cultural and religious values that result from this. For example, Muslim families may work harder at maintaining their relationships with family members in other countries due to pain and/or guilt for the distance. There also may be generational differences in adherence to cultural traditions that may or may not be sources of conflict. The western concept of differentiation may not fit as well for the Muslim values, which are collectivist oriented.

Bowen therapists need to ensure that they don't pathologize a collectivist-oriented family as fused, if their approach is working for the family system. It is also important to consider how one's differentiation is influenced by experiences of privilege, discrimination or marginalization (Mosher et al., 2017). One strength of Bowen Family Systems Theory is that self-of-the-therapist work is a key piece; as a result, therapists can integrate a self-critique related to their own cultural values, knowledge about diverse groups and identities that afford them with privilege and power.

References

Bowen, M. (1978). *Family therapy in clinical practice*. New York, NY: Jason Aaronson.

Friedman, E. H. (1991). Bowen theory and therapy. In A. S. Gurman & D. P. Kniskern (Eds.), *Handbook of family therapy: VII* (pp. 134–170). New York, NY: Brunner Mazel.

Guerin, P. J., Fogarty, T. F., Fay, L. F. & Kautto, J. G. (1996). *Working with relationship triangle*s. New York, NY: Guilford Press.

Hare-Mustin, R. T. (1978). A feminist approach to family therapy. *Family Process, 17*, 181–194.

Kerr, M. E. (1988). Chronic anxiety and defining a self. *The Atlantic Monthly, 3*, 35–58.

Kerr M. E. & Bowen, M. (1988). *Family evaluation*. New York, NY: W. W. Norton & Co.

Klever, P. (2004). The multigenerational transmission of nuclear family processes and symptoms. *American Journal of Family Therapy, 32*(4), 337–351.

Knauth, D. G., Skowron, E. A. & Escobar, E. (2006). Effect of differentiation of self on adolescent risk behavior. *Nursing Research, 55*, 336–345.

Miller, R. B., Anderson, S. & Keala, D. K. (2004). Is Bowen theory valid?: a review of basic research. *Journal of Marital and Family Therapy, 30*, 453–466.

Mosher, D. K., Hook, J., Captari, L. & Davis, D. (2017). Cultural humility: a therapeutic framework for engaging diverse clients. *Practice Innovations, 2*(4), 221–233.

Sabatelli, R. M. & Bartle-Haring, S. (2003). Family-of-origin experiences and adjustment in married couples. *Journal of Marriage & Family, 65*(1), 159–169.

Sauerheber, J. D., Nims, D. & Carter, D. J. (2014). Counseling Muslim couples from a Bowen family systems perspective. *The Family Journal, 22*(2), 231–239.

Schnarch, D. M. (1991). *Constructing the sexual crucible: an integration of sexual and marital therapy*. New York, NY: Norton.

Silverstein, L. B. (2005). Bowen family systems theory as feminist therapy. In M. Harway, (Ed.) *Handbook of couples therapy*. New Jersey, Hoboken, NJ: John Wiley & Sons, 103–118.

Skowron, E. A. (2000). The role of differentiation of self in marital adjustment. *Journal of Counseling Psychology, 47*, 229–237.

Titelman, P. (2003). Emotional cutoff in Bowen Family Systems Theory: an overview. In P. Titelman (Ed.), *Emotional cutoff: Bowen family systems theory perspectives* (pp. 9–66). New York, NY: Haworth Press.

Toman, W. (1993). *Family constellation [electronic resource]: its effects on personality and social behavior*. New York, NY: Springer Pub. Co.

13 Emotionally-Focused Family Therapy

Emily Schmittel

Introduction

Emotionally-Focused Family Therapy (EFT) is one of our most empirically-validated systemic therapy models (Johnson, 2004). As you learn this approach, you will see many similarities between EFT and other systemic models as it was built on many of the same principles. EFT therapists are systemic in that they treat the couple subsystem by focusing the patterns of interaction that occur between partners, or their "dance". The goal of this approach is second-order change, which occurs through experiential methods in which the therapist identifies problematic patterns in the moment and coaches the partners through reprocessing their responses to one another and practicing new, more secure connection and patterns of interaction.

One of the strengths of this model is that it is highly structured and brief (typically completed within 8–20 sessions). Therapists have a clear set of steps (nine to be exact!) for creating change. This same structure also allows the model to be consistently replicated and studied, creating a robust literature of its effectiveness for a variety of presenting issues. EFT can be used with couples, families and individuals who are experiencing a variety of relationship and mental health problems (Wiebe & Johnson, 2016). Like many of our approaches, therapists need to be aware of how to adapt this model for various ethics-related circumstances such as when emotional expression isn't a cultural norm for clients or when emotional vulnerability isn't physically or emotionally safe (Johnson, 2004).

If, after reading this introductory chapter to EFT, you are interested in learning the model more deeply, we recommend Susan Johnson's text: *the practice of emotionally focused couple therapy: creating connection* (2004). This is a comprehensive guide written on the theory, interventions and specific steps of the model. *Hold me tight* is a text that Johnson wrote for the lay population that is a great resource for clients participating in EFT, which you might also find helpful for gaining a deeper understanding of how to explain the approach to clients. There are also various options for additional trainings and certification in this approach that can be found through the International Centre for Excellence in Emotionally-Focused Therapy (ICEEFT).

History

EFT concepts were developed by Susan Johnson and Les Greenberg in the 1980s with a distinct focus on how emotions organize relationships and can be a vehicle for change (Johnson, 2004). Susan Johnson branched off to focus on developing her unique application

DOI: 10.4324/9781003382621-16

of Emotion-Focused Therapy with couples, while her colleague, Les Greenberg focused on a different variation typically applied to individuals and families (e.g., Goldman & Greenberg, 2019). Because Susan Johnson's model is more widely used in MFT and systemically focused, her approach is the core focus of this chapter.

Philosophical underpinnings

Several theoretical frameworks and clinical assumptions about change inform EFT. In this model, both internal emotional processes are explored as well as external interactional patterns, and how internal and external processes influence one another (Johnson, 2004). So, we could identify this clinical model as both **intrapsychic** and **systemic**. The core theoretical frameworks informing this approach are attachment theory, emotional development theory and systems theory. Assumptions about how change occurs are adopted from experiential therapies.

Attachment theory and emotional development

At its core, EFT is an attachment-based approach. Each client's presenting problem is understood in relation to attachment history in their family of origin, past relationships and in their current relationship. Thus, the emotional responses of each partner to one another are considered to be directly related to current or past attachment contexts. In an attachment framework, it is believed to be understandable to experience distress if an attachment figure is unavailable. As a result, clients' reactions to one another are consistently validated and normalized as part of an attachment response. For example, pursuing one's partner is considered an understandable response to distress that their partner may not be available to meet needs for emotional safety and security. We consider EFT a modern model of therapy since it has a clear framework for healthy couple functioning based on attachment theory.

Now that you are aware that attachment is a key organizing theory for EFT, let's review this theory more in-depth. Attachment, especially in infancy, is viewed as a response that humans have developed for survival. Infants are born with innate attachment behaviors such as crying and cooing, which elicit closeness of a caregiver. Think about how these behaviors both draw in a caregiver and help to keep an infant alive. John Bowlby (1969) and other attachment researchers (e.g., Harlow & Zimmermann, 1958) discovered that closeness with a caregiver is just as essential to thriving as other basic needs such as food and water.

Mary Ainsworth built on Bowlby's work through the identification of types of attachment. The three main attachment styles are **secure, anxious-ambivalent** (or anxious-resistant) and **anxious-avoidant** (Ainsworth, Blehar, Waters, & Wall, 1978). A fourth style was later discovered and labeled as **disorganized** (Main & Solomon, 1986). Although originally identified in infants, these types have been translated and validated in adulthood (Main, 2000). It is generally believed that attachment in early childhood with a caregiver provides a template for what individuals can expect from other relationships as they enter adolescence and adulthood (e.g., Quinton, Pickles, Maughan & Rutter, 1993). Although we know that there are often parallels between early and later attachment styles, attachment is not a static trait. If a secure attachment isn't developed during early childhood, it can still be facilitated later in life through subsequent sensitive care (Werner & Smith, 1992). Secure attachments can also be disrupted through later traumas.

It is critical that we view attachment systemically, as a circular relationship between two individuals, in which they both contribute to the quality of the relationship. It is not a uni-directional bond. This is even the case with parents and infants. While a parent has more power in a relationship with a child and is ultimately the most influential in building the attachment through sensitive care, infant qualities also influence the dynamic through their temperament (Vaughn & Bost, 2016). Attachments also exist in a larger context, so we cannot ignore factors like social support, oppression or work stress that have the potential to influence an attachment figure's ability to provide sensitive responsiveness to a child or partner (Shin, Park & Kim, 2006). Keep these factors in mind as you review the different types of attachment styles that are listed in the following sections.

Secure attachment

Individuals with secure attachments experience distress when their attachment figure is not present; however, as soon as their attachment figure returns, they are immediately soothed. They can explore their surroundings when their attachment figure is close by with some checking in with their caregiver, as if they use them as a secure base. It is believed this secure attachment is developed through consistent-sensitive care from the attachment figure. Essentially, they have learned that their caregiver will accurately read their cues for care and then respond appropriately (Ainsworth et al., 1978). Imagine an infant who starts crawling and accidentally ventures too far from their caregiver. A secure infant likely would start crying to signal to the caregiver their need for closeness. A sensitive-responsive parent, if available, will quickly pick up on the cue and meet this need, thus soothing the child and reinforcing their availability as a secure base for the child to explore. We can observe similar dynamics in adulthood. Consider a time where you may have needed closeness or reassur-ance from a partner or close family member that you trust. How did you signal to them you needed this? How did they respond? Were you immediately soothed by their response?

Anxious-ambivalent/resistant attachment

Individuals who have an anxious-ambivalent/resistant attachment have difficulty trusting that their caregiver will consistently meet their needs. When their attachment figure is unavailable, they become distressed and are not soothed by the return of the caregiver. They will display resistance to being soothed by the caregiver. When in the same room as the attachment figure, they will cling to the caregiver rather than freely explore their surroundings (Ainsworth et al., 1978). It is believed this attachment style is related to a caregiver having difficulty reading their cues and responding either intrusively or inconsist-ently. In adulthood, someone with this type of attachment style may struggle to engage in activities independent from their partner and excessively reach out for bids for connection through phone calls or texting. When hurt, attempts to apologize or soothe them may be ineffective.

Anxious-avoidant attachment. Those with avoidant attachment appear as though the individual is indifferent to their attachment figure. They explore their surroundings whether their caregiver is present or not and do not use the caregiver as a secure base. If the caregiver leaves, they are not visibly distressed and do not seek closeness when the caregiver returns (Ainsworth et al., 1978). Although the individual appears as if they do not "need" the caregiver, when their heart rate is monitored during sessions in which the caregiver leaves, their heart rate increases showing a distress response (Sroufe & Waters, 1977). However, its believed that, due to a history of lack of sensitive care, the child learns not to seek out closeness from learning that they won't get their needs met. Adults with avoidant attachment style similarly don't appear to need closeness with others. When in a relationship, they may bottle up their feelings or act as if they don't have any needs from their partner.

Disorganized attachment. A fourth category was discovered by one of Mary Ainsworth's students, Mary Main, who also went on to study adult attachment (Main & Solomon, 1986). Disorganized attachment occurs most commonly in populations who have experienced abuse or neglect. It appears that those with this type of attachment fail to have an organized response to their caregivers. They might initially seek out closeness, but then freeze before doing so as if they are uncertain what type of response they will get from their caregiver.

Here is a succinct list of components of attachment theory that EFT therapists consider when understanding partner interactions (Johnson, 2004):

1. Attachment is an evolutionary motivational force across all stages of the family life cycle.
2. Secure attachment is complementary to autonomy.
3. Attachment provides a sense of safety.
4. Attachment provides a secure base from which we can explore the world.
5. Emotional accessibility/responsiveness of an attachment figure creates a secure bond.
6. Fear and uncertainty activate attachment needs.
7. Separation distress is predictable.
8. There are limited responses to unavailable/unresponsive attachment figures.
9. Attachment informs internal working models of ourselves and others.
10. Isolation and loss are traumatizing.

Emotion

As the name suggests, client emotions are a key focus of EFT. Johnson articulates that, "Emotion is the music of the couple's dance and so organizes key interactions" (2004, p. 31). Emotional experience can be viewed systemically. Emotions give us important information about our environment and ourselves. For example, if we are feeling afraid, our body is sending us a signal that there is something in the environment that it is detecting as unsafe. These reactions help us to determine how to respond to aspects of our environment. Emotions are also important pieces of information that we communicate to others so that they can identify how to best respond to us. As a result, it is critical that we are able to observe our emotions and understand the external and internal triggers for these emotions so that we can determine the best course of action for getting what we need. Clear communication of our emotions also helps others in responding to us in helpful ways. As a result, EFT therapists work to support clients in identifying and expressing their emotional experience. To help in this process, emotions are categorized as primary and secondary.

Primary vs. secondary emotions

Primary emotions are the initial response we have to a circumstance. While they can be any emotion, typically EFT therapists look for primary emotional reactions of hurt and fear in response to partner behaviors.

Secondary emotions are the emotional responses we have to our primary emotions. These can also be any emotion; however, EFT therapists look for secondary emotional reactions such as feeling angry in response to being hurt by a partner's unavailability or jealous from fear that their partner might care about someone else. In EFT, we look for how negative interaction cycles are fueled by the expression of secondary emotions and that lack of attention and expression of more vulnerable primary emotions. Secondary emotions are not seen as "bad", but rather protective mechanisms that help maintain one's emotional survival.

While any emotion can be a primary or secondary emotion, the figure below illustrates common combinations of primary and secondary emotions. In this example, you'll see that partners commonly have a secondary reaction of anger to the primary emotions of hurt or fear of abandonment, betrayal or rejection.

Systems theory

With its focus on attachment and emotion, a picture of how EFT is systemic is likely already emerging, yet there are several other ways in which a systemic framework informs this approach. EFT therapists are "process consultants" (Johnson, 2004, p. 29) who are highly attuned to interactional patterns over the content of problems. They view presenting issues as resulting from circular causality (within the attachment relationship) and seek to support couples in externalizing the problem outside of the individual as a problem of cycles of interaction. They view these cycles of interactions as patterns that couples involuntarily become stuck due to homeostasis.

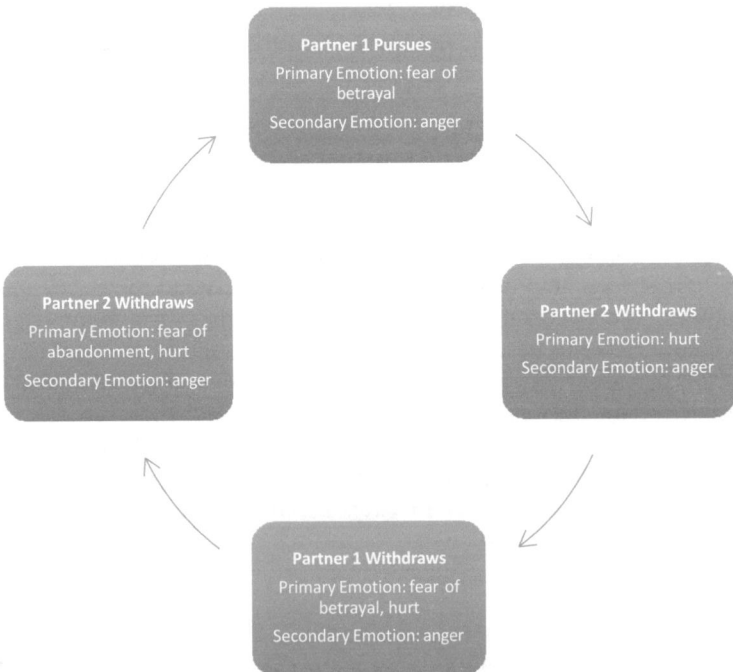

Figure 13.1 Primary and Secondary Emotions.

Second-order change is believed to occur by identifying the homeostatic patterns, understanding how these patterns are related to attachment history and emotions, and engaging in new patterns of interaction in the moment in therapy. Couple and family systems are viewed as a whole, made up of interdependent subsystems that engage in patterned dynamics. So, no one person's behavior is viewed as isolated from the interactions with the other parts of their system. In tracking the cycles of interaction in the whole system, EFT therapists assess quality of boundaries, including closeness and distance between family members, as well as rigidness or flexibility in patterns.

Throughout the process of EFT, we can observe both first- and second-order changes occurring. For example, in the first stage of EFT, we de-escalate the cycle, so there is a decrease in engagement in the negative interactional cycle, although the pattern of interaction may remain the same, indicating more of a first-order change. Second-order changes occur when the cycle shifts, such as when the withdrawing partner seeks out more closeness from the pursuing partner (Johnson, 2004).

Some examples of cycles include:

- pursue-withdraw
- criticize-avoid
- withdraw-withdraw (often occurs after a history of pursue-withdraw)
- attack-attack

Experiential therapy

Stemming from these systemic underpinnings, EFT assumes an experiential lens on how to create change. Consider the classic models of MFT that you learned in your early courses. Each model had its own unique beliefs about how change occurs. Virginia Satir and Carl Whittaker each believed that change occurred through in-the-moment interventions that were disruptive to homeostasis due to introducing chaos into the system, forcing it to re-organize (Satir, Banmen, Gerber & Gomori, 1991). EFT embodies these experiential principles (in the next section, we will outline the specific methods EFT therapists use to create this in-the-moment, second-order change). As a result, EFT therapists are carefully attuned to the internal and external processes that are happening for clients in the present during therapy.

Related to the experiential nature of EFT, it is not a model that teaches skills, facilitates insight; nor is it generally past or future focused (Johnson, 2004). As a result, you won't see EFT therapists exploring a lot of detail about family of origin issues; the exception to this is processing any past attachment injuries that are affecting reactions that occur in the present during session. Additionally, EFT therapists don't regularly give homework outside of sessions like cognitive, behavioral or solution-oriented therapies.

Interventions

As you review the interventions for EFT, think about how these methods align with attachment theory, emotional development, systems theory and experiential assumptions about change. Each framework is present in the therapist's efforts to build therapeutic rapport, to access and reprocess client emotions, and restructure new interactional patterns.

Therapeutic alliance

According to the common factors literature, the therapeutic alliance is one of the most important ingredients in what makes therapy effective (Lambert, 1992; Wampold, 2001). It comes as no surprise, then, that the therapeutic relationship is a central component of EFT. In this model, the therapist and client create an attachment relationship in which the therapist is sensitive and responsive to the client's emotional needs. This sensitive responsiveness is believed to build trust and a sense of safety to explore vulnerable internal processes and external dynamics between partners. To promote safety, EFT therapists are collaborative, genuinely caring, empathic and accepting of each client's emotional experience (Johnson, 2004).

Empathy and acceptance

An empathic stance is one of the most important qualities of an EFT therapist (Johnson, 2004). There are several functions that empathy serves in a therapeutic context. Empathy and acceptance from a therapist provide in-the-moment validation of clients' emotional experiences and models for clients how to be more empathic toward themselves. This approach also slows down clients' conversations about their experiences and makes them sit with those experiences longer to truly examine them and see their emotional responses from a different perspective and make sense of those experiences. Finally, from an attachment perspective, empathy creates a space where it is safe for clients to express and tolerate difficult emotions and experiences.

A challenge for any couple and family therapist is to empathize with each person without invalidating the experience of their partner or other family members. Empathic responses in EFT are typically directed toward emotional responses, particularly those relevant to attachment dynamics (Johnson, 2004). If a husband expresses deep hurt that his wife didn't ask him how a presentation at work went, the therapist should automatically validate this response and help the couple understand how this event fits into their larger attachment dynamic. Along with an empathic stance, EFT therapists also maintain a nonjudgmental position in which they are accepting of client emotions and related responses.

Methods for accessing and reprocessing emotions

Throughout various stages of EFT, the therapist will direct clients to observe and express their past and in-the-moment emotional experience. The goal is that this can help clients better ask for their emotional needs to be met and help their partners better respond to those needs. During attachment-related interactions in session as well as discussion around attachment experiences, the therapist also helps clients find new meanings in their emotional experiences as they are framed in an attachment framework and externalized outside of the individual. Techniques for accessing and preprocessing emotions include reflection, validation, evocative responding, heightening, empathic conjecture and self-disclosure (Johnson, 2004).

Reflection

The first step to accessing and reprocessing emotional experiences occurs through therapist reflection of the experience. This is generally seen as more than reflexive listening, as the therapist is carefully tracking and absorbing themselves in the client's experience. The goal is to slow down the client's experience of their emotions in the moment and create more awareness of their emotions (Johnson, 2004).

Validation

Validation is an intervention that directly results from the therapist's empathy and acceptance toward clients. EFT therapists consistently send the message to their clients that they have a right to their own experiences and emotions (Johnson, 2004).

Evocative responding

One intervention that may sound unfamiliar to you is evocative responding. The purpose of this intervention is to, "vividly capture the quality and implicitly elements of this experience, tentatively expanding such experience, often by the use of evocative imagery" (Johnson, 2004, p. 77). It is used to help clients clarify and engage in emerging aspects of their experience that have yet to be explored. Therapists are cautious with these responses and check-in to see if they fit for the client. Some examples of question prompts that align with this method include, "What happens to you when… How do you feel as you listen to… or as you say… What is it like for you… directly ask the client to expand his or her present experience. The focus here may be on the inner experience or on the process of interaction" (Johnson, 2004, p. 78).

Heightening

The method, heightening, is used to intensify the experience of an interaction that is relevant to the couple's attachment dynamic. Aspects of the old negative interactional cycle or new more secure patterns could be heightened to bring attention to the current state of the couple's functioning. Johnson gives specific examples of heightening (2004, p. 79):

Repeating a phrase to heighten its impact:

- responding while leaning forward and changing tone of voice
- using images or metaphors
- asking partners to enact responses
- maintaining a specific and relentless focus

Empathic conjecture

In empathic conjecture, an EFT therapist pays attention to the nonverbal cues of a client's experience, and will provide support for expressing their emotion if they are struggling to identify their experience. In these moments, therapists use empathic conjecture, in which they make an educated assumption about what the client may be feeling based on their knowledge of attachment and emotional responses. These conjectures are offered carefully, and always checked for fit with the client. We never want to impose assumptions on to the client, so we must be careful about how these suggestions are offered.

Self-disclosure

One way therapists demonstrate empathy and validation is through self-disclosure of their own emotional experience during therapy sessions or when they've been in situations similar to the client. For example, if a client shares about a time their parent told them to shut up and stop crying, an EFT therapist might share how sad they felt during the story or how they would feel hurt in a similar situation.

Methods for restructuring interactions

Once the therapist has de-escalated the intensity of a couple's negative interactional cycle (a first-order change), they will begin to use methods to restructure new interactions (a second-order change). The main methods for restructuring interactions are tracking, reframing and enactments, which will sound familiar from other models you've learned (Johnson, 2004).

Tracking and reframing

To restructure interactions, therapists first need to carefully track the circular patterns in which partners are entrenched. Two negative cycles commonly present in couple therapy are "blame-defend" and "pursue-withdraw". Cycles are described generally and as they occur during the session.

Describing the problem as a cycle also helps to externalize the problem outside of the people in the relationship. The cycle is the problem, and no one person is to be blamed for it. Johnson explains, "The experience of a common external enemy creates a pull towards cohesion in the couple" (2004, p. 85).

Tracking and identifying the cycle creates an opportunity to reframe each partner's behavior as part of the cycle and in the context of the attachment dynamic.

Reframes help partners to better understand and empathize with each person's responses and make sense of how their responses are linked to one another (Johnson, 2004).

Enactments

You'll recall that you learned about enactments in the chapter on structural family therapy. This is also a hallmark intervention of EFT. The main premise of this method is that the therapist has clients turn toward each other and coaches them on having a past conversation in a new manner. While structural therapists inform their directions with a theoretical base on boundaries and hierarchy, EFT therapists direct interactions based on their knowledge of attachment theory to increase expression of vulnerable primary emotions and sensitive responses from partners. Because of the experiential philosophy of this approach, a key method is for the therapist to direct clients in interacting with each other in new ways during the session (Johnson, 2004). Therapists direct clients for several reasons:

1. to emphasize their present positions in the relationships to move beyond these positions
2. to use a new emotional response to inform a new response to one's partner to facilitate a change in the negative interactional cycle
3. to heighten a new response that can also influence the other partner's current position in the cycle
4. to create new moments for change (Johnson, 2004)

Techniques for implementing interventions: RISSSC

Johnson provides a list of suggested techniques for implementing interventions that can easily be remembered by the acronym, RISSSC (2004). Use these techniques when you observe clients taking emotional risks (this should help you remember the acronym!):

- Repeat: restate key words or phrases to emphasize their importance.
- Image: describing experiences using imagery can heighten the experience.
- Simple: explain ideas or respond to clients as concisely as possible.
- Slow: a slow pace helps clients also slow down their emotional experience, allowing for greater processing.
- Soft: keeping a soft voice helps enhance the safety in the therapy room allowing for greater vulnerability.

Three stages and nine steps

The techniques we just reviewed are used throughout the entire therapy process; however, EFT is organized into nine steps that span three stages. Although they are distinctly delineated here, keep in mind that progress through these stages is not always linear. Sometimes couples may return to previous stages.

There are three overarching stages (Johnson, 2004):

1. de-escalation of negative cycles of interaction
2. changing interactional positions
3. integration and consolidation

During these stages, we look for three major signals of change. First, we want to see that the negative interactional cycle has reduced by the end of step three. Next, in the second stage, we want to see the withdrawn partner more engaged and seeking connection with the pursuing partner. Also, in this stage, we want to see the blaming partner soften and respond to the withdrawn partner with more empathy and understanding (Johnson, 2004).

Stage 1: de-escalation of negative cycles (Steps 1–4)

Step 1: create alliance and delineate conflicts related to attachment struggle.
Step 2: identify negative interaction cycle.
Step 3: access primary attachment emotions that underlie the cycle.
Step 4: reframe the problem in terms of a cycle, underlying emotions and attachment needs.

Stage 2: changing interactional positions (Steps 5–7)

Step 5: promote identification with disowned emotions/needs and integrate into the relationship.
Step 6: promote acceptance of one another's experience and new responses.
Step 7: facilitate expressions of needs and wants; create emotional engagement and new bonding moments that redefine attachment.

Stage 3: consolidation and integration (Steps 8–9)

Step 8: facilitate emergence of new solutions to old relationship problems.
Step 9: consolidate new positions and cycles of attachment behaviors. (Johnson, 2004, p. 33)

De-escalation

Stage 1 (Steps 1–4). In the first stage of EFT, the therapist is focused on joining and assessing the negative interactional cycle the couple is stuck in.

Typically, the therapist will meet with the couple both conjointly and individually to complete an assessment of the problem and to determine if EFT is an appropriate fit for the couple and their presenting issue. Later in this chapter, we will discuss some contraindications (which are indicators that this model is not safe to use) that the therapist will look for in their assessment. Assessment occurs both by gathering historical information about the couple and problem, as well as observing couple interactions during session. Once the therapist understands the couple's goals, attachment history and cycle of interaction, they will work to help the couple identify the cycle and how it relates to their attachment needs (Johnson, 2004).

Toward the end of Stage 1, the therapist focuses on supporting clients to identify primary and secondary emotions that relate to their attachment security and the negative interactional cycle. Emphasis is on identifying the primary emotions that are related to the secondary emotional responses that are often more visible and fuel the interactional cycle. Once these components are identified, the problem is labeled and externalized as a cycle. Externalizing the cycle helps to promote the couple to unite together to fight against the cycle that they have fallen into. These components together ideally lead to a de-escalation in the presenting problem, which we would consider to be a first order change (Johnson, 2004).

Changing interactional positions

Stage 2 (Steps 5–7). Once couples understand their cycle and how it relates to their security in the relationship and attachment-related emotions, they move into Stage 2. This stage involves a deeper exploration of emotions and needs that have gone unacknowledged or disowned that underlie the attachment negative interactional cycle. The role of the therapist is to coach partners toward more authentic expression of their primary emotions and attachment needs, as well as helping partners to better understand and respond to their partners' needs.

Often the focus encompasses a partner's beliefs about self, including how much they deserve their partner's love (Johnson, 2004). The hope is that, through expression of vulnerable needs and new, sensitive responses to those needs from partners, the couple can begin to rebuild a stronger sense of security and bond in their relationship as well as test new patterns of relating to one another. It is important for the therapist to be aware that, after much time engaging in a negative cycle, partners may have difficulty trusting one another's new responses. It's important that this mistrust is validated and reframed in terms of the negative attachment cycle. Johnson (2004) highlighted how this stage illustrates the social constructionist nature of our reality – particularly how emotional communication and interactions with our partner construct our views of self and others.

Step 7 particularly focuses on supporting clients in expressing their needs and wants and eliciting sensitive responses to those needs/wants from partners (Johnson, 2004). The two main milestones of this stage when successful are that the blaming partner softens and the withdrawn partner re-engages.

Integration and consolidation

Stage 3 (Steps 8–9). The final stage of EFT consists of finding solutions when previous negative interactions re-emerge, consolidating the new responses that emerged in Stage 2 and ultimately terminating therapy. Hallmarks of these new positions include flexibility and accessibility to one's partner (Johnson, 2004). Because, at this point, larger attachment-related issues are resolved, therapists will see partners being more willing to take ownership of how they can resolve specific problems. Consider the following example:

> A husband states that he understands his wife's concerns over finances and is ready to take care of this, so he has arranged to deposit an amount of money each month in the family account. He then intends to run his business on his own terms without his wife's interference.

When instances like this occur, the therapist's role is to support these initiatives and foster openness from their spouse to these actions. The therapist also draws attention to how a couple's ability to discuss these issues successfully reinforces relationship security and intimacy (Johnson, 2004).

In this final stage, any time the therapist observes the couple engaging in their new, positive interactional cycle, the therapist brings attention to it and uses this information to help to construct a new narrative of their relationship and therapy experience.

Construction of new narratives helps to solidify the couple's sense of security in their relationship. As the process moves toward termination, progress, strengths and future desires are reviewed. It's also important to discuss fears about termination and discuss strategies for addressing fears and any other potential future problems, such as the re-emergence of old negative patterns (Johnson, 2004).

Emotionally-Focused Family Therapy (EFFT)

EFT was primarily developed for use with couples; however, the philosophies and methods can transfer to family therapy as well. Just as with couples, family conflicts are conceptualized through an attachment lens and the focus is to rebuild secure bonds between family members. Consider a family moving through the family cycle. Often transition points can be the most challenging for families, such as when a child moves into adolescence or an adolescent emerges into adulthood. Often these transitions require a shift in family structure, including boundaries related to closeness and autonomy. When families have secure attachments, they can be more flexible and move through these transitions more smoothly (Aquilino, 1999). So, an attachment-based approach to family therapy can be critically helpful for families during transitions, when they often come in for therapy. Rather than dyadic, this approach is triadic in which it involves both parents (when applicable) and the child subsystem.

There are several considerations when adapting this approach for family therapy. A main difference from traditional EFT is that all family members do not have equal power and responsibility for the attachment relationship. In parent-child relationships, parents are responsible for providing sensitive responsiveness that is age appropriate. For example, when assessing the relationship between a parent and adolescent, in a secure relationship, we will find the parent has empathy for the emotions and desires of the adolescent, can communicate expectations clearly and is flexible when responding to conflict. Insecure attachment in the parent-adolescent subsystem can be indicated when the parent has assumed a rigid view of the adolescent that is negative and lacks understanding of their underlying emotions behind problematic behaviors (Stavrianopoulos, Faller & Furrow, 2014).

Evidence-base

EFT is considered an evidence-based practice. It has been studied across presenting issues and populations using a wide variety of methods (Wiebe & Johnson, 2016). Efficacy research has been conducted in which couples were randomly assigned to treatment and non-treatment groups, the model has been compared to many other types of couples therapy, and couples who've completed EFT have been studied both pre- and post-intervention. Once it was determined that EFT was effective in clinical trials, researchers started looking more closely at its use with specific presenting issues. Some specific presenting issues that EFT is effective in reducing symptoms include depression (Denton, Wittenborn & Golden, 2012), posttraumatic stress disorder (Greenman & Johnson, 2012) and couples coping with illness (Kowal, Johnson & Lee, 2003). It should also be noted that the effects of EFT have been found to remain stable over time (Halchuk, Mackinen & Johnson, 2010)

Special topic: infidelity

Because infidelity is one of the most difficult presenting issues to treat in couples therapy, we will take some extra time to discuss the recommendations in the literature on how EFT can be used to treat infidelity. A partner's affair may be one of the most painful attachment injuries that can be experienced within a marriage. It is often experienced as a traumatic event by the hurt partner who will re-experience the event during the recovery period. These flashbacks will likely trigger attachment-based emotions and secondary emotional reactions such as anger that can then lead to defensiveness by the partner who had an affair, which creates a missed opportunity to serve as a secure base, soothing the hurt partner's emotions.

Each time a re-experiencing episode occurs, a couple can spiral into a negative interaction cycle of blame-defend (Cluff Schade & Sandberg, 2012).

One of the first goals of an EFT approach to infidelity will be to support the hurt partner in identifying primary, attachment-based emotions such as hurt, abandonment and betrayal in a manner that can be better heard by their partner. The offending partner is then coached on sensitive responses to this hurt and toward identifying their own primary emotions that arise related to the affair such as shame or guilt. The hope is that the hurt partner's reactions can be understood as a result of how significant their partner is to them and how much they need them as a secure base. It is important for the offending partner to take ownership of the affair and express remorse. After this occurs, the therapist will coach the hurt partner to ask for comfort and soothing that they have not yet been able to receive. Together, partners need to construct a new narrative around the affair and the immediate aftermath of the affair, including the offending partner's unavailability to soothe the pain from the affair. After this injury is addressed, a more positive cycle of interaction can be constructed and consolidated (Cluff Schade & Sandberg, 2012).

Special topic: trauma

EFT, by nature, is an emotionally intense approach.

Therapists using this model intentionally heighten emotions of clients to create second-order change. Most clients will find this experience uncomfortable and difficult, yet will be able to tolerate these emotions in order to experience meaningful change.

However, clients with a trauma history sometimes experience interpersonal and emotion regulation difficulties that could be exacerbated by EFT interventions if not implemented carefully (Johnson, 2004). Despite these concerns, EFT is considered an effective treatment for trauma symptoms (e.g.,; Greenman & Johnson, 2012; MacIntosh & Johnson, 2008; Weissman et al., 2018).

Because trauma disrupts one's sense of safety, ability to regulate emotions and sense of security in interpersonal relationships, EFT, a model that targets these areas, is a clear fit for clients with this history. Targeting one's primary attachment relationship, the couple offers an opportunity to rebuild one's sense of safety, security and ability to vulnerably connect in an experiential manner. This approach also allows the partner to be an ally and active participant in the healing process (MacIntosh & Johnson, 2008). EFT is truly a systemic, relationally-based approach to healing trauma symptoms.

There are some trauma symptoms that child sexual abuse survivors have identified as arising during the EFT process that therapists need to consider. These include emotional flooding, numbing, dissociation, constricted or dysregulation of emotions, hypervigilance toward one's partner and shame related to sexuality (MacIntosh & Johnson, 2008). Assessment of trauma symptoms at the beginning of therapy can help the therapist identify which symptoms may be most likely to arise in therapy and strategies for supporting clients in managing those symptoms. Some specific clinical recommendations with survivors include going slow in the therapy process to ensure a "therapeutic window" (Briere, 1997) is always maintained in which a client is not over-exposed or under-exposed to trauma – both of which can be unhelpful. To maintain this window, therapists should be especially careful with heightening emotions to ensure that it does not lead to flooding, which could trigger trauma symptoms of dysregulation or numbing responses (MacIntosh & Johnson, 2008). Psychoeducation on trauma symptoms and attachment, as well as externalizing trauma symptoms outside the relationship are also critical components to integrate. To accommodate a slower process and integration of trauma-education, treatment should be extended to 30–35 sessions (Johnson, 2002).

Ethical and diversity considerations

Gender

Many classic MFT models have been criticized for being male-centric or having traditionally masculine traits viewed as healthy with more feminine traits pathologized (Vatcher & Bogo, 2001). For example, consider the concept of differentiation, which privileges autonomy and independence over dependence and emotionality. EFT, conversely, views interdependence, connection and emotional expression as strengths and healthy ways of being in relationships (Johnson, 2002).

Cultural variance in emotional expression

According to the AAMFT Code of Ethics (2015), therapist must ensure that therapy relationship is beneficial to the client and practice non-discrimination. These two codes direct us to consider if the original application of this model is always appropriate for diverse populations. While emotion is a generally universal experience, culturally competent therapists should be aware of variances in how cultures express and experience emotions (Karakurt & Keiley, 2009). As a result, EFT therapists are encouraged to employ a not-knowing stance in exploring clients' culturally-informed beliefs and values related to emotion identification and expression at the outset of therapy. For example, the original application of EFT will need to be adapted for cultures that practice limited emotional expression and vulnerability. Therapists training to use this model should also consider their own cultural perspective on emotional expression to understand personal reactions to both the model and their expectations with applying the model to diverse clients.

Contraindications

All therapists need to be aware that there are times where certain models or interventions could be potentially unhelpful or even harmful. We often refer to indicators that a model should not be used as "contraindications". Contraindications should be assessed at the beginning of treatment to avoid applying the model at a time that would be unethical. For EFT, two major contraindications are when the couple is experiencing active domestic violence (DV) and when the couple has at least one partner who is ambivalent about staying committed to the relationship.

Domestic violence

All couples in therapy should be adequately assessed for DV. It is generally agreed that couple therapy is never safe when active DV is occurring. This holds true for EFT as well. While this can be obvious to determine if a couple is engaged in recent physical violence, therapists should also consider the use of other forms of power and control tactics when determining if couples therapy is safe. Using couples therapy, especially EFT, when active DV is occurring asks a person who is already unsafe to be emotionally vulnerable, which has the potential to leave them more at risk of violence. Couples therapy is also contraindicated as these vulnerable interactions have the potential to escalate to violence after the couple leaves. It's recommended that EFT therapists meet with partners separately early on in the assessment process to adequately assess for violence. Keep in mind that assessing clients on DV together will likely prevent an honest disclosure about violent history.

Ambiguous commitment

Like most couples therapies, in order for EFT to be a useful process, both partners must be committed to working on the relationship (Johnson, 2004). Imagine asking someone to share their vulnerable emotions with their partner who isn't sure they want to stay together. This has the potential to have detrimental effects in which the sharing partner has taken a risk and can get further hurt if their partner isn't willing to work toward becoming a secure base. So, in the initial assessment of the couple, we must determine if both partners are committed to staying in and improving the relationship. If one or both partners is unsure if they want to continue the relationship, we first need to complete another type of therapy before EFT can begin. One option might be discernment counseling, which is often used with what we call "mixed agenda couples". Discernment counseling generally helps couples decide if they would like to stay together and work on their relationship or separate. It honors that more intensive therapy, which typically cannot occur if one partner is interested in separating (Doherty, Harris & Wilde, 2016). If, after discernment counseling, both partners are willing to invest in their relationship and work on improving it, then EFT can be used.

Case example

Jay and Jewel have been together for three years. They are both MFT graduate students about to enter the clinical training portion of their programs, so they are working a lot of hours as they build their careers. Jewel was recently offered an out-of-state internship in Wisconsin for one year, which will cause the couple to be in a long-distance relationship for the year. They come to therapy as they have been fighting a lot and neither trust that the other partner is fully invested in the relationship. The couple describe that any time a small issue happens, their interactions escalate quickly into arguments during which Jay is often very dysregulated in that he is tearful, anxious and has difficulty calming down. Jewel describes wanting to run away in this moment and that her empathy for Jay is very low, in that she feels he overreacts to everything and turns everything into a bigger deal than it should be. While she wants to stay in the relationship, she's not sure if she can "keep doing this". She wonders if she will always have to reassure Jay that she isn't leaving him, which is exhausting and makes her want to leave (even though she has no plans to).

In their first sessions, the therapist spends time getting to know each partner, their relationship histories and validating their experiences to build a relationship with each of them. She asks them questions to understand the cycle of interaction they are caught in and emphasizes that each partner's response is understandable.

Then, several sessions in, the therapist works with Jay and Jewel to map out the negative cycle that they are stuck in, which is a pursue-withdraw cycle. The pattern is generally characterized by Jay pursuing and Jewel withdrawing. She allows them to discuss the weekly challenges in session, which inevitably leads to the cycle occurring in session. This gives her the opportunity to help the couple identify when they are in their pattern and use enactments to practice stopping the cycle. The therapist notes that usually the couple sits as far apart as possible on the couch with Jewel holding a pillow in her lap, as if it were a shield. During enactments, she uses empathic conjecture to assist Jay and Jewel in identifying the primary emotions that underlie their reactions to each other.

During one particular session, the therapist interrupts the cycle as Jay begins pleading with Jewel not to move. He begins accusing her of throwing away their relationship and not caring about him. The therapist quietly asks Jay to pause and observe his emotions. When the therapist asks him what he's feeling in the moment, he quickly expresses he is angry. The therapist reframes his anger by emphasizing that he must truly be invested in the relationship if it is so painful to imagine living apart. She then connects his anger to a more vulnerable emotion that anger often protects, fear. Using empathic conjecture, she offers that, if she were in his position, she might feel very afraid that she would lose her partner forever and then checks in to see if that fits for him. When he agrees, the therapist turns to Jewel and asks her what it is like to hear him share his fears. She responds that she feels like a wall is up right now and she can't really connect to it because she is so tired of telling him she's not leaving. The therapist asks her, what would you need to bring down the wall a bit to hear what he's saying? She shares that she feels pretty hopeless, but that it would help if he could tell her he believes her when she reassures him, because it is frustrating and hurtful that he doesn't believe her. The therapist then asks her to share more about the hurt part, because it seems like the frustrated part is louder and comes out more. She goes more in-depth about how it feels to not be trusted and that he must not think all that highly of her that she would lie to him about her commitment. The therapist explores this further, asking what it's like to not be trusted, which leads Jewel to share her experience of feeling alone, which reminds her of growing up with her family, when she often felt alone. She explained that as a child she often felt she could only depend on herself and so avoided asking for help from others. She found that when she took charge of her own life and stopped expecting others to be there for her, she stopped feeling so disappointed all the time. She then shared she was most drawn to Jay in the beginning because he had a strong presence, a lot of his own interests and when she needed something, like when her car broke down, he could be there. He was strong; but now it just seemed like he was weak and dependent on her for everything, which makes her feel lonely and smothered at the same time. While recounting this information, Jewel started crying. The therapist again paused Jewel to ask her to reflect on what was behind the tears they were seeing. She shared that as she told this story, she just felt sad about the point their relationship had gotten to, and that she missed the old Jay she fell in love with. The therapist validated her emotions and highlighted how hard it must be to have this secure base feel as though she's lost it, that it must also feel quite unsteady for her after she finally found a rock to depend on. When Jewel confirmed this fit, the therapist checked in with Jay about his reactions to Jewel's experiences. He admitted he was shocked and that he didn't know what was going on for her. This immediately led to blaming her for their problems because she always shuts him out. To again interrupt their cycle, the therapist asked him to slow down and take a moment to observe what's going on for him emotionally. She used empathic conjecture as she hypothesized that he must be feeling powerless in not knowing how to fix the problem when he doesn't understand what's going on for her. When she checked in with him about the fit of her conjecture, he disagreed that powerless didn't quite fit; but rather he felt more hurt that she didn't feel like she could share this with him before. He then said he was sorry he hadn't been there for her lately in a way that she's needed and that he'd acted like her parents, who he knows she can't depend on.

The therapist thanked both of the partners for being so vulnerable in the session and highlighted that both have been feeling hurt, scared and alone. She asked them if each can identify one small action that would help them feel less alone. They both agreed that sitting more closely together on the couch and holding hands would help. Even if they weren't sure what would happen next, just sitting by each other, as if they are at least in it together, could lessen some of the fear. The therapist then asked them to share what it was like to sit a bit closer. After probing this further, the therapist closed the session by highlighting the couple's strengths, including their vulnerability and commitment to the relationship. She normalized their experiences through an attachment framework by explaining that when we don't feel close to our partners or when we feel that they are not accessible when we need them, it is terribly painful. This pain can cause us to react in ways to try to regain that closeness that are unhelpful and ultimately push us further away. She asked them to commit to at least trying to recreate the moment of sitting closer when they are stuck, so that they can know they are at least in the struggle together, united against the cycle.

A couple of months later, the therapist notes that the couple is in the closing stages of therapy as they can now identify when they are caught in their cycle and interrupt it. Now when Jay becomes escalated, he is able to go to a more vulnerable place and express his fears, which are then soothed by Jewel who can respond in an empathic way and reassure him. Additionally, when Jewel feels an impulse to withdraw, she can express that she is afraid they will never get out of this cycle, to which now Jay can reassure her that he ultimately does trust her, which is signaled by the fact that they have these instances less frequently than a few months prior, even though Jewel's departure date is approaching. The couple decides to have one more session before Jewel leaves for Wisconsin. In this session the therapist reviews their progress and skills that have developed over the last year.

Summary

In EFT, therapists will find a well-researched, systemic approach that builds on our classic MFT models. The model also addresses feminist critiques as it provides an alternative to traditional gender role expectations and can be adapted to fit diverse cultural contexts. Therapists learning this approach should be particularly considerate of assessing clients to ensure that the model is a good fit for clients, as it cannot be used with couples who are experiencing a lack of commitment or DV.

Although originally developed for couples, the utility of the model with families and even individuals cannot be overstated.

References

AAMFT (2015). Code of ethics. Retrieved from www.aamft.org/Legal_Ethics/Code_of_Ethics.aspx

Ainsworth, M.D., Blehar, M., Waters, E. & Wall, S. (1978). *Patterns of attachment: a psychological study of the strange situation.* Hillsdale, NJ: Lawrence Erlbaum.

Aquilino, W. S. (1999). Two views of one relationship: comparing parents' and young children's reports of the quality of intergenerational relations. *Journal of Marriage and Family*, 61(4), 858–870.

Bowlby, J. (1969). *Attachment. Attachment and loss: Vol. 1. Loss.* New York, NY: Basic Books.

Briere, J. (1997). Psychological assessment of adult posttraumatic states. APA. https://doi.org/10.1037/10267-000

Cluff Schade, L. & Sandberg, J. G. (2012). Healing the attachment injury of marital infidelity using emotionally focused couples therapy: a case illustration. *The American Journal of Family Therapy*, 40(5), 434–444.

Denton, W. H., Wittenborn, A. K. & Golden, R. N. (2012). Augmenting antidepressant medication treatment of depressed women with emotionally focused therapy for couples: a randomized pilot study. *Journal of Marital and Family Therapy*, 38, 23–38.

Doherty, W. J., Harris, S. M. & Wilde, J. L. (2016). Discernment counseling for "mixed-agenda" couples. *Journal of Marital and Family Therapy*, 42(2), 246–255.

Goldman, R. N. & Greenberg, L. S. (2019). *Clinical handbook of emotion-focused therapy.* Washington, DC: American Psychological Association.

Greenman, P. S. & Johnson, S. M. (2012). United we stand: emotionally focused therapy for couples in the treatment of posttraumatic stress disorder. *Journal of Clinical Psychology, 68*(5), 561–569.

Halchuk, R., Makinen, J. A. & Johnson, S. M. (2010). Resolving attachment injuries in couples using emotionally focused therapy: a three-year follow up. *Journal of Couple and Relationship Therapy, 9*(1), 31–47.

Harlow, H. F. & Zimmermann, R. R. (1958). The development of affective responsiveness in infant monkeys. *Proceedings of the American Philosophical Society, 102,* 501–509.

Johnson, S. (2004). *The practice of emotionally focused marital therapy: creating connection* (2nd ed.). New York, NY: Brunner/Routledge.

Karakurt, G. & Keiley, M. (2009). Integration of a cultural lens with emotionally focused therapy. *Journal of Couple & Relationship Therapy, 8*(1), 4–14.

Kowal, J., Johnson, S. M. & Lee, A. (2003). Chronic illness in couples: a case for emotionally focused therapy. *Journal of Marital and Family Therapy, 29*(3), 299–310.

Lambert, M. (1992). Psychotherapy outcome research: implications for integrative and eclectic therapists. In J. C. Norcross & M. R. Goldfried (Eds.), *Handbook of psychotherapy integration* (pp. 94–129). New York, NY: Wiley.

Main, M. (2000). The organized categories of infant, child, and adult attachment: flexible vs. inflexible attention under attachment-related stress, *Journal of the American Psychoanalytic Association, 48*(4), 1055–1096.

Main, M. & Solomon, J. (1986). Discovery of a new, insecure-disorganized/disoriented attachment pattern. In M. Yogman & T. B. Brazelton (Eds.), *Affective development in infancy* (pp. 95–124). Norwood, NJ: Ablex.

McIntosh, H. B. & Johnson, S. (2008). Emotionally focused therapy for couples and childhood sexual abuse survivors. *Journal of Marital and Family Therapy, 34*(3), 298–315.

Quinton, D., Pickles, A., Maughan, B. & Rutter, M. (1993). Partners, peers and pathways: assortative pairing and continuities in conduct disorder. *Development and Psychopathology, 5,* 763–783.

Satir, V., Banmen, J., Gerber, J. & Gomori, M. (1991). *The Satir model: family therapy and beyond.* Palo Alto, CA: Science and Behavior Books.

Shin, H., Park, Y.-J. & Kim, M. J. (2006). Predictors of maternal sensitivity during the early post-partum period. *Journal of Advanced Nursing, 55*(4), 425–434.

Sroufe, L. A. & Waters, E. (1977). Heart rate as a convergent measure in clinical and developmental research. *Merrill-Palmer Quarterly of Behavior and Development, 23,* 3–27.

Stavrianopoulos, K., Faller, G. & Furrow, J. L. (2014). Emotionally focused family therapy: facilitating change within a family system. *Journal of Couple & Relationship Therapy, 13*(1), 25–43.

Vatcher, C. A. & Bogo, M. (2001). The feminist/emotionally focused therapy practice model: an integrated approach for couple therapy. *Journal of Marital and Family Therapy, 27*(1), 69–83

Vaughn, B. E. & Bost, K. K. (2016). Attachment and temperament as intersecting developmental products and interacting developmental contexts throughout infancy and childhood. In J. Cassidy & P. Shaver (Eds.), *Handbook of attachment: theory, research, and clinical applications* (3rd ed., pp. 202–222). New York, NY: Guilford Press.

Wampold, B. E. (2001). *The great psychotherapy debate: models, methods, and findings.* Mahwah, NJ: Erlbaum.

Weissman, N., Batten, S. V., Rheem, K. D., Wiebe, S. A., Pasillas, R. M., Potts, W., Brown, C. H. & Dixon, L. B. (2018). The effectiveness of emotionally focused couples therapy with veterans with PTSD: a pilot study. *Journal of Couple and Relationship Therapy, 17*(1), 25–41.

Werner, E.E. & Smith, R.S. (1992). *Overcoming the odds: high risk children from birth to adulthood.* Ithaca, NY: Cornell University Press.

Wiebe, S. A. & Johnson, S. M. (2016). A review of the research in emotionally focused therapy for couples. *Family Process, 55*(3), 390–407.

14 Gottman Method Couple's Therapy

Amanda Veldorale-Griffin

Introduction

The Gottman Method is a model of couple therapy that is based on the research of John and Julie Gottman. It emphasizes the importance of building a strong foundation of friendship and positive sentiment in relationships (Gottman & Gottman, 2017). The model is directive and includes a strong focus on assessment, psychoeducation and skills training. It is an active therapeutic model that engages clients in experiential learning and practice of new skills and ways of interacting with their partner (Penner, 2017). However, that is outside the scope of this chapter, which will focus exclusively on the Gottman Method for working with couples.

Founders

The Gottman Method was founded by Dr. John Gottman. Dr. Gottman is a clinical psychologist with a degree from The University of Wisconsin (The Gottman Institute, 2019a) and the co-founder of the Gottman Institute, with his wife and fellow clinical psychologist, Dr. Julie Gottman. He began working with and conducting extensive research with couples in the 1980s and founded the Gottman Institute, focused on couples therapy work, in 1996. In 2002, he also became the Executive Director for the Relationship Research Institute in Seattle, Washington (The Gottman Institute, 2019a). He has published numerous journal articles and books on the subject of marriage and creating strong marital bonds.

Dr. Julie Gottman, the co-founder of the Gottman Institute, is also a clinical psychologist (The Gottman Institute, 2019a). She began to work and conduct research with couples in 2004. In 2002, she became the Clinical Director of The Relationship Research Institute and began to train therapists in Gottman Method Couple's Therapy. She also is a Clinical Assistant Professor at the University of Washington and has published many research articles and co-authored several books on marital relationships (The Gottman Institute, 2019a).

Systemic foundation

Although not derived out of marriage and family therapy theories, the Gottman Method is at its core a dyadic approach. As such, it lends itself well to a systemic viewpoint. There are several systemic concepts that we can see inherent in this model. These are interdependence of subsystems, wholism, circular causality and context (Watzlawick, Weakland & Fisch, 1974).

DOI: 10.4324/9781003382621-17

Circular causality

Couples develop patterns of interacting, as well as both implicit and explicit rules for how they communicate and manage conflict. These tend to develop over time and are reinforced by the responses each partner receives from the other. As a result, interactions are circular in nature, with no single behavior causing another. This can create both positive interactions, as well as negative ones. On the positive side, couples may develop family rules to bring them closer together, such as setting aside time each day to share positives and talk about concerns. On the negative side, couple interactions can reinforce negative patterns and create problems for the couple. For example, if there is a couple where one partner tends to be distant and one tends to criticize, they may inadvertently reinforce the negative patterns of interaction in one another. In this scenario, Partner A may feel distant from Partner B and criticize him for this, which may lead to further distancing and defensiveness by Partner B, which leads to increased criticism and lashing out by Partner A. This cycle continues to be perpetuated in patterns of circular causality (Watzlawick et al., 1974). Neither partner is the sole cause of the issue, which helps to remove blame from the discussion.

Wholism

Viewing each person and their behaviors as part of a larger system (wholism) helps the Gottman therapist to shift couples from criticizing or contemptuous language aimed at personality characteristics (e.g., lazy, disrespectful, selfish) to focusing on specific behavioral concerns.

Context

The idea of context is another crucial concept in the Gottman Method. Context is considered both internally and externally. That is, it is important to consider what is going on with a couple at both an interpersonal level, as well as an intrapersonal level. It is this idea that provides the basis for the extensive assessment process that is part of this approach. Therapists must consider the history of each member of the couple, understand their hopes, dreams and fears, and assess for their level of "emotional flooding" or physiological overload they are experiencing in a particular moment (Penner, 2017).

Main concepts and philosophical underpinnings

The Gottman Method is based on the research conducted by John and Julie Gottman and the Gottman Institute on couple interactions. From their research, Drs. Gottman developed the Sound Relationship House Theory. This theory undergirds the therapeutic model. This theory posits that there are **seven key elements** in creating a strong relationship or "sound relationship house" and that these elements are supported by trust and commitment. The seven building blocks of the sound relationship house are: (a) building love maps; (b) sharing fondness and admiration; (c) turning toward instead of away; (d) the positive perspective; (e) managing conflict; (f) making life dreams come true; and (g) creating shared meaning (Gottman & Gottman, 2017).

Building love maps is about helping partners understand one another's interests and inner world and to help partners to feel known by one another. The second part of the relationship house focuses on helping couples to value their partner's qualities. The third portion, turning toward, is about building emotional connections between partners and expressing needs to one another.

When those three levels of the relationship house are solid, it creates a positive perspective or positive sentiment override. That is, partners view one another in a positive light, highlight their partner's good qualities, minimize partner's less desirable traits and engage in relationship reinforcing thoughts (Gottman & Gottman, 2017). When it comes to dealing with conflict, Gottman posited that the majority of conflicts between partners were unsolvable and that what mattered in maintaining a positive relationship was not how those problems were solved, but the way they were discussed when they came up (Gottman & Gottman, 2017).

The sixth part of the sound relationship house is making life dreams come true. This is about partners connecting to each other's dreams. Even within conflict, dreams exist (and can often be at the core of a conflict). It is important for couples to discuss and validate the dreams of their partner (Gottman & Gottman, 2017). The last level of the sound relationship house is creating shared meaning. This is about making connections and can include both formal and informal rituals that bring partners close to one another. It is also about helping couples to support each other in their roles, discussing their values and creating mutual goals (Gottman & Gottman, 2017). Trust and commitment are seen as forming the sides of this house that help to hold it all up. Trust is the idea of knowing that your partner has your best interests in mind. Commitment refers to acting in accordance with a belief that your relationship is lifelong (Gottman & Gottman, 2017).

Basic assumptions and conceptualization of issues

The Gottman Method is a couple's therapy approach. It is grounded in the assumption that a couple's issues are relational and need to be treated within the context of the dyad (Gottman, 1999). The model is also heavily influenced by cognitive behavioral therapy (CBT) and its underlying assumption that cognitions, affect and behavior are all inherently linked and are mutually influential (Epstein & Baucom, 2002; Dattilio, 2010). Because of its roots in CBT, the Gottman model focuses on having couples act differently with one another in order to shift their thoughts about their partner and their relationship. Related to this, it is assumed that therapy should be a positive emotional experience for couples and that the Gottman therapist should model non-critical or blaming language in their approach (Gottman, 1999).

In addition to being heavily influenced by CBT, the Gottman Method also has a strong experiential component. The main assumption of experiential therapy is that change occurs when people have new emotional experiences with one another in the moment during the therapy process (e.g., Napier & Whitaker, 1967; Satir & Bitter, 1991). In this vein, one underlying assumption of the Gottman Method is that couples need to engage in conversations where emotions are heightened and that they need to institute new skills during these conversations in order for change to occur (Gottman, 1999). Related to this is the assumption that all emotions and needs are valid and should be expressed and understood. It is the way in which this is done that determines whether an interaction is productive or unproductive (Penner, 2017).

How change occurs

Change occurs primarily through increasing couples' positive interactions during conflict (Gottman, 1999). Gottman's (1999) research with couples suggests that one of the key factors that differentiates couples who stay together from couples who divorce is the ratio of positive to negative interactions they experience in their relationship. This work is done through the practice of skills related to becoming aware of negative interactional patterns, improving communication and problem-solving, increasing positive affect and creating shared meaning in the relationship (Gottman & Gottman, 2017). The assumption is made that no other change can occur if couples are engaging in negative sentiment override (i.e., hyperfocusing on negative aspects of their partner or their relationship), making addressing this a vital component of the change process (Penner, 2017). Gottman therapists provide psychoeducation to clients around the research on the positive to negative interaction ratio and work with them to increase the positive interactions they have with one another during conflict (Penner, 2017).

Role of the client

Clients are expected to take an active role in their treatment. Couples are expected to practice the skills they are being taught and to generalize what they are learning to other areas of conflict within their relationship. They are expected to be committed to the relationship and willing to do the work required of them. Another role of the client is also to express their emotions and be open to the affective process of therapy.

Role of the therapist

The Gottman therapist acts as a coach for the couple. The therapist's job is to provide the couple with the tools they need to improve their communication and relationship intimacy. The Gottman therapist seeks to empower couples to use these tools on their own and to generate their own solutions based on the skills they have learned (Gottman, 1999). The Gottman Method starts with an in-depth assessment of the couple's strengths, challenges, presenting problem and history. This initial intake is done with the couple conjointly. After that, the therapist will meet with each partner individually to further assess important family history, each partner's level of commitment, any betrayals (including infidelity or abuse) and to administer questionnaires (Penner, 2017). From there, the therapist will bring the couple back together for ongoing conjoint sessions. The therapist will discuss the assessment with the couple and give them feedback on areas of strength and areas of growth.

Additionally, the therapist introduces the couple to the research base for the model and the Sound Relationship House Theory (Penner, 2017). At this point, the couple works with the therapist to create treatment goals and therapy proceeds into the intervention stage.

Interventions

Gottman Method interventions each have a specific structure. If you'd like to learn more about the unique way these methods are laid out, a great resource is Gottman's text, The marriage clinic: a scientifically based marital therapy.

Love maps

This intervention consists of the therapist asking the couple a series of questions designed to generate conversation about one another and help couples to get to know each other better. Some couples may already know each other well, leading the therapist to move past this intervention to focus on other areas first (Penner, 2017). Love map questions may touch on subjects such as getting to know about one another's friends, hobbies, important life events, stresses, worries and hopes (Gottman, 1999).

Addressing the Four Horsemen of the Apocalypse

Problems with couples are conceptualized as occurring due to a breakdown or failure to build a strong friendship base. When this occurs, couples can begin to engage in negative patterns of interaction known as the Four Horsemen because of their strong correlation with relationship dissolution (The Gottman Institute, 2019b). An important part of Gottman Couple's Therapy is to identify and label these destructive patterns as they occur. The Four Horsemen are criticism, contempt, stonewalling and defensiveness. Criticism refers to attacks couples make against who their partner is.

Contempt, which Gottman has identified as the most toxic of the Four Horsemen (The Gottman Institute, 2019b), refers to insults or other attacks that are designed to wound a partner's sense of self. Defensiveness means taking on the role of victim and shifting the blame from one's self to one's partner. Stonewalling is withdrawal from conflict and creating distance between one's self and one's partner.

Once couples are able to identify the negative patterns in which they are engaging, they can work to ameliorate them. Each of the Four Horsemen has an accompanying antidote

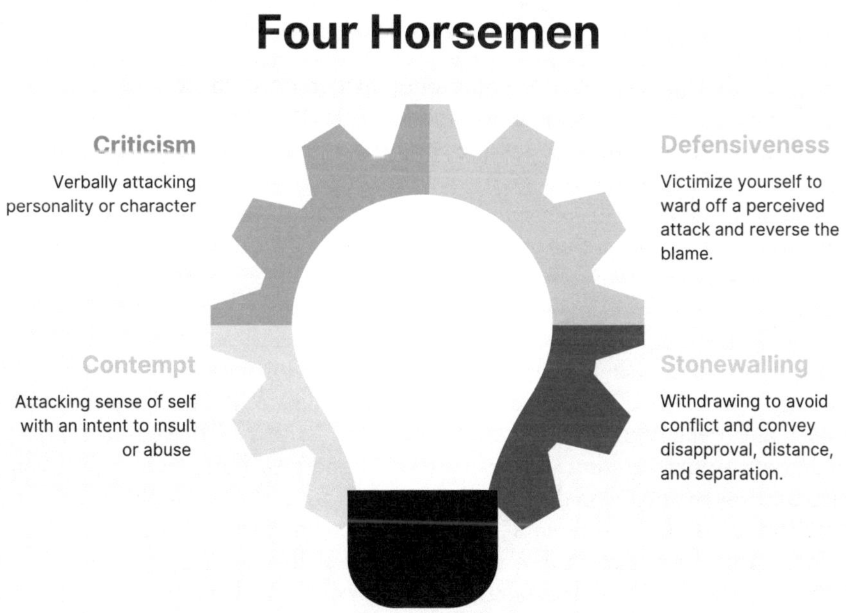

Four Horsemen

Criticism
Verbally attacking
personality or character

Defensiveness
Victimize yourself to
ward off a perceived
attack and reverse the
blame.

Contempt
Attacking sense of self
with an intent to insult
or abuse

Stonewalling
Withdrawing to avoid
conflict and convey
disapproval, distance,
and separation.

Figure 14.1 Four Horsemen Infographic.

(Gottman Institute, 2019b). To combat criticism, couples need to employ a gentle or softened start up. This was described in further detail above. To stop contempt, couples need to create an atmosphere of regard in their relationship. That is, they need to focus on the positive characteristics and behaviors of their partner and express gratitude for those. To work against defensiveness, couples need to take responsibility for their actions, be open to their partner's viewpoint and apologize for any transgression. Finally, to combat stonewalling, couples need to engage in "physiological self-soothing" (2019b, para 4). That is, they need to take a time-out and engage in relaxing activities.

Soften startup

Engaging in harsh startup is one of the key variables noted by Gottman (1999) that can accurately predict the likelihood of a couple divorcing. In heterosexual marriages, Gottman found that the use of harsh startup by wives was particularly likely to lead to divorce. Given this data, one area that Gottman therapists are apt to focus on is teaching couples how to engage in softened startup. There are eight key components to a softened startup: (a) be concise; (b) eliminate blame; (c) begin with the positive; (d) speak from your own point of view; (e) be specific in what happened; (f) be specific about what you need; (f) be kind and appreciative; and (g) expressing primary emotions (Gottman, 1999). Taken together, couples engaging in softened startup begin conversations with something they appreciate about their partner or something that is going well, are brief in explaining specifically what their complaint is and what they wish their partner would do differently, and explain how they feel in the current situation. This should all be done using "I" statements and avoiding placing judgment or blame on their partner.

Gottman-Rapoport exercise

This is a speaker-listener exercise in which one partner must show understanding of the other's position before they can take on the speaker role (Penner, 2017). Within the exercise, there are defined roles for both the speaker and listener. It is the speaker's job to express her thoughts, feelings and needs in a gentle way without resorting to the Four Horsemen. It is the listener's job to engage in focused listening in order to truly understand her partner's experience and then to express this understanding to her partner (Penner, 2017).

Dreams-within-conflict

This intervention is used when couples become stuck (Gottman, 1999). This is likely to occur with particular "gridlock issues" (Penner, 2017, p. 35). These are issues that are revisited over and over without any conclusion. Discussions of these issues are typically devoid of humor, understanding, warmth or willingness to compromise (Penner, 2017). Rather than address the problem directly, the therapist focuses the couple on understanding each other's "hopes, dreams, and fears" (2017, p. 36) related to that particular area of contention. This is done by engaging in a modified speaker-listener activity in which partners are prompted to interview one another about their core values and needs that are driving their unwillingness to budge on the issue. It is important to note that the goal here is not necessarily to "solve" the problem, but instead to seek a compromise, which can then be evaluated and adjusted.

Negotiating marital power

Gottman (1999) has a comprehensive checklist related to gender roles and division of labor (pp. 298–300). This checklist is used to help the therapist assist the couple in understanding and appreciating one another's roles and responsibilities. It can also be used to help the couple develop their own agreement of the division of labor and arrive at a shared meaning of what is fair in their relationship.

Case example

A couple, Joe (38) and Arthur (42), present for couples therapy. They report they have been together for 12 years and married for five years. They have two children, Jessie age 8 and Page age 4. They state that, since the birth of their younger child, they have struggled to connect with one another and that, in the past few months, they "fight all the time". Arthur describes Joe as "always too busy with other stuff to care about what I need". He seems to blame Joe for their problems and tends to describe Joe's behaviors in terms of "always" and "never". Joe frequently rolls his eyes and shakes his head while Arthur is talking.

Questions:

1. What Horsemen can you identify in this case?
2. How might the birth of their second child have affected the marital power in their relationship?
3. What interventions might you use to help this couple address their concerns?

Example intervention approach:

Throughout the first several sessions, the therapist gathers a detailed relationship history from clients from when they first met until present. They are asked to identify first impressions and significant events in their relationship. The therapist asks them about their roles within the relationship, division of labor and their hopes, dreams and fears about their relationship and their communication. An in-depth family history is also gathered during this assessment process. Additionally, the therapist asks the couple to spend about ten minutes discussing an issue in their relationship. They choose to talk about household chores. The conflict escalates quickly, and the pattern of blame and defensiveness is readily apparent. The therapist then provides feedback to the couple about the assessment and results from measures administered during this phase, as well as psychoeducation to the couple about the Four Horsemen. The therapist instructs Joe not to engage in eye rolling or head shaking while Arthur is talking and tells Arthur to focus on single complaints with requested solutions, rather than engaging in the use of "always" and "never". The therapist then leads the couple in a "dream within conflict" exercise. The therapist explains that they will be engaging in a speaker-listener exercise and that the therapist will only intervene to keep the dialogue progressing. The therapist lets them know that the purpose of the exercise is to help them better understand each other and the meanings surrounding the problem for each of them. They are instructed not to problem-solve at this time.

Joe is given a sheet of questions to ask Arthur and the therapist helps to keep him on track, as needed. Arthur expresses that he feels abandoned by Joe and thinks Joe must not really care about him because he "never makes time" for him. Joe quickly becomes defensive, and the therapist refocuses them both on the task. Joe is able to uncover that Arthur's dream is that he and Joe will be able to spend quality time together and enjoy each other's company like they used to. The therapist has them switch roles, so that Arthur is now asking questions of Joe. Arthur's questions begin to come off as overly harsh or blaming and the therapist intervenes to keep him to the list. In this process, Joe expresses that he feels hurt that he can't do anything to make Arthur happy and hopeless about even trying. He tells Arthur that his dream is that they will be able to smile and laugh together again. The therapist highlights their shared dreams as the foundation of their sound relationship house.

Termination of therapy

Termination of therapy is deemed appropriate with couples able to show a consistent ability to apply the problem-solving and communication tools they have learned in therapy, not necessarily when they are done working on improving their marriage (Gottman, 1999). Couples should be able to develop their own methods of addressing conflict based on their work in therapy. Other markers that a couple is ready for termination include (Gottman, 1999):

- they are having more positive interactions with one another than negative ones
- the Four Horsemen of the Apocalypse have significantly reduced
- they are using communication tools to deal with solvable problems (e.g., using softened startups, accepting influence from one another)

They are able to engage in dialogue about perpetual problems rather than feeling stuck.

Key legal and ethical considerations

The Gottman Method is a therapeutic model that has its own certification.

Therapists can become Certified Gottman therapists by completing specialized training through the Gottman Institute. There are four levels of training required in order to complete certification (The Gottman Institute, 2019a). Because of the intensive training required to become a Certified Gottman therapist, it is important that therapist who have not undergone this training do not promote or advertise themselves as Gottman therapists. This is not to say that therapists who are not certified cannot make use of Gottman's methods. However, adhering to Standard 9.1 of the AAMFT Code of Ethics (AAMFT, 2015) regarding accurately presenting ones competencies, education and training, it is important that therapists do not claim certifications they have not obtained.

As with any model, it is important to address situations in which the Gottman Method may be contraindicated. This model is not recommended for couples where there is an ongoing extramarital affair (Gottman & Gottman, 2016) or in situations of domestic violence where power and control tactics are pervasive (Stith, McCollum, Amanor-Boadu & Smith, 2012). Additionally, further research is needed into the model's utility in working with couples from lower socioeconomic backgrounds, as some research suggests that these couples may interpret interactions differently than is suggested by Gottman's model (Kim, Capaldi & Crosby, 2007) and thus the Gottman Method might not be appropriate or may require modifications to be useful to these clients.

Use with a diversity of clients

The current literature on the Gottman Method supports its use with diverse couple populations. Garanzini et al. (2017) demonstrated the effectiveness of using Gottman Method Couples Therapy with gay and lesbian couples. Their research showed that couples experienced significantly enhance relationship satisfaction over the course of 11 weeks of therapy. In their work with gay, lesbian and heterosexual couples, Gottman et al. (2003a; 2003b) observed some differences in the ways that couples approached conflict, which have important ramifications for therapists working with same-sex couples. One dynamic they noted was that same-sex couples tend to be more positive in broaching issues with one another. Related to this, same-sex partners also tended to use more humor than heterosexual partners. Furthermore, when both partners are positive in what they are communicating, lesbian partners tended to be more stable in their interactions with one another than were gay or heterosexual couples. When it came to making repair attempts, gay male couples tended to be less effective than did lesbian or heterosexual couples. Finally, same-sex couples were more effective at decreasing inappropriate levity in a situation. These results suggest that therapists employing the Gottman Method may be more effective by focusing more heavily in certain areas (such as repair work for gay male couples) depending on their populations.

In addition to working with sexual minority clients, the Gottman Method has been shown to be effective in improving marital relationships with couples from other diverse backgrounds. It has been used with success in non-U.S. populations (Davoodvandi, Nejad & Farzad, 2018;), where it has been demonstrated to be effective in improving relationship satisfaction. Bermúdez and Stinson (2011) created five additional couple typologies for Latino couples based on Gottman's Marital Conflict Scale. This suggests that there may be other aspects of couple relationships for some populations, which are not sufficiently addressed by Gottman's model. More research needs to be conducted with diverse populations to determine the efficacy of the model with these populations, as well as to explore adjustments that would support more effective work with diverse populations.

The Gottman Method does not overtly integrate components of cultural competence and humility, so there are several principles that need to be integrated in the implementation of this model. Because of this, therapists working from this model need to be especially intentional about engaging in self-of-the-therapist work. Therapists need to be mindful of how couple dynamics can be influenced by cultural values and experiences of discrimination, marginalization or privilege (Falicov, 2007). Therapists also need to be aware of their personal beliefs about couple or relationship dynamics and how this might be similar or different to the beliefs of their clients (Fisher-Borne et al., 2015; Mosher et al., 2017). This may include exploring beliefs about intimacy, sex, gender, same-sex relationships, polyamory and many other topics relevant to intimate relationships. When clients and therapists have differences, extra care should be taken in building and maintaining the therapeutic alliance. Particularly, therapists need to address any ruptures that may occur when navigating differences (Mosher et al., 2017). This may look different depending on the clients and the type of rupture but involves acknowledging the wound and discussing with clients their experience of the situation and how they would like to address it.

Self-of-the-therapist reflection questions

1. What do healthy boundaries look like in intimate relationships?
2. What are your beliefs about gender roles in couples/partnerships?
3. Who were your role models for intimate relationships? What did you learn from those?
4. What are your beliefs about sex and sexuality? How comfortable are you discussing these topics in therapy?

Research support

Somewhat uniquely in the therapy world, the Gottman model was born out of research rather than theory. As such, it has a strong research base. Founders John and Julie Gottman began studying couples in the Gottman Lab in the 1970s (Gottman Institute, 2019a). This research helped determine what distressed couples looked like compared to nondistressed couples, which led to the development of Gottman Method Couples Therapy (Gottman, 2008). So, the specific interventions were designed based on what they learned about couples who stay together vs. those who do not.

While interventions are based in research on couple dynamics, the model is not considered an empirically supported treatment since research on the implementation of the interventions with couples is limited. However, some research has been conducted to examine the effectiveness of the model in creating long-lasting change.

Gottman Method Couples Therapy has been shown to improve marital adjustment and relationship intimacy and research suggests that these improvements endure over time (Davoodvandi, et al., 2018). It has also been shown to be effective in decreasing marital burnout and improving couples' approach to conflict resolution (Havaasi, Kaar & MohsenZadeh, 2018). Additionally, while the model is not recommended for cases of domestic terrorism, it has been shown to be effective in treating couples who engage in mutually violent or situational violence (Bradley, Drummey, Gottman & Gottman, 2014; Bradley & Gottman, 2012). The Gottman Method has also been incorporated in couples' workshops, which have shown to be effective in improving marital satisfaction and decreasing conflict (Babcock, Gottman, Ryan & Gottman, 2013). Another area in which the Gottman Method has been shown to be effective is improving communication and increasing positive sentiment in couples following the birth of their first child (Shapiro, Gottman & Fink, 2015).

References

AAMFT (2015). *Code of ethics*. [online] Available at: www.aamft.org/iMIS15/AAMFT/Content/Legal_Ethics/Code_of_Ethics.aspx

Babcock, J. C., Gottman, J. M., Ryan, K. D. & Gottman, J. S. (2013). A component analysis of a brief psycho-educational couples' workshop: one-year follow-up results. *Journal of Family Therapy, 35*, 252–280.

Bermúdez, J. M. & Stinson, M. A. (2011). Redefining conflict resolution styles for Latino couples: examining the role of gender and culture. *Journal of Feminist Family Therapy, 23*, 71–87.

Bradley, R. P. C., Drummey, K. Gottman, J. M. & Gottman, J. S. (2014). Treating couples who mutually exhibit violence or aggression: reducing behaviors that show a susceptibility for violence. *Journal of Family Violence, 29*(5), 549–558.

Bradley, R. P. C. & Gottman, J. M. (2012). Reducing situational violence in low-income couples by fostering healthy relationships. *Journal of Marital and Family Therapy, 38*, 187–198.

Dattilio, F. M. (2010). *Cognitive-behavioral therapy with couples and families*. New York, NY: Guilford Publications.

Davoodvandi, M., Nejad, S. N. & Farzad, V. (2018). Examining the effectiveness of Gottman Couple Therapy on improving marital adjustment and couples' intimacy. *Iranian Journal of Psychiatry, 13*(2), 136–142.

Epstein, N. B. & Baucom, D. H. (2002). Enhanced cognitive-behavioral therapy for couples: a contextual approach. APA: APA PsycNet. https://doi.org/10.1037/10481-000

Falicov, C. J. (2007). Working with transnational immigrants: expanding meanings of family, community, and culture. *Family Process, 46*(2), 157–171.

Fisher-Borne, M., Cain, J. M. & Martin, S. L. (2015). From mastery to accountability: cultural humility as an alternative to cultural competence. *Social Work Education, 34*(2), 165–181.

Garanzini, S., Yee, A., Gottman, J., Gottman, J., Cole, C. Preciado, M. & Jasculca, C. (2017). Results of Gottman Method Couples Therapy with gay and lesbian couples. *Journal of Marital and Family Therapy, 43*(4), 674–684.

Gottman, J. M. (1999). *The marriage clinic: a scientifically based marital therapy*. New York, NY: Norton.

Gottman, J. M. (2008). Gottman method couple therapy. *Clinical handbook of couple therapy, 4*(8), 138–164.

Gottman, J. & Gottman, J. (2016) *Treating affairs and trauma: a Gottman approach for therapists on the treatment of affairs and posttraumatic stress*. Seattle, WA: The Gottman Institute.

Gottman, J. & Gottman, J. (2017). The natural principles of love. *Journal of Family Theory and Review, 9*, 7–26.

Gottman, J. M., Levenson, R. W., Gross, J., Frederickson, B. L., McCoy, K., Rosenthal, L., Ruef, A. & Yoshimoto, D. (2003a). Correlates of gay and lesbian couples' relationship satisfaction and relationship dissolution. *Journal of Homosexuality, 45*(1), 23–43.

Gottman, J. M., Levenson, R. W., Swanson, C., Swanson, K., Tyson, R. & Yoshimoto, D. (2003b). Observing gay, lesbian, and heterosexual couples' relationships. *Journal of Homosexuality, 45*(1), 65–91.

The Gottman Institute (2019a). *John and Julie Gottman*. Retrieved February 28, 2019 from www.gottman.com/about/john-julie-gottman/

The Gottman Institute (2019b). *The Four Horsemen*. Retrieved March 7, 2019 from www.gottman.com/blog/category/column/the-four-horsemen/

Havaasi, N., Kaar, K. Z. & Mohsen Zadeh, F. (2018). Compare the efficacy of emotion focused couple therapy and Gottman couple therapy method in marital burnout and changing conflict resolution styles. *Journal of Fundamentals of Mental Health, 20*(1), 15–25.

Kim, H. K., Capaldi, D. M. & Crosby, L. (2007). Generalizability of Gottman and colleagues' affective proves models of couples' relationship outcomes. *Journal of Marriage and Family, 69*(1), 55–72.

Mosher, D. K., Hook, J. N., Captari, L. E., Davis, D. E., DeBlaere, C. & Owen, J. (2017). Cultural humility: a therapeutic framework for engaging diverse clients. *Practice Innovations, 2*(4), 221–233.

Napier, A. Y. & Whitaker, C. A. (1967). *The family crucible: the intense experience of family therapy*. New York, NY: Bantam Books.

Penner, D. R. (2017). Clinical application of "the natural principles of love." *Journal of Family Theory and Review, 9*, 33–38.

Satir, V., & Bitter, J. (1991). The therapist and family therapy: Satir's human validation process model. In A. M. Horne & J. L. Passmore (Eds.), *Family therapy and counseling*. Itasca, Illinois: F.E. Peacock, 13–45.

Shapiro, A. F., Gottman, J. M. & Fink, B. C. (2015). Short-term change in couples' conflict following a transition to parenthood intervention. *Couple and Family Psychology, Research, and Practice, 4*(4), 239–251.

Stith, S. M., McCollum, E. E., Amanor-Boadu, Y. & Smith, D. (2012). Systemic perspectives on intimate partner violence treatment. *Journal of Marital and Family Therapy, 38*(1), 220–240.

Watzlawick, P., Weakland, J. H. & Fisch, R. (1974). *Change: principles of problem formation and problem resolution.* New York, NY: W. W. Norton & Company.

15 Contextual Therapy

Aurélia Bickler

Introduction

As a psychiatrist with psychoanalytic training, Ivan Boszormenyi-Nagy (pronounced: *Bah-zor-men-yee Nahj*) aimed to understand the biochemical elements of Schizophrenia. However, after multiple unsuccessful attempts, he and his colleagues shifted their focus to psychological and behavioral components and found resonance in the core of a system throughout multiple generations. In other words, this model focuses on the idea that we may be products of the cross-generational impacts of our family system. If you can, think about who you are and how you came to that… Do you possibly fight a cause as a response to an ancestor's battle (for the same cause)? Do you remember encountering a sense of injustice in your upbringing and perhaps find it challenging to focus on how to make it just for the one to come? Nagy found that so much of who we are is to be explored through this systemic and cross-generational lens.

After emigrating from Hungary in 1948, Nagy founded the Eastern Pennsylvania Psychiatric Institute (EPPI) in Philadelphia in 1957 as a way to research Schizophrenia. After a funding freeze from the State, the EPPI closed its doors in 1980 and Nagy and his colleagues continued their development of this model at the Hahnemann University Medical School (Goldenberg & Goldenberg, 2013).

Nagy's father was a judge, making the concept of fairness and balance of significant importance to him. As one of the developing models and pillars of Marriage and Family Therapy (MFT), Contextual Therapy centered around the idea of reciprocity, fairness, connectedness and justice within relationships (Ewijk, 2017). According to this model, individuals maintain a ledger throughout their lives that helps them keep track of the fairness in give and take between themselves and their family members. This plays a role in their sense of entitlement in relation to what they deem is due to them from others within the system, both objectively (in comparison to others and the world) and subjectively (in comparison to what they've "given" to others in the system) (Boszormenyi-Nagy, 1987; Boszormenyi-Nagy & Krasner, 1986). According to this model, cases should be conceptualized, assessed and treated, with the intention to bring back fairness and balance within families (Boszormenyi-Nagy, 1987).

Founders

Nagy (1920–2007), a psychoanalytically trained psychiatrist, emigrated from Hungary to the U.S. in the late 1940s. He is considered one of the pioneers of Contextual Therapy

DOI: 10.4324/9781003382621-18

(Boszormenyi-Nagy, 1987; Watson, 2007; Wilburn-McCoy, 1993. Nagy was the founder of the Institute for Contextual Growth and provided training in the Contextual Therapy Approach. For some time, he and his colleagues worked on figuring out the psychological and behavioral elements of Schizophrenia until they turned their focus to transgenerational issues within systems (Goldenberg & Goldenberg, 2013). Psychologist David Ulrich (1998), and the founder's wife Catherine Ducommun-Nagy (1999), also contributed to the model.

Brief history of the model

Contextual Therapy has been influenced by several earlier models and concepts.

Mainly, Fairbairn's object relations theory, which focuses on the process of psyche formation in relation to others, and Sullivan's interpersonal psychiatry, which focuses on how interactions provide insight on both causes and treatment for mental disorders (Fairbairn,1952; Sullivan, 1953). These two theories played a significant role in the foundation and construction of this model (Boszormenyi-Nagy, 1987; Goldenberg & Goldenberg, 2013). The essence of the model focuses on the equilibrium of give and take within relationships across generations, and it emphasizes ethics, trust, fairness, loyalty, entitlements and indebtedness between family members across generations (Boszormenyi-Nagy, 1987). On a more holistic level, the founder defines the focus of the model as "the dynamic foundation of viable, continuing, close relationships" (Boszormenyi-Nagy & Krasner, 1986, p. 417).

Philosophical underpinnings

Contextual Therapy focuses on the balance between the individual psychology (intrapsychic) of each family member and the relational and intergenerational elements that connect them to one another. According to Boszormenyi-Nagy, Grunebaum and Ullrich, (1991):

> The contextual orientation assumes that the "leverages" of all psychotherapeutic interventions are anchored in relational determinants, and that a comprehensive approach addresses these determinants in terms of the four interlocking dimensions of (1) facts, (2) individual psychology, (3) behavioral transactions, and (4) relational ethics. While we speak of relational determinants for therapy, the contextual approach never loses sight of the goal of benefiting persons, as well as promoting change within systems.
>
> (p. 201)

Let's take a closer look at these four dimensions:

Facts: gender, ethnicity, potential birth defects and life experiences, such as divorce within the family, abuse, illness, etc.

Individual psychology: thoughts, emotions, dreams, fantasies and any other internal processes that take place within a person's mind, along with the meaning behind those in relation to the context of their lives.

Behavioral transactions: within a family, there are patterns that contribute to the system's sequence. For example, triangles and hierarchy have a significant role in the system's transactional sequence.

Relational ethics: each family member's interests being considered by each family member in order to maintain a long-term level of fairness within the family system. This promotes a sense of connectedness and consideration within the system.

Integrating these promotes connectedness and accountability for each family member, keeping each member ethically responsible for their contributions to the system. This also promotes a sense of balance between **entitlements** (what they feel is due to them) and **indebtedness** (what they feel they owe others). (Boszormenyi-Nagy, 1987). Throughout a life, each family member keeps tab of what she or he owes the other family members and what she or he is owed from them. The process of keeping account of such exchanges, according to this model, is known as the **family ledger**.

Another important concept is **loyalty**. This occurs when a family member internalizes expectations or obligations based on how others in the family have treated her or him (Boszormenyi-Nagy, 1987). When unspoken or denied, these loyalties are known as **invisible loyalties**. These often lead to repetition of injustices and unfairness in future generations (Knudson-Martin, 1992). This model also assumes that parents are obligated to take care of their child(ren). In response, children are to have **filial loyalty** toward their parents. This allows children to feel they were fairly cared for and they, therefore, grow to care for their partners and children adequately as an act of indebtedness to their parents (Boszormenyi-Nagy, 1987). At times, children experience what is known as **split filial loyalty**, where they feel their loyalty to one parent is at the expense of the other. This often causes the child to become additionally symptomatic as she or he struggles to get his parents back together. In contrast, when a family member feels that he has given what others needed, he gains merit (Boszormenyi-Nagy, 1987). If children find their parents' degree of care was different but of equal value as that of their siblings, their experience is known as **equitable asymmetry**.

A child that was unloved and perhaps had to care for her parents may in turn expect a partner to nurture her in a parental way. She also may place this role on her own child(ren). This is known as **parentification**. When a child; perhaps abused, manipulated or neglected, feels like he did not receive what he feels was owed to him, he seeks it through other means. Often, the person feels unequally treated and, as a result, acts destructively toward completely unrelated or undeserving victims. For example, a child that was neglected or harmed may want to find a scapegoat to blame or cause distress to. This is known as **destructive entitlement**. This is often seen as a cause for dysfunction (Boszormenyi-Nagy, 1987). At times when these issues go unresolved for generations, the system goes through what is known as the **revolving slate of injustice**, where each generation continues to cause damage to the next innocent generation (Boszormenyi-Nagy, 1987).

As you can see, the contextual model focuses heavily on the relational aspect within families. Through these concepts, Nagy evoked the "innate tendency to care about other people" (Boszormenyi-Nagy & Krasner, 1986; p. 78).

Systemic foundation

A system is defined as a set of entities that are connected to each other through their interactions (Laszlo, 1972). Yet, approaching therapy from a systemic perspective does not mean that you have to work with couples or families in order to apply the concept. Instead, systemic thinking means that you will take into consideration the context of each presenting situation or client no matter how many people are in the room. With this in mind, you can easily observe the world from a systemic perspective by simply paying attention. For example, watching nature around you allows you to see the interactional patterns between beings. This approach allows you to think of each member's individual contribution to the system as a whole, while understanding the interaction itself is an entity of the system. Let's take a closer look at some systemic concepts in relation to the contextual model.

Open system

As a transgenerational and more specifically contextual therapist, taking into consideration the powerful influences of past generations are important to understand the presenting "problem". Specifically, the relationships between the presenting system (the client) and the ones that preceded them (previous generations) allows the client to better understand and improve the relationships both in the present and the future. This communication process between the system and the surrounding **suprasystems** (or contextual entities), allowing information to flow in and out of it, define an **open system** (Minuchin, 1985). The relational element is key as the core of the model speaks of "ethical give and take" that occurs between members within a system. Nagy promoted a sense of fairness and balance across the generations, requiring the system to be open (Boszormenyi-Nagy, 1987).

Rules

Family systems all have rules that help both stabilize the system and manage change (Watzlawick, Bavelas & Jackson, 1967). This implies that there is a certain sense of order within a system that contributes to each participating role. From a contextual perspective, these roles can be seen in several concepts, such as **loyalties**. Those bring upon the family members a sense of indebtedness based on family placement or previously received care (Boszormenyi-Nagy, 1987).

Homeostasis

Specific to MFT, homeostasis speaks of seeking a desired stability, but even at the expense of the system's needed or desired change (Jackson, 1957). For example, a family may come into therapy, requesting help with their troubled daughter. However, as the therapeutic journey begins and the daughter begins to shift, the family may resist the daughter's positive changes as this means a shift for all participants within the system. According to the Contextual Therapy lens, a **destructive entitlement** can easily become a **revolving slate of injustice** if not addressed or processed, making it extremely difficult for the system to break the multigenerational **homeostasis**.

The whole is greater than the sum of its parts

Whether you are witnessing the different roles that each animal takes on to make the group function or whether you are seeing how a specific animal helps the environment as a whole, by just following its instincts, the systemic idea of **the whole is greater than the sum of its parts** is present (Watzlawick et al., 1967). For example, female lions work as a team to hunt for prey. When the prey is too large (like an elephant or a zebra), the male lions come to help them finalize the task. In contrast, the male lions are responsible to fight for and maintain their territory and protect their females. This requires them to use their strength and size to fight off competition.

Together, the members of the lions' pride and the interactions that keep them connected allows them to achieve greater outcomes, than if each of them worked independently from one another (Lion Facts: 20 Interesting Facts About Lions, 2018). A systemic therapist thinks of the interactions within a system as an entity in itself – one that is not orchestrated by any single system member, thus making the whole greater than the sum of its parts (Bertalanffy, 1968; Davison, 1983; Watzlawick et al., 1967).

Contextual therapy is inherently systemic. The core of this model relies on ethical foundations that are exchanged both within the system and outside of it – even across multiple generations (Boszormenyi-Nagy et al., 1991).

Assessment, treatment and interventions

You may want to note that Contextual Therapy is not about removing any of the presented symptoms or relational interactions. Instead, this model focuses on the ethical consideration and relational balances between family members. To do so, the therapist is responsible for building a level of trust with the family to then explore and utilize family resources in the assessment process. A contextual therapist's goal is to assess possible **invisible loyalties**, in order to address them and rebalance the system. Further, the assessment process of this model encourages open negotiations of ledger issues and explores the loyalty and ledger impasses that may lead to **destructive entitlements**. If the assessment reveals a parent's exploitation of their child's loyalty to the point of **parentification**, the therapist should then guide treatment toward **de-parentification**, allowing the child to return to the intended and preferred role. As the therapeutic process progresses, family members are encouraged to acknowledge and overcome any guilt they may hold onto that stands in the way of their relationships and the balance between the "give and take". By taking ownership of them, the ledgers get reassessed and relationships, hopefully, shift accordingly (Boszormenyi-Nagy, 1987). "The lack of trustworthiness in one's relational world is the primary pathogenic condition of human life" (Boszormenyi-Nagy, 1987, p. 230). Therefore, the ultimate goal of treatment is to help the family move toward regaining mutual trust and rebalancing the system.

Bringing theory into practice

Now that you have an idea about the way this model works, let's do a short exercise. I invite you to think about your own family system, and place some of these concepts within the scale below, based on whether they currently **serve you, owe you** or are of **neutral value** in your life. Let's begin together with a few examples: Have you experienced or witnessed **invisible loyalties** within your family system? Have you witnessed or experienced any **destructive entitlements** or instances of **parentification**? If so, do you believe those might have evoked feelings of **indebtedness** or **entitlement** for you or the person(s) involved?

Let's keep going. I invite you to reflect on the rest of the Contextual Therapy concepts you've learned about and think about how they might impact the systems you currently belong to or are surrounded by.

Is the scale tipping over more heavily on either side? Do specific experiences weigh more heavily than others and therefore tip the scale significantly? How might your personal scale impact your daily interactions with the people in your life? Do you imagine your interpretation matching one or other members of your family? If so, in what ways might that impact your relationships with them, presently? Could that shift in the future? If so, what kind of processing might it take to make a change in your experience?

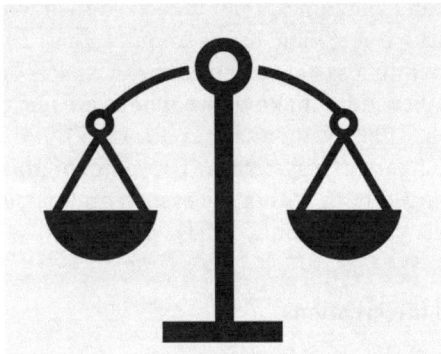

Figure 15.1 Image Illustrating the Concept of the Family Ledger.

I hope you found this exercise helpful. Seeing the impact of our experiences through this exercise can promote clarity for ourselves and the way we interact with other members of our respective systems.

Role(s) of a therapist

The therapist's stance is one that advocates for each family member, including the absent or deceased. The therapist is not to be impartial or neutral, but instead they aim to maintain ***multidirectional partiality***, allowing each member to be heard and advocated for. "Keeping both partners in mind when addressing either of the two" is what allows each partner to feel heard, validated and taken into consideration (Boszormenyi-Nagy, 1987; Friedman, 1989). The therapist's roles also include encouraging negotiations regarding ledger issues, exploration of loyalty and ledger impasses (by exploring personal accountability that results in destructive entitlement), de-parentification and addressing inequities within the system. The therapist is an active guide in helping each individual become aware and accountable for their actions and positions within the system, in relation to fairness. In addition, the therapist pays attention to the political, social and historical contexts of the family. Remembering the personal stance of the therapist is necessary. According to Boszormenyi-Nagy & Krasner (1986):

> Like other therapists, the contextual therapist may well feel sympathy with the victim in a situation. Deep sympathy for other people's suffering probably connects the professional therapist with her own moments of helpless pain, despair and shame. Her alliance with a suffering person is thus likely to be real and honest. It would seem to follow, then, that an alliance with the victim implies an alliance against the victimizer.
>
> (p. 405)

These values come into play as they help the therapists understand their view of fairness and give and take. For example, if a history of abuse or illness exists in the family system, the value system of each family member is likely to have shifted. This is to be taken into consideration (by the therapist) and explored in order to better understand and guide the family system toward their desired goals.

Self of the therapist

Contextual therapists might find it helpful to reflect and process personal ideas around fairness and balance through consultation and supervision. Given that clinicians likely have their own experiences of unfairness and inadequacies within their own family system, processing those feelings and (potential) corresponding biases might be helpful in maintaining the focus on the client's experience.

Contextual family therapy is cerebral in nature and asks for each participant to address the therapist instead of other members of the family, to minimize emotional reactivity. This allows for each partner to internalize the content of the conversation and stay away from blame, while focusing on the personal experience of each family member. Inevitably, that places additional pressure on the therapist to remain centered and neutral through the conversation. Thus, asking of the therapist to reduce facial responses or body language that might evoke judgment or pain onto the clients in the room.

*Let us take the scale exercise a step beyond. I invite you to put your therapist hat on and think about the following: How do you imagine your own experiences and feelings might impact your therapeutic role and position in the therapy room? If the scale is heavier on the side that **serve you**, is it fair to assume you will likely approach the case, feeling confident that fairness or satisfaction are reachable? What if your scale is significantly heavier on the "**owes me**" side? Do you envision as optimistic an outcome? How might these personal feelings shape your questions? And how might those questions then shape the direction of therapy?

Hopefully, this short exercise gave you a sense of how easily therapists might impact the therapeutic process. More importantly, this should be a good reminder that ongoing supervision is essential to ethical and meaningful practice.

Ethical considerations

This model relies heavily on the concept of ethics. After all, Contextual Therapy is largely influenced by the founder's father being a judge. Each person's specific position within the family plays a significant role in the concept of **relational ethics**. Specifically, a contextual therapist needs to remember that fairness may be subjective, and loyalty has multiple meanings. When working with a family system, it is the therapist's responsibility to explore each family member's experience and definitions of these concepts, by maintaining **multidirectional partiality** and take all of these nuanced definitions into consideration. While multidirectional partiality is an essential component in Contextual Therapy, therapists also should be willing to challenge the use of power and privilege to control or marginalize others (Fisher-Borne et al., 2015; Mosher et al., 2017).

As a contextual therapist explores different interactional patterns across generations, they need to consider the cultural shifts that have taken place along the way. For example, gender roles, birth order, abuse or neglect have different meanings based on history and culture. Exploring those meanings within the system allows for the therapist to have greater insight into the particular system.

Cultural/diversity considerations

In addition to considering the more obvious cultural differences such as race, background, language and gender, a therapist needs to remember that each family has a unique culture and identity unto itself. Taking the unique culture of the client system into consideration, a contextual therapist takes time to get to know the specifics of the particular system in order to avoid generalizing based on specific academic concepts. Let's take, for example, a blended family and think about how children from the first marriage may assess their ledger when new children join the newly formed family. How can a therapist take into consideration the multigenerational elements and ensure the relational ethics are taken into consideration? This concept speaks to the ability for each family member to expect their position to be respected and equitable to others in the family. Now that a new parental figure has entered and another may have exited or moved to the side, the therapist may want to help the family members renegotiate what they deem to be fair. It is also important to note that our current society encompasses varying types of family entities. Some historically accepted "norms" may no longer apply. Families' legacies and sense of justice may also be influenced by the larger social context. Therapists should consider how strengths or entitlements are created through experiences from being part of a majority or minority group. Additionally, contextual therapists need to explore how their own cultural context influences their perceptions of fairness and justice in a family system and how their background will affect their perceptions of their clients' systems (Fisher-Borne, Cain, & Martin, 2015; Mosher et al., 2017).

Research support

While several peer-reviewed articles on the topic of Contextual Therapy have been published, there is a limited number of studies that have been conducted on the effectiveness of Contextual Therapy. Because the model is mostly theory with limited instruction for implementing intervention, some recent articles have analyzed tapes of Nagy's sessions and surveyed contextual therapists (van der Meiden, Noordegraaf & van Ewijk, 2019) to get a better sense of how the model is implemented.

While not a direct test of the model, one study found that adolescent mothers in foster care experienced a negative correlation between relational ethics and depression symptoms and physical health symptoms. This highlights that relational ethics may be an important clinical focus for this population (Wilson, Glebova, Davis & Seshadri, 2017).

Summary

The contextual model explores experiences from the past in relation to the present-day functioning within a system. This model allows for each family member to explore their experience of balance and fairness within their family unit across generations. By doing so, family members can revisit their experiences and reconstruct a balanced level of "give and take" within their family unit. Thus, allowing fairness, trust and accountability to be established or reestablished.

References

Bertalanffy, L. V. (1968). *General system theory: foundations, development, applications.* New York, NY: Braziller.

Boszormenyi-Nagy, I. (1987). *Foundations of Contextual Therapy: collected papers of Ivan Boszormenyi-Nagy, MD.* New York, NY: Brunner/Mazel.

Boszormenyi-Nagy, I, Grunebaum, J., Ulrich, D. (1991). Contextual therapy. In A. S. Gurman & D. P. Kniskern (Eds.), *Handbook of family therapy.* New York, NY: Routledge.

Boszormenyi-Nagy, I. & Krasner, B. R. (1986). *Between give and take: a clinical guide to contextual therapy*. New York, NY: Brunner/Mazel.

Davison, M. (1983). *Uncommon sense: the life and thought of Ludwig von Bertalanffy (1901–1972), father of general systems theory*. Los Angeles, CA: J. P. Tarcher.

Ducommun-Nagy, C. (1999). Contextual Therapy. In D. M. Lawson & F. F. Prevatt (Eds.), *Casebook in family therapy*. Pacific Grove, CA: Brooks/Cole.

Ewijk, H. V. (2017). Applying the paradigm of relational ethics into Contextual Therapy. Analyzing the practice of Ivan Boszormenyi-Nagy. *Journal of Marital and Family Therapy, 44*(3), 499–511.

Fairbairn, W. R. D. (1952). *Psychoanalytic studies of the personality*. London, UK: Routledge and Kegan Paul, 1981.

Fisher-Borne, M., Cain, J. M. & Martin, S. L. (2015). From mastery to accountability: cultural humility as an alternative to cultural competence. *Social Work Education, 34*(2), 165–181.

Friedman, M. (1989). Martin Buber and Ivan Boszormenyi-Nagy: the role of dialogue in Contextual Therapy. *Psychotherapy, 24*(3), 402–402.

Goldenberg, H. & Goldenberg, I. (2013). *Family therapy: an overview* (8th ed.). Belmont, CA: Brooks/Cole.

Jackson, D. D. (1957). The question of family homeostasis. *Psychiatric Quarterly Supplement, 31*, 79–90.

Knudson-Martin, C. (1992). Balancing the ledger. An application of Nagy's theories to the study of continuity and change among generations. *Contemporary Family Therapy, 14*(3), 241–258.

Laszlo, E. (1972). *Introduction to systems philosophy*. New York, NY: Gordon and Breach.

Lion Facts: 20 Interesting Facts about Lions Answers Africa. (2018). Retrieved from: https://answersafrica.com/interesting-lion-facts.html

Minuchin, P. (1985). Families and individual development: provocations from the field of family therapy. *Child Development, 56*(2), 289.

Mosher, D. K., Hook, J. N., Captari, L. E., Davis, D. E., DeBlaere, C. & Owen, J. (2017). Cultural humility: a therapeutic framework for engaging diverse clients. *Practice Innovations, 2*(4), 221.

Sullivan, H. S. (1953). *The interpersonal theory of psychiatry*. New York, NY: Norton.

Ulrich, D. N. (1998). Contextual Family Therapy. In F. M. Dattilio (Ed.), *Case studies in couple and family therapy: systemic and cognitive perspectives*. New York, NY: Guilford Press.

van der Meiden, J., Noordegraaf, M. & van Ewijk, H. (2019). How is contextual therapy applied today? An analysis of the practice of current contextual therapists. *Contemporary Family Therapy, 41*, 12–23.

Watson, M. F. (2007). Ivan Boszormenyi-Nagy, MD: a testimony to life. *Journal of Marital and Family Therapy, 33*(3), 289–290.

Watzlawick, P., Bavelas, J. B. & Jackson, D. D. (1967). *Pragmatics of human communication: a study of interactional patterns, pathologies, and paradoxes*. New York, NY: Norton.

Wilburn-McCoy, C. (1993). Rediscovering Nagy: what happened to contextual therapy? *Contemporary Family Therapy: An International Journal, 15*(5), 395–404.

Wilson, K. L., Glebova, T., Davis, S., & Seshadri, G. (2017). Adolescent mothers in foster care: relational ethics, depressive symptoms and health problems through a contextual therapy lens. *Contemporary Family Therapy, 39*, 150–161.

16 Cognitive Behavioral Family Therapy

Amanda Veldorale-Griffin

Cognitive Behavioral Therapy (CBT) is widely practiced across a range of mental health professions. CBT has its roots in early behavioral psychology, pioneered by Ivan Pavlov, John Watson and B. F. Skinner. CBT was introduced by Joseph Wolpe (1948) in the form of systematic desensitization for the treatment of phobias. The use of CBT for other anxiety disorders was further developed in the 1970s and 1980s by Childress and Burns (1981). More recently, systems orientation was incorporated into CBT to form Cognitive Behavioral Family Therapy (CBFT). This shifted the focus from individuals to exploring how people's behaviors and cognitions are reinforced by those they are in relationships with. Since its inception, CBFT has been particularly impactful in the area of parenting and the development of parent training programs. Most therapists who work with children incorporate aspects of CBFT, especially ideas of reinforcement and consistency, into their work (e.g., Patterson & Forgatch, 1987).

Other, related approaches, such as Integrative Behavioral Couples Therapy, Gottman Method Couple Therapy (see Chapter 14 in this text) and Functional Family Therapy are also often included as part of the larger umbrella of systems-focused CBT models. While these approaches do derive from much of the same theoretical foundation and while their contributions are important to acknowledge, they are outside of the scope of this chapter.

Founders

The behavioral family therapy movement, which began to take shape in the 1970s, was influenced largely by three key figures: Gerald Patterson, Robert Liberman and Richard Stuart. Patterson was a psychologist credited with developing behavioral parent training based on social learning theory (1971). Liberman was a psychiatrist who published a paper focused on the use of behavioral techniques in family and couple therapy, in which he addressed problems such as depression and marital discord (1970). He also introduced the idea of modeling into the family therapy field. Finally, Stuart was a social worker who shifted the focus of behavioral family therapy from reduction of undesired behaviors to the maximization of positive behaviors (1969).

Cognitive Behavioral Therapy began to truly take shape in the 1980s, adding cognitions to the longstanding behavioral approach, as a key part of treatment. This therapy model is based largely on the work of Albert Ellis and Aaron Beck, who stressed the importance of creating attitudinal change in order to promote change and maintain behavioral modifications (Beck, 1976; Ellis, 1979). The separate paths of CBT and behavioral family

DOI: 10.4324/9781003382621-19

therapy were brought together as a systemic model known as CBFT. One of the major contributors in this integration was Frank Dattilio, a clinical psychologist who trained in Cognitive Therapy with other founders such as Joseph Wolpe and Aaron Beck. Norman Epstein was also a key figure in expanding cognitive and cognitive behavioral approaches to working with couples and families (e.g., Epstein & Baucom, 2007; Epstein, Schlesinger & Dryden, 1988).

Systemic foundation

In formulating a systemic version of CBT to apply with couples and families, Frank Dattilio (2010) acknowledged that early criticisms of CBT when used with these populations were valid. As a result, his updated approach integrates the concept of circular causality and an increased consideration of the role of emotions in familial dynamics. We also see these concepts in Epstein and Baucom's (2007) Cognitive Behavioral Couple's Therapy (CBCT). Chief among the systemic assumptions of CBFT is the idea that family members are simultaneously influencing, and being influenced by, one another (Dattilio, 2010). In other words, it is assumed that the behaviors of one member of the system will trigger thoughts, feelings and behaviors in the other members of the system. These, in turn, will trigger reactions in the original member, creating a **circular causality**. In addition to circular causality, **homeostasis** and **context** also play important roles in CBFT.

Families are viewed as maintaining homeostasis through patterns of thinking and behavior that reinforce one another through **negative feedback** loops. These concepts are clearly illustrated in CBFT through **family schemas**. Family schemas are the internal working structures that allow people to make sense of the world around them and which are passed down through generations (Dattilio, 2010). These are seen as being formed by the experiences in one's family of origin, and they are also the frameworks with which people engage in other relationships. Each partner will bring with them their schema from their family of origin. Over time, they will combine the ideas from their own schemas to create a new family schema that will be passed on to their children (Dattilio, 2010). This combining of schemas and creation of a new family schema can be a source of conflict for couples and is one area addressed by CBFT in order to create **second-order change**.

Dattilio's model of CBFT is also systemic in that it recognizes important roles of attachment and affect in problem formation and treatment (2010). Rooted in the theories of John Bowlby and Mary Ainsworth, this model acknowledges that relationship problems can stem from a lack of insecurity within a present relationship or may also be related to insecure attachment relationships in one's childhood or previous romantic relationships. The model also acknowledges that the marital system is a smaller unit embedded in larger social contexts. In CBFT, attachment is thought to be organized based on both emotional and cognitive processes. For example, if one developed a schema that they were unlovable based on their family of origin, they may carry that schema into future romantic relationships. As a result, CBFT seeks to address attachment problems through challenging maladaptive schemas and enhancing emotion regulation skills.

Main concepts and philosophical underpinnings

CBT and its subsequent systemic formulations are rooted in behaviorism and cognitive theory. As a result, CBT and CBFTs include both behavioral interventions and cognitive interventions.

Behaviorism

In particular, it has been influenced by the ideas of **classical** and **operant conditioning**. **Classical conditioning** refers to the process by which an unconditioned stimulus is paired with a conditioned stimulus to produce a desired result. This concept was developed by Ivan Pavlov during experiments with dogs. Pavlov noticed that the dogs naturally salivated when food was present. He hypothesized that he could train them to salivate to the sound of a bell. He did this by ringing a bell whenever the dogs saw food. After repeating this process, Pavlov was able to remove the food and the dogs would salivate solely at the sound of the bell (Pavlov, 1932).

The basic premise of operant conditioning is that when a behavior is accompanied by an enjoyable experience it is more likely to be duplicated, whereas a behavior that is accompanied by a disagreeable experience is less likely to be duplicated. **Reinforcement and punishment** are key concepts from Skinner's theory that shaped CBFT. Reinforcement rewards desired behaviors whereas punishment seeks to reduce undesirable behaviors. Both reinforcement and punishment have two types: positive and negative (Skinner, 1953).

Positive reinforcement refers to the adding of a desired item or event in order to increase a preferred behavior. For example, giving a child a treat for completing their chores. **Negative reinforcement** refers to the removal of an undesired item or event in order to increase a preferred behavior (Skinner, 1953). For example, lifting the curfew on the weekends as a reward for getting good grades. Positive punishment refers to the adding of something unwanted as a consequence of an undesired behavior. For example, adding an evening curfew as a result of a teen drinking at a party. Negative punishment refers to the removal of something wanted as a consequence of an undesired behavior. For example, taking away a teenager's phone after violating their curfew.

Skinner went on to highlight the importance of frequency in reinforcing or punishing a behavior in determining success in having a particular behavior reinforced or extinguished. Specifically, he noted three key points related to frequency: (a) immediacy, (b) consistency and (c) intermittent reinforcement (Ferster & Skinner, 1957; Skinner, 1953). Immediacy means that the shorter the length of time between behavior and consequence, the faster the desired behavior will be learned. Consistency is the idea that rewarding or punishing a behavior each time it happens (or on a predictable schedule) helps increase the speed at which the desired behavior is learned. Finally, **intermittent reinforcement** refers to unpredictable reinforcement of behavior.

Intermittent reinforcement of preferred behaviors can have the opposite effect as desired, by leading to an increase in undesirable behaviors. For instance, if a parent inconsistently reinforces the rule that chores must be finished before watching TV, a child is more likely to watch TV before completing their chores. However, intermittent reinforcement of ingrained desirable behaviors helps to maintain them (Ferster & Skinner, 1957; Skinner, 1953). For example, if a parent randomly treats their child for continued good grades.

Cognitive theory

While the previous section focused on behavioral theory, the next section shifts to look at theories about cognition and how we change cognitions. One key cognitive theory that is now part of CBFT is Albert Ellis' (1962) ABC Theory, which helps us understand how problematic thoughts develop and the effects on a person. The acronym ABC stands for:

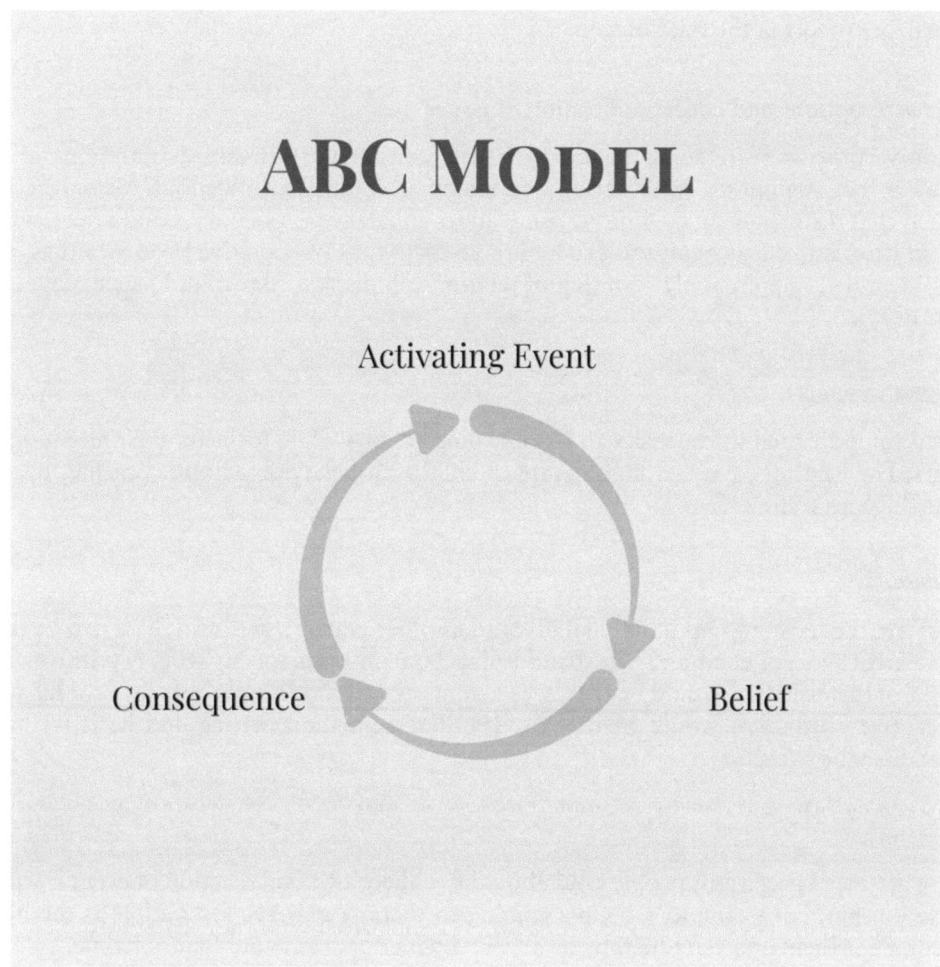

Figure 16.1 Infographic ABC Model.

Often, clients fail to attend to their belief about the event, and instead view A as the cause of C. When the belief is ignored or is irrational, it can create problems for the individual and the family. Moreover, family members may have different beliefs about an activating event, which in turn produce a variety of behavioral consequences throughout the family. As a result, CBFT often helps families map out their beliefs about events and focuses on changing those beliefs to create new emotional and behavioral responses to the event.

Social exchange theory

A final important theory that helps to form the foundation of CBFT is social exchange theory (Thibaut & Kelley, 1959). This theory posits that people engage in behaviors designed to increase "rewards" and limit "costs" in their relationship. When families are doing this well, all parties are working toward mutual increase of rewards (reciprocity). However, this can get out of balance when one person starts looking for ways to protect themselves and fails to consider others in the relationship.

Basic assumptions and conceptualization of issues

Cognitive processes are fundamental to CBFT. One of the primary assumptions of the model is that cognitions, behavior and emotions are mutually influential. Moreover, it is posited that distortions in cognitions can lead to imbalances in behavior and affect, which can, in turn, influence cognitions. There are several types of cognitive processes that have been identified as commonly resulting in relationship distress (Baucom, Epstein, Sayers & Sher, 1989).

Selective attention

This is an individual's propensity to ignore some actions while focusing their attention on others. For example, parents highlighting a child's misbehavior without praising her for what she does well.

Attributions

These are the meanings an individual gives to another person's actions. These can be positive or negative. For example, a husband brings home flowers for his wife. A positive attribution of this behavior would be that he is acting out of kindness to show love for his wife. A negative attribution would be that he has done something wrong and he is trying to soften his wife's reaction.

Expectancies

These are the expectations people hold about how likely a certain reaction of event is within a relationship. For example, a couple coming to therapy may see separation as the likely outcome for them and view therapy as a "last ditch effort" to avoid that outcome.

Assumptions

These are general beliefs about others. In family and couple contexts, these are the beliefs about what type of person each member of the system is. When a person takes an action that goes against these assumptions, this can cause problems within the system. For example, an affair can lead one spouse to doubt what they know about their partner and create a sense of betrayal.

Standards

These are beliefs about how people "should' behave or what a relationship "should" look like. These are used to determine if a family member's behavior is deemed "appropriate" or not. For example, if the standard is that family should care for one another, then a daughter failing to check on her injured parent would be viewed as unacceptable.

While these five types of cognitions are all normal parts of the human thought process, they are prone to distortions that can lead to issues. There are **ten common cognitive distortions that affect couples and families** (Dattilio, 2010).

Arbitrary inference

These are unsupported conclusions. For example, when one partner stays out late, the other assumes they must be seeing someone else.

Selective abstractions

This is when people hone certain information or details of a situation, while ignoring others. For example, a father notices that his teenage daughter has been quiet at dinner and thinks that she must be mad at him.

Overgeneralization

This is when one or few events are assumed to represent the whole. For example, a child forgets to do his chores after school one day and his caregivers tell him that he is irresponsible because he never does what he is told.

Magnification and minimization

This is when a particular incident is valued or devalued to an inappropriate degree. An example of magnification is when one spouse finds that the other didn't take out the garbage, they yell "this is going to be the end of us!" On the opposite side of the spectrum, one spouse engages in an affair, but downplays it by saying it "wasn't a big deal and didn't mean anything".

Personalization

This is when one assumes personal connection to an event, even when there is no evidence one exists. For example, a young adult decides to move out of state for college and their parent thinks this is because their child doesn't want to be around them.

Dichotomous thinking

This is black or white, either/or thinking. It allows no room for ambiguity. For example, a child with divorced parents thinks she can either love her mom or her dad and that loving one means that she cannot love the other.

Labeling and mislabeling

This is when a person builds their identity around their missteps or flaws. For example, a woman forgets to buy something at the store that her partner asked for several times. This leads her to view herself a "worthless partner" instead of recognizing that mistakes happen and that this is relatively minor.

Tunnel vision

This is the notion of viewing everything through a narrow lens that allows only for the confirmation of pre-existing ideas. For example, a dad who views his child as "lazy" may blame the child's poor grades on lack of effort without exploring other possibilities.

Biased explanations

This is an assumption of negative motivations on behalf of others. For example, a woman brings her girlfriend flowers and her girlfriend thinks she must be trying to make up for something negative she did.

Mind reading

This refers to the idea that one person can know what another is thinking without them expressing their ideas verbally. This can often result in negative attributions. For example, a parent may say of their children, "I know what they are thinking; they think I'm stupid."

How change occurs

In CBFT, there are three primary entry points for therapists to make change; these are in the areas of **affect, behavior and cognition**. In CBFT, these three domains are viewed as creating a cycle of interaction in which each affects the other (Dattilio, 2010).

Affect

It is a common misconception of CBFT that emotions are not addressed in therapy (Dattilio, 2010). In actuality, however, they play a key role in understanding the experience of clients and addressing their problems. One way that CBFT therapists can intervene in the domain of affect is through emotional regulation. This refers to a person's ability to influence their experience of their emotions and manage and express their emotions in appropriate ways (Cavanagh, Quinn, Duncan, Graham & Balbuena, 2014). CBFT therapists can teach clients skills to help them enhance their emotional regulation.

Another way in which CBFT therapists intervene in the domain of affect is by helping clients to examine their thoughts and beliefs about experiencing and expressing emotions (Dattilio, 2010). For example, an individual may have a family schema built around the idea that men do not show sadness because sadness is weakness. The therapist will explore this idea with the client, including how this belief interacts with the beliefs of other family members, and help the client to create a more adaptive relationship to their emotional experience.

Behavior

CBFT therapists attend to both macro- and micro-level behaviors couples and families engage in. Micro-level behaviors are those that occur in a specific situation, whereas macro-level behaviors are those patterns of behavior that occur across contexts (Dattilio, 2010). CBFT therapists may intervene in this area by helping clients to create meaningful rituals, define the boundaries of their relationships and attend to their social exchange process. This last, which has been dubbed by John Gottman (1999) as a "bank account", refers to the idea that family members, and couples particularly, operate in relationship via social exchange. That is, positive behaviors accumulate in the "account" over time and are "spent" during times of conflict. CBFT therapists can help couples to make more positive "investments" in their relationship.

Cognition

The final area in which CBFT therapists can intervene is cognition. CBFT therapists conduct thorough assessments with their clients, which help them to understand clients' family schemas and any cognitive distortions that may be affecting their relationships (Dattilio, 2010). The CBFT therapist then works with clients to first acknowledge the need for change and then to make shifts in their beliefs. This can be achieved in a variety of ways, including Socratic questioning, psychoeducation, evaluation of family schemas and keeping a thought record. These specific interventions will be discussed in more depth later in this chapter.

Role of the client

The client involved in CBFT is there as a learner. It is the client's job to listen to the information the therapist provides and to practice the techniques that are prescribed. This may include keeping thought records, engaging in role-plays, practicing communication techniques and reading books assigned by the therapist. Another important role of the client is to create goals for therapy. These goals need to be measurable and focused on specific behaviors.

Role of the therapist

The Cognitive Behavior Family Therapist operates from the stance of the expert and takes the role of educator and director (Dattilio & Epstein, 2016). Historically, little emphasis was placed on the role of the therapeutic relationship. However, in light of more recent research on common factors (Davis, Lebow & Sprenkle, 2012), many CBFT therapists are moving toward a warmer and more empathic model in order to foster the therapeutic alliance (e.g., Epstein & Baucom, 2007). There are several ways in which CBFT therapists can enhance the therapeutic alliance:

(a) maintaining a collaborative stance
(b) creating safety through empathy
(c) offering flexibility in therapeutic style
(d) demonstrating effectiveness and credibility
(e) providing a structure to therapy, including setting clear goals
(f) seeking feedback at the end of each session (Beck, 2005; Epstein & Baucom, 2007)

It is important to note that this use of empathy is not seen as an intervention in itself, as it would be in a more humanistic model of therapy, but rather as a means for fostering client confidence in the therapy process, which will then allow the therapist to more effectively deliver the interventions associated with the model (Epstein & Baucom, 2007).

Another key role of the therapist is that of assessor. CBFT requires extensive assessment to identify strengths and problems at multiple levels of the system, including individual, family and larger context (Dattilio, 2010). Cognitions, emotions and behaviors are all evaluated to inform case conceptualization. The assessment should consider the context of the family's stage of development within the family life cycle and ultimately identify which aspect of the family interaction should be the focus of therapy. Dattilio highlights that assessment, while most predominant in the beginning of therapy, is an ongoing process until termination (2010). There are several main areas of assessment in CBFT: (a) defining the problem;

(b) identifying a baseline; (c) identifying the factors that contribute to the problem or are part of the sequence of events occurring before or after the problem; (d) identifying client resources and strengths that can be utilized to address the problem; and (e) determining the appropriateness of CBFT in treating the problem (Epstein & Baucom, 2007).

Interventions

CBFTs use a wide range of interventions that seek to change behaviors and cognitions. Most interventions are focused on teaching new skills such as regulating emotions, communicating more effectively or challenging unhelpful thought patterns (e.g., Dattilio, 2010; Epstein & Baucom, 2007; Patterson & Forgatch, 1987). Clients are typically given homework, which they are expected to complete outside of sessions to practice the skills learned (e.g., Epstein & Baucom, 2007.

Behavioral interventions

Behavior exchange and quid pro quo

Behavior exchange agreements are contracts designed to increase desired behaviors among family members. This is when family members agree to exchange behaviors desired by one another (Dattilio, 2010). However, this can result in individuals being unwilling to make a change before they see change in others. Thus, it is important that family members are encouraged to take positive steps regardless of the actions taken by others. Without this, they may engage in a cycle of negative reciprocity, which exacerbates the relational distress and leads to lower levels of marital satisfaction (Gottman, 1999). Thus, while engaging in a quid pro quo (this for that) contract can be helpful, it has been recommended that this technique is used in conjunction with interventions aimed at increasing positive affect and understanding that people focus on what they can change versus what they would like others to change (Dimidjian, Martell & Christensen, 2002).

Contingency contracts

Contingency contracts are aimed at getting family members to make changes in their behavior contingent on other family members making changes (Stuart, 1969; Dattilio, 2010). This is generally used more with adolescents and adults than with young children. When implementing contingency contracting, therapists introduce the idea of compromising and coming to a mutually agreed upon and beneficial contract. To do this, the therapist needs to facilitate clear communication between family members (both about what is going on and how they feel about it), help them to present their ideas and requests clearly, and engage in give-and-take regarding the desired outcome (Stuart, 1969). It's also recommended that family members or partners agree to make changes in their behavior first (Dattilio, 2010).

Communication and problem-solving training

One common area of intervention for CBFT couples' therapists is communication. Poor listening and problem-solving skills, as well as difficulty with encoding (expressing one's own thoughts effectively) and decoding (interpreting other's thoughts appropriately), have all been pinpointed as common areas of concerns in couple communication (Dattilio, 2010).

Communication training has been the focus of a number of programs aimed at enhancing couple relationships, as well as improving parenting. Many recommendations exist on the principles to teach in communication training. Here is a list of common principles that are taught for both the speaker and the listener in a conversation (Epstein & Baucom, 2007; Holtzworth & Jacobson, 1991):

Speaker:

- engages in softened startup (i.e., start with a positive before discussing a problem)
- focuses on one problem at a time
- identifies specific behavioral concerns (rather than global statements, such as "he never helps")
- expresses your emotions related to the problem
- takes responsibility for your part in creating and/or maintaining the problem
- avoids any kind of verbal abuse, including insults and threats
- takes pauses to allow the other person to respond

Listener:

- reflects what they have heard from others
- uses words and body language that communicate understanding and respect
- attempts to place yourself in your partner's shoes to understand their perspective
- avoids making assumptions about other people's thoughts, feelings or motivations
- asks questions only for clarifications
- avoids offering judgments, opinions or solutions

The therapist will redirect client interactions in order to help them adhere to these communication rules. Overall, therapists will try to stay focused on improving the process of how clients communicate, rather than getting stuck in the details of the content (Dattilio, 2010).

Point charts and token economies

Point charts and token economies are often used in parent training (Kazdin, 2005). It is focused on using a point-system to reward children for a desired behavior. Children can earn points based on engaging in an agreed upon behavior or set of behaviors.

These points are usually exchanged for a larger reward upon the accumulation of a particular number of points (e.g., ten points) or at the end of a set period of time (e.g., one week). One author on child and adolescent interventions notes that token economies and point systems are just as much for parents as they are children. Structured systems help parents be more consistent in following through with rewards and tracking the frequency of rewards (Weisz & Kazdin, 2017). Rewards should be developmentally appropriate and approved by the parent to ensure the child will be motivated by the reward and the parent will consistently follow through (Kazdin, 2005).

Role-play

Research on parent training shows that one of the ingredients that makes it effective is the use of role-play (Wyatt Kaminski, Valle, Filene & Boyle, 2008). In this intervention, the therapist will instruct family members on how to interact with one another and then have them act out those behaviors in session. Role-plays can also be done between an individual client and therapist with the therapist acting as a child or partner (e.g., Patterson & Forgatch, 1987).

Role reversal

This technique involves having a couple or two members of a family discuss an issue while role-playing as their partner. In this way, each can gain some insight into the other's perspective and avoid engaging in the negative attributions that often go along with relational stress. This intervention also allows the therapist a chance to correct any misperceptions each family member may have about the other (Dattilio, 2010).

Shaping

This intervention is designed to help people reach a closer and closer approximation of the preferred behavior until it becomes well-established. At each step, the bar is raised for reinforcement until the desired behavior is achieved. At that point, the intermittent reinforcement is begun to help maintain the new behavior (Kazdin, 2005).

Time-out

Time-out is perhaps one of the best-known methods of disciplining children, and it is one that is often recommended as part of behavioral therapy (Weisz & Kazdin, 2017). It is based on the ideas of operant conditioning and involves separating a child from others immediately following an unacceptable behavior. Studies have consistently shown time-outs to be one of the most effective methods for increasing behavioral compliance in children (Leijten, Gardner, Melendez-Torres, Knerr & Overbeek, 2018; Pendergrass, 1971). However, some recent literature suggests that the use of time-outs may lead to increased anger and emotional dysregulation in children (Siegel & Bryson, 2014).

Based on a descriptive analysis of 30 years of research, Everett, Hupp and Olmi (2010) suggest that time-outs are beneficial in addressing externalizing behaviors (specifically, non-compliance with parental directives) in children aged 3–7. They also suggest that time-outs be used when other more positive interventions have been unsuccessful and that time-outs should be used in conjunction with other interventions, including praise. Along with including more positive interventions, Everett and colleagues (2010) also warn against the use of holding, spanking or other "physical guidance" in implementing time-outs. Finally, they note that practitioners who are training parents in the use of time-outs need to make sure they are "consistent with widely recommended behavior management principles" (p. 252), including: (a) implementing the time-out in a calm manner; (b) employing the time-out consistently and immediately following the undesired behavior; and (c) following up after the use of the time-out to assess its effectiveness (Everett et al., 2010).

Cognitive interventions and psychoeducation

Psychoeducation refers to the process by which CBFT therapists teach their clients about issues and techniques used to address them. Psychoeducation falls broadly into two categories: problem-oriented and change-oriented (Gehart, 2013). Problem-oriented psychoeducation is focused on providing clients information about their presenting problem or diagnosis. Change-oriented psychotherapy is aimed at educating clients on ways to reduce symptoms by introducing clients to new skills, which they can begin to implement in small, manageable steps. Bibliotherapy is another type of psychoeducation, which can be problem-oriented or change-oriented. It involves providing clients with books, articles or other literature to clients to read in order to help motivate them toward their goals and provide them further information about their presenting problem. Resources can also be in audio or video form such as a podcast or YouTube video (Epstein & Baucom, 2007).

Challenging cognitive distortions

Recall the list of cognitive distortions listed earlier in this chapter. In cognitive-based therapies, one of the primary interventions is to help clients identify these thoughts, challenge them and replace them with new, more helpful thoughts. This intervention is designed to challenge the cognitive distortions clients have that are maintaining problems. Challenging of thoughts can be done either through direct confrontation (telling the client the belief is irrational) or indirect confrontation (employing questioning to help guide the client to an understanding of the belief as irrational and part of the problem or psychoeducating the client generally on cognitive distortions) (Epstein & Baucom, 2007). This type of indirect communication is often done via the Socratic method, which is when the therapist uses a series of open-ended questions to help clients think logically about their maladaptive beliefs in order to see them either as irrational or dysfunctional (Beck, 2005). In CBFT, the main focus is on cognitive distortions that are related to the responses between family members; they might also explore distortions related to one's family of origin (Dattilio, 2010).

Thought records are one tool commonly used to help clients identify and challenge cognitive distortions (Beck, Rush, Shaw & Emery, 1979). They are typically demonstrated during session, and then assigned as homework for clients to complete outside of session. They are designed to help clients analyze their thought processes and behaviors and to brainstorm more functional responses (Beck et al., 1979; Dattilio, 2010; Persons, Davidson & Tomkins, 2001). Thought records generally tend to follow a standard format, which includes: (a) the triggering event; (b) the initial or "automatic" thought; (c) emotions related to what happened; (d) evidence supporting the automatic thought; (e) evidence against the automatic thought; (f) identification of any cognitive distortions present; and (g) a "corrected" thought, which incorporates the evidence for and against to create a whole and balanced picture of the situation (Beck et al., 1979; Dattilio, 2010).

Case study

Marlene (50) and Alan (47), a White, middle-class, Christian, married couple present for therapy following the disclosure by their 18-year-old son Paul about his sexual orientation. They report that Paul talked to them about a month ago when he was home on vacation from college and told them that he thinks he might be gay. Marlene and Alan state that they were "surprised" and spent most of their time over dinner asking him questions about how long he'd known and if he was sure. Marlene reports that she has been doing "okay" since then and just "hasn't been thinking about it". Alan expresses feeling "angry" and "confused". Both state that they love their son and want to be able to support him.

Questions:

1. What automatic thoughts might be at play for Marlene and Alan?
2. What contextual factors might be important to assess in this case?
3. Which interventions would be appropriate for this family?

Example intervention approach

The therapist begins by identifying automatic thoughts, attribution, expectancies and family schemas present within the system. The therapist reflects some of Marlene and Alan's words to them from the intake session as part of identifying their automatic thoughts. These include statements such as "he's going to be bullied", "maybe this is just a phase", "people experiment all the time in college" and "this is my fault". The therapist asks follow-up questions to drill down to the core fears and beliefs that these statements represent. This process revealed three main core beliefs: that being gay will create problems for Paul, that heterosexuality is more natural and preferable to homosexuality, and that Paul's sexual orientation represented a failing as parents. Alan was able to identify that, in his family of origin, homosexuality was viewed as a sin and gay people were frequently the butt of jokes. Marlene reported that her family didn't talk much about sexual orientation, but there was an idea that if people were gay they should "keep it to themselves". The therapist validates their emotions, reframing them as understandable given their context. The therapist also provides them with readings on sexual orientation and a referral to the local chapter of PFLAG, an organization dedicated to supporting, educating and advocating for LGBTQ+ people and their families. In following sessions, the therapist will explore these automatic thoughts again and challenge them with the information that Marlene and Alan have learned about sexual orientation.

Termination of therapy

Therapy ends when the client and therapist decide jointly that it is an appropriate time for termination. Because of CBFT's focus on setting concrete behavioral goals, there is generally a clear measure of "success" in therapy. Termination is likely to be considered when the family's initial goals have been met for the period of time set forth in the treatment plan. The therapist and clients will consider if meeting those goals has sufficiently resolved their concerns or if additional goals need to be created.

Key legal and ethical considerations

One of the key ethical considerations in the use of CBFT is that of maintenance of competency. While this is an important ethical principle regardless of the model of therapy used, it is especially salient with CBFT. This is because it is a highly technical model and, as such, requires extensive training and practice both in cognitive-behavioral principles and systemic ones. If a therapist ignores the latter part in favor of a more linear and traditional CBT approach, they may fail to address key areas of circular causality and mutual influence, thereby limiting the effectiveness of treatment (Dattilio, 2010). To incorporate a cultural humility stance, therapists must also pay careful attention to the power dynamics of therapy, as CBFT places the therapist in an "expert" role. In this situation, therapists must be careful that they are not imposing their own beliefs of what constitutes "logical" or "rational" thinking upon their clients (Dattilio, 2010).

Use with a diversity of clients

As with all models of therapy, it is important to address cultural diversity and practice with a sense of cultural humility. This is heightened with CBFT because of its focus on challenging patterns of thinking, which are often borne out of cultural norms. CBFT must make sure to carefully assess the cultural context of the clients with whom they are working and be willing to adjust their approach to meet their clients' needs (Dattilio, 2010). This may occur in many different ways depending upon the cultural context of the clients. For instance, therapists may need to be less directive and work to decrease the hierarchy when working with those who are likely to be either overly compliant in these situations or prone to rebel against this authority (Gehart, 2013; Gehart & Lyle, 2001).

Because the methods of CBFT can put a therapist at risk of reinforcing dominant cultural ideas, therapists need to educate themselves on working with minority populations who may be harmed by society's view of what is "rational" or "normal". For example, transgender individuals may be viewed by society at large, or by a specific segment of the population in which the client resides, as having irrational thinking regarding their gender. It is important for therapists not to promote these harmful beliefs and instead explore how cognitions and behaviors are influenced by the larger social context (Austin & Craig, 2015). Exposure to transphobic attitudes may influence negative attitudes toward self. As a result, cognitive interventions can work toward retraining cognitions to be more trans-affirming for both the trans individual and their family members. Psychoeducation on the effects of a transphobic environment on mental health and creating the space to discuss personal experiences with transphobia are key cognitive interventions It is also important that CBFT therapists familiarize themselves with the research on working with the variety of populations they are working with. CBFT does not explicitly promote self-of-the-therapist reflection regarding therapist background and dynamics of power and privilege that may be present in the therapist-client dynamic. Therefore, clinicians practicing this model will need to integrate this reflexive component to ensure that they are considering how social justice issues may be influencing not only the client's presenting problem, but also the therapy process.

Research on CBFT with diverse populations suggests a few important points for CBFT therapists to consider. When working with Latinx clients, research points to the importance of translating both language and concepts when working with Spanish-speaking clients and being informed regarding the process of acculturation (Piedra & Byoun, 2012). It is further suggested that it may be helpful to focus more on doing than on talking. Research also indicates that there are several key cultural ideals that need to be understood and respected, namely familismo, personalismo, machismo and respecto (Duarté-Vélex, Bernal & Bonilla, 2010; González-Prendes, Hindo & Pardo, 201l; Organista & Munoz, 1996).

Another group with whom research has been conducted is African American clients. Adjustments suggested for these clients include maintaining a specific focus on addressing discrimination, rejecting stereotypes (McNair, 1996) and empowering clients, especially by increasing client agency through the use of a collaborative therapeutic relationship (Kelly, 2006). One way to help CBFT therapists avoid imposing implicit bias on their clients is through a focus on behaviors and skills and the use of a functional analysis, which will examine the problem in behavioral terms (Kelly, 2006).

Social justice considerations

Parker and McDowell (2017) provide considerations for CBFT therapists wanting to use their model to treat the effects of social injustices clients experience. They argue that CBFT therapists could potentially do harm to minority clients by reinforcing thoughts and beliefs that maintain oppression and marginalization. To remedy this, they recommend that CBFT be integrated with principles from critical social theory, which seeks to challenge ideologies and social structures that maintain social inequities.

Primarily, they suggest that CBFT therapists expand their focus to include societal schemas, such as those on race, gender and sexual orientation. Therapists are encouraged to explore how societal schemas affect family functioning and challenge families to adopt equity-based schemas (Parker and McDowell, 2017). In this approach, self-of-the-therapist work is critical to provide culturally competent care. Specifically, therapists need to be able to identify how their own schemas and their clients' schemas are influenced by socially constructed norms on race, gender, class, sexual orientation and other aspects of identity, particularly as they provide differences in the power and privilege people are afforded. Based on this integration, CBFT therapists challenge problematic social schemas, identify how individual and family schemas are influenced by social schemas and co-create new schemas that clients are encouraged to use to change thoughts and behaviors.

Self-of-the-therapist reflection questions

1. What have you learned about race, gender, class, sexual orientation, etc. from society?
2. What comes to mind for you when you think about people who have different identities from your own?
3. What identities do you hold that are privileged (e.g., White, educated, male, cisgender)?
4. What identities do you hold that are minoritized (e.g., Black, Muslim, gay)?
5. How have your identities shaped what you think of as "healthy" or "normal"?

Research support

CBFT is perhaps the most researched model of family therapy especially as it shares components with traditional CBT, which has been widely validated in hundreds of outcome studies (Butler, Chapman, Forman & Beck, 2006). This is likely due to its origins in experimental psychology. In particular, there is a vast wealth of literature on the use of CBFT with couples and with parents. Dattilio (2010) notes that CBT with couples has been the subject of more controlled outcome studies than any other method or model. This does not, however, mean that CBFT is superior to other models. Indeed, research indicates that no particular model of therapy consistently produces better outcomes than any other (Sprenkle & Blow, 2004).

Research focusing on Cognitive Behavioral Couple Therapy has shown general increases in marital satisfaction, functioning and attachment, as well as couple problem-solving skills (Belanger, Laporte, Sabourin & Wright, 2015; Benson, Sevier & Christensen, 2013; Fischer, Baucom, & Cohen, 2016). It has been shown to be as effective as individual CBT in treating psychological issues, such as anxiety and substance use disorders and significantly more effective in treating relational issues (Fischer et al., 2016). Conjoint therapy using CBT has also been found to be effective in treating PTSD (Monson et al., 2012; Wagner, et al., 2016).

Research on the use of CBT with children has indicated its effectiveness in reducing symptoms of anxiety in children with high-functioning autism spectrum disorders (Ung, Selles, Small & Storch, 2015). Moreover, research has suggested that parental involvement plays a key role in helping children to maintain gains. In a three-year follow-up study of children treated for anxiety disorders using CBT, Walczak, Esborjn, Breinholst and Reinholdt-Dunne (2017) found that children whose parents had only limited involvement with treatment were at higher risk for a resurgence of problems, whereas those whose parents were actively involved in treatment were more likely to remain without anxiety symptoms.

References

Austin, A. & Craig, S. L. (2015). Transgender affirmative cognitive behavioral therapy: clinical considerations and applications. *Professional Psychology: Research and Practice*, 46(1), 21.

Baucom, D., Epstein, N., Sayers, S. & Sher, T. (1989). The role of cognitions in marital relationships: definitional methodological, and conceptual issues. *Journal of Family Psychology*, 10, 72–88.

Beck, A. T. (1976). *Cognitive therapy and emotional disorders*. New York, NY: International Universities Press.

Beck, A. T. (2005). The current state of cognitive therapy: a 40-year retrospective. *Archives of General Psychiatry*, 62(9), 953–959.

Beck, A. T., Rush, A. J., Shaw, B. F. & Emergy, G. (1979). *Cognitive therapy of depression*. New York, NY: Guildford Press.

Belanger, C., Laporte, L., Sabourin, S. & Wright, J. (2015). The effect of cognitive- behavioral group martial therapy on marital happiness and problem solving self-appraisal. *The American Journal of Family Therapy*, 43, 103–118.

Benson, L. A., Sevier, M. & Christensen, A. (2013). The impact of behavioral couple therapy on attachment in distressed couples. *Journal of Marital and Family Therapy*, 39 (4), 407–420.

Butler, A. C., Chapman, J. E., Forman, E. M. & Beck, A. T. (2006). The empirical status of cognitive-behavioral therapy: a review of meta-analyses. *Clinical Psychology Review, 26(*1), 17–31.

Cavanagh, M., Quinn, D., Duncan, D., Graham, T. & Balbuena, L. (2014). Oppositional defiant disorder is better conceptualized as a disorder of emotional regulation. *Journal of Attention Disorders*, 1–9.

Childress, A. R. & Burns, D. D. (1981). The basics of cognitive therapy. *Psychosomatics*, 22(12), 1017–1027.

Dattilio, F. M. (2010). *Cognitive behavioral therapy with couples and families*. New York, NY: Guilford Press.

Dattilio, F. M. & Epstein, N. B. (2016). Cognitive-behavioral couple and family therapy. In T. L. Sexton & J. Lebow (Eds.), *Handbook of family therapy* (pp. 89–119). New York, NY: Routledge/ Taylor & Francis Group.

Davis, S. D., Lebow, J. L. & Sprenkle, D. H. (2012). Common factors of change in couple therapy. *Behavior Therapy*, 43(1), 36–48.

Dimidjian, S., Martell, C. R. & Christensen, A. (2002). Integrative behavioral couple therapy. In A.S. Gurman & N.S. Jacobson (Eds.), *Clinical handbook of couple therapy* (pp. 251–277). New York, NY: The Guilford Press.

Duarté-Vélez, Y., Bernal, G. & Bonilla, K. (2010). Culturally adapted cognitive-behavioral therapy: integrating sexual, spiritual, and family identities in an evidence-based treatment of a depressed Latino adolescent. *Journal of Clinical Psychology*, 66(8), 895–906.

Ellis, A. (1962). *Reason and emotion in psychotherapy*. New York, NY: Lyle Stuart.

Ellis, A. (1979). *Rational-emotive therapy*. In R. J. Corsini (Ed.), *Current psychotherapies* (2nd ed.). Itaska, IL: Peacock.

Epstein, N. B. & Baucom, D. H. (2007). Couples. In: N. Kazantzis & L. L'Abate, (Eds.), *Handbook of homework assignments in psychotherapy*. Boston, MA: Springer. https://doi.org/10.1007/978-0-387-29681-4_12

Epstein, N. E., Schlesinger, S. E. & Dryden, W. E. (1988). *Cognitive-behavioral therapy with families*. New York, NY: Brunner/Mazel.

Everett, G. E., Hupp, S. D. A. & Olmi, D. J. (2010). Time-out with parents: a descriptive analysis of 30 years of research. *Education and treatment of children, 33*(2), 235–259.

Ferster, C. B. & Skinner, B. F. (1957). *Schedules of reinforcement*. Englewood Cliffs, NJ: Prentice Hall.

Fischer, M. S., Baucom, D. H. & Cohen, M. J. (2016). Cognitive-behavioral couple therapies: review of the evidence for the treatment of relationship distress, psychopathology, and chronic health conditions. *Family Process, 55*(3), 423–442.

Gehart, D. (2013). *Mastering competencies in family therapy: a practical approach to theories and clinical case documentation*. Belmont, CA: Cengage Learning.

Gehart, D. & Lyle, R. R. (2001). Client experience of gender in therapeutic relationships: an interpretive ethnography. *Family Process, 40*, 443–458.

González-Prendes, A., Hindo, C. & Pardo, Y. (2011). Cultural values integration in cognitive-behavioral therapy for a Latino with depression. *Clinical Case Studies, 10*(5), 376–394.

Gottman, J. M. (1999). *The marriage clinic: a scientifically based marital therapy*. New York, NY: Norton.

Holtzworth-Munroe, A. & Jacobson, N. S. (1991). Behavioral marital therapy. *Handbook of Family Therapy, 2*, 96–133.

Kazdin, A. E. (2005). *Parent management training: treatment for oppositional, aggressive, and antisocial behavior in children and adolescents*. New York, NY: Oxford University Press.

Kelly, S. (2006). Cognitive-behavioral therapy with African Americans. In P. A. Hays & G. Y. Iwamasa (Eds.), *Culturally responsive cognitive-behavioral therapy: assessment, practice, and supervision* (pp. 97–116). Washington, DC: American Psychological Association.

Liberman, R. P. (1970). Behavioral approaches to family and couple therapy. *American Journal of Orthopsychiatry, 40*, 106–118.

Leijten, P., Gardner, F., Melendez-Torres, G. J., Knerr, W. & Overbeek, G. (2018). Parenting behaviors that shape child compliance: a multilevel meta-analysis. *PLOS One, 13*(10), 1–15.

McNair, L. D. (1996). African American women and behavior therapy: integrating theory, culture, and clinical practice. *Cognitive and Behavioral Practice, 3*(2), 337–349.

Monson, C. M., Fredman, S. J., Macdonald, A., PUkay-Martine, N. D., Resick, P. A. & Schnurr, P. P. (2012). Effect of cognitive-behavioral couple therapy for PTSD: a randomized controlled trial. *The Journal of the American Medical Association, 306*(7), 700–709.

Organista, K. C. & Muñoz, R. F. (1996). Cognitive behavioral therapy with Latinos. *Cognitive and Behavioral Practice, 3*(2), 255–270.

Parker, E. O. & McDowell, T. (2017). Integrating social justice into the practice of CBFT: a critical look at family schemas. *Journal of Marital and Family Therapy, 43*(3), 502–513.

Patterson, G. R. (1971). *Families: application of social learning to family life*. Champaign, IL: Research Press.

Patterson G. R. & Forgatch, M. (1987). *Parents and adolescents: living together: Part 1: the basics*. Eugene, OR: Castalia.

Pavlov, I. P. (1932). The reply of a physiologist to psychologists. *Psychological Review, 39*(2), 91–127.

Pendergrass, V. E. (1971). Effects of length of timeout from positive reinforcement and schedule of application in suppression of aggressive behavior. *Psychological Record, 21*, 75–80.

Persons, J. B., Davidson, J. & Tompkins, M. A. (2001). Using the thought record. In *Essential components of cognitive-behavior therapy for depression* (pp. 129–169). Washington, DC: American Psychological Association.

Piedra, L. M. & Byoun, S. (2012). Vida Alegre: preliminary findings of a depression intervention for immigrant Latino mothers. *Research on Social Work Practice, 22*(2), 138–150.

Siegel, D. J. & Bryson, T. P. (2014) *No drama discipline: the whole brain way to calm the chaos and nurture your child's developing mind*. New York, NY: Random House.

Skinner, B. F. (1953). Some contributions of an experimental analysis of behavior to psychology as a whole. *American Psychologist, 8*(2), 69.

Sprenkle, D. H. & Blow, A. J. (2004). Common factors and our sacred models. *Journal of Marital and Family Therapy, 30*, 113–129.

Stuart, R. B. (1969). Operant-interpersonal treatment of marital discord. *Journal of Consulting and Clinical Psychology, 33*, 675–682

Thibaut, J. & Kelley, H. H. (1959). *The social psychology of groups*. New York, NY: Wiley.

Ung, D., Selles, R., Small, B. J. & Storch, E. A. (2015). A systematic review and meta-analysis of cognitive-behavioral therapy for anxiety in youth with high-functioning autism spectrum disorders. *Child Psychiatry and Human Development, 46*, 533–547.

Wagner, A. C., Torbit, L. Jenzer, T., Landy, M. S. H., Pukay-Martin, N. D., Macdonald, A., Fredman, S. J. & Monson, C. M. (2016). The role of posttraumatic growth in a randomized controlled trial of cognitive-behavioral conjoint therapy for PTSD. *Journal of Traumatic Stress, 29*, 379–383.

Walczak, M., Esbjorn, B. H., Breinholst, S. & Reinholdt-Dunne, M. L. (2017). Parental involvement in cognitive behavior therapy for children with anxiety disorders: 3-year follow-up. *Child Psychiatry and Human Development, 48*, 444–454.

Weisz, J. R. & Kazdin, A. E. (Eds.). (2017). *Evidence-based psychotherapies for children and adolescents* (3rd ed.). New York, NY: The Guilford Press.

Wolpe, J. (1948). *An approach to the problem of neurosis based on the conditioned response* [Unpublished M.D. thesis]. University of Witwatersrand, Johannesberg, South Africa.

Wyatt Kaminski, J., Valle, L. A., Filene, J. H. & Boyle, C. L. (2008). A meta-analytic review of components associated with parent training program effectiveness. *Journal of Abnormal Child Psychology, 36*, 567–589.

17 Psychoanalytic Family Therapy

Siva Perera and Emily Schmittel

Introduction

Traditional psychoanalysts such as Sigmund Freud worked with individuals and focused on their individual mental processes and the relationship between the analyst and patient (as they were typically referred to rather than the now-preferred term – client). However, over time, certain psychoanalysts decided to examine further than the individual mind and began to consider the interaction between individuals and their families and how these relationships influenced relationships in later life. This overlap in relational thinking between psychoanalysis and the interactional perspective in family therapy led to the development of the Psychoanalytic Family Therapy approach.

Psychoanalytic Family Therapy is an approach to therapy that bridges the gap between the traditional analytical way of thinking and the relational nature of family systems and interactions. Social and cultural aspects that influence these systems especially in terms of personality development and functioning play a large role in this approach to therapy. Object relations family therapy (Scharff & Scharff, 1987), contextual therapy (Boszormenyi-Nagy & Krasner, 1985) and family of origin therapy (Framo, 1992) are all approaches to therapy that have developed from Psychoanalytic Family Therapy. In an editorial, Lebow points out that, while psychoanalytic approaches in their pure form are less commonly practiced, many concepts from these models are present in integrative approaches and common factors concepts (2017).

Key players

While the field of family therapy itself evolved from unlikely theoretical sources such as cybernetics, mathematics and communications, several family therapy pioneers such as Ivan Boszormenyi-Nagy, Nathan Ackerman, Don Jackson, Carl Whitaker, Salvador Minuchin and Murray Bowen were all trained psychoanalysts. This form of therapy was tremendously influenced by the works of numerous neo-Freudian theorists such as Karen Horney, Carl Jung and Alfred Adler. Ackerman, a classically trained psychoanalyst, is perhaps one of the earliest proponents of Psychoanalytic Family Therapy. He incorporated traditional psychoanalytic therapy with systems theory and argued that the well-being of an individual is directly tied to the nature of the relationships in one's family of origin (Ackerman, 1938). Over time, object relations family therapy (Scharff & Scharff, 1987) developed into the more dominant form of Psychoanalytic Family Therapy being practiced.

DOI: 10.4324/9781003382621-20

Main concepts of Psychoanalytic Family Therapy

Psychoanalytic therapists believe that **unconscious forces** present in an individual's psyche influence the individual and the interactions and relationships they have with others. These unconscious forces include negative intrapsychic conflicts generated from interactions with one's family of origin that are now impacting current relationships. The family is considered to be the link between the individual's relationships and they either support or hinder the healthy development of the individual. Therefore, psychoanalysts attempt to understand these unconscious forces and how they are impacting the individual and their relationships.

Drawing from this understanding, psychoanalytic family therapists apply these same traditional principles when working with individuals, their clients more specifically, to make sense of these unconscious forces so that they are better able to deal with those forces that impact their day-to-day life and interactions at the present time.

Interpersonal interactions and social interactions will also be explored, especially in family setting. Like traditional psychoanalytic approaches, Psychoanalytic Family Therapy revolves around examining intrapsychic and interpersonal factors and developing insight into how to relate to one another better. Carmel Flaskas (2005) argues that several core concepts of psychoanalytic theory are relevant to systemic family therapy practice, including the unconscious, transference/countertransference, attachment and conditions for thinking/emotional containment. Transference, countertransference, conditions for thinking and emotional containment are discussed in more detail in the following sections. We also expand on object relations theory, since it is a subset of psychoanalytic theory that is most often used in systemic applications.

Transference and countertransference

Transference refers to how clients recreate their patterns with the therapist, while counter-transference refers to the therapist's reactions to clients based on their own emotional and relationship history (Scharff & Scharff, 1987). These observations are identified during sessions and reflected back to clients to help promote insight about these processes. The hope is that insight about how the client and therapist interact with one another based on their own relational history will help the client to engage in new patterns of interactions in their relationships moving forward.

Conditions for thinking/emotional containment

In psychoanalytic theory, thinking is viewed as an emotional and relational process.

In order to engage in thinking, we need to be able to contain emotions (Bion, 1967). Thinking also helps us to contain emotions. In order for an infant to learn how to think, they need to interact with a caregiver who is interested in knowing the infant and their internal experience. So, ultimately, the ability to think is established through this relationship. This concept can be translated to the therapy process, in which the therapist, through their relationship with the client, creates the capacity for thinking or creating insight about the client's presenting problem (Flaskas, 2005).

Object relations theory

Object relations theory, a type of psychoanalytic theory often used in systemic therapy, posits that the main driving force for people is the need for an attachment relationship

(Scharff & Scharff, 1997). It is believed that family of origin patterns influence intrapsychic dynamics, which in turn influence current interpersonal relationships (Framo, 1992). As an attachment figure meets a child's needs or doesn't meet their needs, the child develops various internal states in response to feeling rejected or cared for by the figure (Scharff & Scharff, 1997). Pleasure is a result of the relationship with an object (e.g., parent), while aggression is a result of the rejection by the object (Fairburn, 1952; Framo, 1992). As an infant gains experiences with both a responsive caregiver and rejecting caregiver, mental objects are created that are then models for what to expect from other relationships (Fairburn, 1952). These mental figures are referred to as introjects (Scharff & Scharff, 1997). When a caregiver is experienced as rejected, the child splits off the image of the caregiver as a rejecting object from the image of the caregiver as an ideal figure. This image of the caregiver (also referred to as the rejected object) is then repressed. One consequence of this process is what's referred to as **splitting**, in which people and their relationships are viewed as all good or all bad.

Scharff and Scharff (1997) summarize the core parts of personality that are developed through the early attachment relationship (Fairburn, 1952):

1. a central self, attached with feelings of satisfaction and security to an ideal internal object
2. a craving self longingly, but satisfyingly, attached to an exciting internal object
3. a rejecting self angrily attached to a rejecting internal object (p. 142)

In object relations therapy, therapists are curious about the relationships between one's self and their internal objects and how these dynamics influence interpersonal relationships. Drawing from Dicks' Model of Marital Interaction (1967), it's believed that people are drawn to potential partners who display lost parts of self, which could in turn be expressed vicariously through a relationship with the person.

The concept of **projective identification** helps to connect intrapersonal and interpersonal processes (Dicks, 1967; Scharff & Scharff, 1997). This is the process by which we defend against anxiety by projecting aspects of self onto others (Klein, 1948; Scharff & Scharff, 1997). Ideally, the early splitting of people as all good or all bad is replaced by an ability to tolerate the fact that objects can have both good and bad traits (Scharff & Scharff, 1997). The early relationship in a marriage is believed to mimic the relationship between infant and caregiver regarding the development of the internal self in relation to the responses from an attachment figure.

The goals of object relations family therapy are best summarized in the following quote:

As we help the family explore its defensive structures, basic assumptions, and under-lying anxieties, we build skills for dealing with the current problem and for future developmental challenges.

(Scharff, 2004, p. 260)

Including children in therapy

The object relations family therapy approach emphasizes that children should be included in family therapy with play as the key modality of treatment (Scharff, 2004). During a play session, therapists listen for unconscious communication patterns between family members and their own countertransference reactions to these observations.

Special topic: Mentalization and family violence

Psychoanalytic Family Therapy is rarely a focus of publications in systemic marriage and family therapy journals. Yet, recently, two companion articles were published on the concept of mentalization in conceptualizing and treating family violence. Asen and Fonagy (2017a; 2017b) define mentalizing as "a form of imaginative mental activity that entails perceiving and interpreting human behavior in terms of intentional mental states" (2017a, p. 8). In other words, it is one's ability to reflect on the mental states of others that underlie their behavior, including their thoughts and feelings (2017a). **Mentalization** is believed to be developed through attachment-based interactions with a caregiver, providing a good example of how psychoanalytic family therapists consider the interactions between the interpersonal and intrapersonal factors (Framo, 1992). Asen and Fonagy (2017a) hypothesize that families who perpetuate violence do not engage in mentalization, particularly when a violent interaction occurs; or if mentalization does occur, it is of poor quality, leading to inaccurate assumptions about a family member's intentions. Mentalization is difficult to engage in when a person is in a heightened arousal state. If attachment relationships are insecure and violent, then it is difficult to develop mentalization skills, increasing the potential for transmitting violence across generations. As a result, interventions seek to improve family members' mentalization skills (2017a; b), particularly when interactions that triggered heightened arousal occur.

How change occurs

Psychoanalysts believe that unconscious forces, including thoughts, feelings, emotions and childhood events, contribute to current difficulties that clients face. In Psychoanalytic Family Therapy, the goal is to help individuals free themselves by gaining insight into these unconscious forces so that they can learn new ways to relate. The hope is that the therapist can provide a safe environment in which a couple or family's defenses can be observed in session. By helping clients to view and understand these unconscious forces, therapists can help facilitate change in current thoughts, behaviors and motions that will impact future relationships (Scharff & Scharff, 1997).

Psychoanalytic family therapists hope that, by altering the ways in which these inner conflicts are understood and expressed, they will thereby alter its influence on the individual and their current and future relationships. Ideally, the therapeutic process will help family members identify their own projections onto others and view one another as separate people from their projections. Hopefully, then family members can begin to love one another based on who they truly are, rather than as a result of seeking lost parts of self in one another (Scharff & Scharff, 1997)). This autonomy in a marriage or other family relationships should ideally promote a more mature love of one another and of self.

Change, therefore, occurs internally when clients are able to gain better awareness and resolve old conflicts.

Role of the therapist

Psychoanalytic therapists, while considered the expert in the room, are non-directive as they remain neutral in allowing the clients to decide how they would prefer to use the therapeutic process (Scharff, 2004; Scharff & Scharff, 1997). They rely heavily on transference and countertransference experiences while family therapists on the other hand rely very little or not at all on transference and countertransference. In fact, family therapists are not necessarily trained extensively on how to incorporate transference and countertransference in therapy. Also, while a psychoanalyst will seek to learn and understand the unconscious forces that exist within the individual, a family therapist does not. Family therapists focus on understanding interpersonal relationships, interactions and observable behaviors, and how they impact the individual, their relationships and their family system.

From a Psychoanalytic Family Therapy approach, the therapist will establish a warm and safe working environment and create a space in which clients can explore individual and interpersonal factors and family members can interact with each other freely. The therapist often will take on the role of an expert and guide the client toward gaining insight into the unconscious forces from the past that are impacting their current relationships and thought patterns. Unconscious forces from early relationships, including feelings of love, hate, jealousy, etc., are often believed to cause conflicts within individuals and their relationships often hindering healthy growth and development. A psychoanalytic family therapist will work toward bringing awareness to the presence of these feelings and encourage family members to relate to each other based on current circumstances rather than previous relationships. Ultimately, the goal is increased self-understanding thereby leading to relief and well-being within the individual and their family system.

Interventions

Although psychoanalysis and family therapy have very different foundations and developed and evolved from very different ideas and concepts, there are some techniques common to both approaches that psychoanalytic family therapists draw on when working with clients. These techniques, designed to promote insight, include listening, empathy, interpretations and analytic neutrality (Nichols & Schwartz, 1991; Scharff & Scharff, 1997).

a. **Non-directive listening.** Psychoanalytic therapists' main intervention is listening and observing for the emergence of interpersonal cycles that are driven by unconscious processes. They are particularly attentive to how each family member's family history is influencing current family patterns (Scharff & Scharff, 1997). They listen not only for patterns between clients, but also the transference/countertransference patterns between client and therapist. The therapist needs to avoid commenting or reassuring the clients on their story and also ensure that they do not say anything to direct attention to anything in particular. One key aspect to being able to listen for clients' unconscious processes is being aware of one's own unconscious. As a result, it is critical for psychoanalytic therapists to engage in their own therapy and self-analysis.

b. **Empathy and holding environment.** Many family therapists will agree that empathy is the cornerstone of the therapeutic relationship and is crucial in order to facilitate an honest and open relationship with the client. The hope is that empathy creates a holding environment that encourages unconsciously driven patterns to emerge (Scharff & Scharff, 1997). Empathy also allows psychoanalytic family to connect with their clients when sharing their interpretations in therapy.

c. **Interpretations.** When applying the technique of interpretation, the psychoanalytic family therapist shares with the client his or her understanding or interpretation of the unconscious forces acting on the individual or family. These interpretations are offered to the client by the therapist so that they can better understand these forces and thereby be liberated from its negative influences (Scharff & Scharff, 1997).

d. **Analytic neutrality.** In many models of family therapy, including structural therapy, the therapist works actively to become part of the family system and to help facilitate change. In contrast, psychoanalytic family therapists take on a neutral position and avoid becoming a part of the family system. Neutrality means they do not take sides, judge life-styles choices or show preference for a treatment outcome such as whether or not a couple should stay to together (Scharff & Scharff, 1997). Neutrality also allows them to remain aware of the process happening within themselves as well as the family. When a therapist feels influenced to move away from neutrality, this is interpreted as an influence of transference or countertransference and is used to promote insight about unconscious processes.

Case example: second session

Guillermo is a 59-year-old Hispanic male who has been married to Julie, a 46-year-old White female, for 7 years. The couple report loving each other very much, but lately they have been struggling to tolerate each other's behavior. Guillermo reports that Julie is always in some sort of pain and sometimes cannot even get out of bed. Julie retorts that she believes she has long Covid and that Guillermo does not listen to her and is always just trying to fix things. Guillermo counters that Julie has had aches and pains long before she got Covid and that sometimes she just needs to get moving in the morning and she usually feels better. He emphasizes, "I'm just trying to help!"

Julie, who has been in therapy for years, explained that she is doing much better than her mother, who suffered from significant depression when she was a child and Julie believed that she was prisoner to her mother and her depression (**influence of family patterns**). Julie reported that things got so bad that her mother would threaten to kill herself if Julie did not acquiesce to her requests and demands. Consequently, Julie was afraid, well into her young adulthood, that she would kill her mother if she did not do what she asked. The therapist could see that Julie was alternating between being visibly teary-eyed and at other times looking enraged at the ridiculous things she had to do for her mother, to which the therapist used non-verbal cues to encourage Julie to talk more about those feelings (**non-directive listening**). Julie shared that growing up she was scared, enraged and guilty about the things she had to do as a young child. She learned at this time if she was physically ill that her mother, albeit reluctantly, would take her to the doctor, even though her mother thought she was doing it to spite her. It was at the doctor's office that she found someone who would listen to her, and she found some relief when she went to the doctor and felt heard. The therapist acknowledged how difficult and risky it must have been to share those painful experiences and thanked Julie for doing that. The therapist then reflected that finding someone who could hear and accept her pain seems to be something she has been searching out for a very long time (**empathy and holding environment**).

Julie shared that she left home in her 20s at the advice of a psychiatrist to get as far away from her mother as possible, but she would still talk to her mother by phone and her mother would visit when she could. It was at this time that Julie started to misuse substances, particularly alcohol, to soothe herself, which she reported provided some temporary relief. The interactions with her mother would invoke intense rage, which led to more substance use and bingeing on food up until her mother died (**identifying unconscious forces**).

Julie reported after her mother's death that she began to attend AA and the self-medication she had engaged in ceased, and she attends weekly AA to date. The therapist pointed out that there seemed to be a relationship between Julie's mother's persecutory behavior, Julie's rage, substance use, physical symptoms, and her guilt and regret (**analytic neutrality**). The therapist pointed out that if she had experienced some of the things that Julie did for much of her life that she too would have been enraged both for the sheer amount of time her mother consumed, but also because she sacrificed so much for her mother. "It makes total sense that on the one hand you were furious that you had to give so much to your mother and that you would regret your outbursts and rage, after all, it was not your mother's fault that she was so depressed." (**transference/countertransference**). Initially, Julie did not see the connection between her suppressing the rage she had for her mother and her substance misuse, physical symptoms and behavior (**acknowledging unconscious forces from the past**).

As Guillermo listened to Julie tell her story, he was taken back as how different Julie's childhood was relative to his own. Guillermo was living a comfortable and affluent life in a South American country when, due to political strife, he was forced to move to the U.S. at the age of 12 to live with a relative and did not see his parents for another decade. Consequently, he learned to avoid feelings and focused on the future with little reflection. Problem-solving was his strength and he was able to build a successful career as a highly sought-out organizational consultant. However, those skills did not serve him as well in his personal life and, after leaving his first wife, he met Julie and they married. Upon reflection he said, "Julie had the ability to emote, which I lack, and I found that appealing at first. Now every time I try to help her, things just get worse." (**identifying unconscious forces**)

The therapist worked with the couple to explore how their current ways of interacting might be evoking in the other a response that was less than desirable (**interpretations/using the therapeutic process**). Julie thought there may be a way that she could share her pain with Guillermo that would be less likely to evoke his need to fix things (**bringing awareness to the present**). Julie's vulnerability and offer to change also evoked in Guillermo a willingness to recognize and share the pain, anger and loss he experienced as a child and connect it to his current behaviors (**developing insight**).

Research support

Psychoanalytic models have limited research support for their theories and interventions, and peer-reviewed presentations and publications have waned on this topic as many therapists are drawn to postmodern models and those concerned with rigorously testing models are drawn to models that are more easily studied such as cognitive behavioral approaches (Lebow, 2017). However, it should be noted that psychoanalytic family therapists draw heavily from attachment theory, which has been well studied across behavioral and social fields and has been found to be a useful foundational concept in therapy (e.g., Johnson, 2004).

Heather MacIntosh systematically reviewed 50 years of publications on couple therapy in the psychoanalytic literature. While reviewing 113 peer-reviewed articles on couple's therapy from a psychoanalytic stance, she found that nearly 80% of articles were case studies and slightly less than 20% were descriptions of conceptual frameworks with no research (MacIntosh, 2018). Only two of the studies reviewed used empirical methods (Cohen, Fisher & Clulow, 1993; Lanman, Grier & Evans, 2003), emphasizing the need for more rigorous methods in this field.

Cultural and ethical considerations

One concerning finding from MacIntosh's (2018) systematic review on psychoanalytic couples therapy is that clients and therapists in the studies were predominantly White and middle class. Therefore, the literature is lacking in research and recommendations for adapting the model for diverse populations.

Since there is little research providing recommendations on adapting psychoanalytic therapy for diverse populations, we need to follow general guidelines regarding cultural competence and humility when using this model. This involves being curious to understand each client's unique cultural context and mindful of how social inequalities can influence presenting problems as well as the therapist-client relationship (Fisher-Borne et al., 2015). Psychoanalytic therapists would want to explore cultural values related to relationships and mental health to ensure that therapy goals are in alignment. If there is a stigma regarding seeking therapy services, the therapist needs to explore what cultural values and family dynamics relate to any hesitancy a family might have to engage in therapy. Using a cultural humility lens, the psychoanalytic therapist will want to reflect upon their own cultural context and how this will influence their relationships with clients, whether they are similar or different (Fisher-Borne et al., 2015; Mosher et al., 2017). This can be integrated as part of the reflection psychoanalytic therapists already engage in related to transference and countertransference.

Psychoanalytic family therapists are strong advocates of neutrality, which has clear therapeutic and ethical advantages. For example, this neutrality can help them to maintain a nonjudgmental stance as they do not take a position on lifestyle choices (Scharff & Scharff, 1997). However, in order to ensure adherence to marriage and the family therapist's code of ethics, they will need to consider times in which they need to break from a neutral stance. This could be related to safety concerns or issues in which neutrality could reinforce marginalization and discrimination. For example, a therapist must take a clear stance against all forms of intimate partner violence; or, if a family member is rejecting of an adolescent who identifies as transgender, the therapist needs to take a clear transaffirmative stance.

References

Ackerman, N. W. (1938). *The unity of the family*. Archives of Pediatrics, 55, 61–62.

Asen, E. & Fonagy, P. (2017a). Mentalizing family violence part 1: conceptual framework. *Family Process*, 56(1), 6–21.

Asen, E. & Fonagy, P. (2017b). Mentalizing family violence part 1: techniques and interventions. *Family Process*, 56(1), 22–44.

Bion, W. R. (1967). *Second thoughts*. London, UK: Karnac.

Boszormenyi Nagy, I. & Krasner, B. (1985). *Between give and take: a clinical guide to contextual therapy*. New York, NY: Brunner-Routledge.

Cohen, N., Fisher, J. & Clulow, C. (1993). Predicting engagement with psychoanalytical couple psychotherapy. *Sexual and Marital Therapy*, 8(3), 217–230.

Dicks, H. V. (1967). *Marital tensions: clinical studies towards a psycho-analytic theory of interaction*. London, UK: Routledge and Kegan Paul.

Fairburn, W. R. D. (1952). *Psychoanalytic study of the personalities*. London, UK: Routledge and Kegan Paul.

Fisher-Borne, M., Cain, J. M. & Martin, S. L. (2015). From mastery to accountability: cultural humility as an alternative to cultural competence. *Social Work Education*, 34(2), 165–181.

Flaskas, C. (2005). Psychoanalytic ideas and systemic family therapy: revisiting the question 'why bother?'. *Australia and New Zealand Family Therapy Journal*, 26, 125–134.

Framo, J. (1992). *Family-of-origin therapy: an intergenerational approach*. New York, NY: Routledge.

Johnson, S. M. (2004). Attachment theory: a guide for healing couple relationships.

Klein, M. (1948). *Contributions to psycho-analysis, 1921–1945*. London, UK: Hogarth Press.

Lebow, J. L. (2017). Mentalization and psychoanalytic couple and family therapy. *Family Process*, 56(1), 3–5. https://doi.org/10.1111/famp.12277

Lanman, M., Grier, F. & Evans, C. (2003). Objectivity in psychoanalytic assessment of couple relationships. *The British Journal of Psychiatry*, 182(3), 255–260.

MacIntosh, H. B. (2018). From application to approach: a systematic review of 50 years of psychoanalytic couple therapy. *Psychoanalytic Inquiry*, 38, 331–358.

Mosher, D. K., Hook, J. N., Captari, L. E., Davis, D. E., DeBlaere, C. & Owen, J. (2017). Cultural humility: a therapeutic framework for engaging diverse clients. *Practice Innovations*, 2(4), 221.

Nichols, M. P. & Schwartz, R. C. (1991). *Family therapy: concepts and methods*. Allyn and Bacon.

Scharff, D. & Scharff, J. (1987). *Objects relations family therapy*. Lanham, MD: Rowman and Littlefield.

Scharff, J. S. (2004). Play and very young children in object relations family therapy. *International Journal of Applied Psychoanalytic Studies*, 1(3), 259–268.

Scharff, J. S. & Scharff, D. E. (1997). Object relations couple therapy. *American Journal of Psychotherapy*, 51(2), 141–173.

Part III

Postmodern Models of Family Therapy

18 Postmodernism and Social Constructionism in Family Therapy

Valerie Q. Glass

Introduction

In Chapter 4, we began to connect to the ideas of postmodernism and social construction. This chapter will continue to make the connection to postmodernism as it is related to family therapy theories. Postmodernist and social constructionist ideas have their roots in philosophy. This chapter will explore the way that postmodernism and social constructions have provided a foundation for the postmodern models of marriage and family therapy (MFT). Essentially, postmodernism and social constructions seek to identify the meaning behind what the clients bring to therapy. Burr (1995) discusses the role of social construction as a primary factor in the current understanding of psychology and mental health. This connection is primary due to the languaging that occurs between therapist and client. Freedman and Combs (1996) attribute postmodern therapy to "meaning" and the understanding and presentation of meaning within clients' lives. The conversation and collaboration that exist between client and therapist generate new realities and new social constructions. This chapter will present the link to the constructs and their role in MFT specifically. Note that, in this chapter, I often used the constructs of postmodernism and social construction interchangeably to better understand the differences; please see the other resources provided to you and/or refer to Chapter 4.

Postmodernism and mental health

Mental health workers have developed their own constructions around diagnosis that play a role in their own work. Consider our identity as systemic therapists and how this might differ from psychiatrists, social workers or counselors who primarily explore cases from an individual perspective. Systemic thinkers (like MFTs) are going to explore how the diagnosis plays out in the family context, while psychiatrists are going to look at the medical background and consider medication. These are professional identities, both supported by research; however, they differ in their constructions of both assessment and change processes of mental illness.

One important contribution that social construction and postmodernism have provided mental health communities is the understanding that every family, every individual, is different. Each person has a different construction, a different reality. In general, mental health fields have begun to better embrace families with different structures, values and morals. There is a sense that, despite a clinician's approach, there is not a "one size fits all" way of assessing or treating specific presenting problems. The incorporation of social

DOI: 10.4324/9781003382621-22

construction and postmodernist ideas in the field of MFT has led to new "constructions" for defining family, defining therapy and defining the role of clinicians.

Considering language

The primary "tool" used by postmodernist and social constructionist ideologies are tied to the understanding of language and the role of language in how we understand the world. Hoffman (1992) shared that our understanding "evolves in the space between people" (p. 8). At the core of what therapists and most mental health workers do is process clients' language and understanding of that language (Mills & Sprenkle, 1995). We work to better understand the worldview of the client, as well as the meaning they place on the presenting ideas that are part of therapeutic work. This expression of language and the language we, as therapists, present back, influences change or direction. Language is a crucial part of all models. In postmodern models, the primary focus is better understanding the client's meaning rather than infusing our understanding of the world by pushing our language. Consider a moment in time where you had a discussion with a teacher, physician, friend or relative where they just did not "get" what you were trying to explain while also pushing their own reality. In many ways physicians do this, they have the diagnosis in mind before entering the exam room. Many modernist therapists projected an understanding of "healthy family" onto the client before noting the client's understanding of a "healthy family".

Language is the way we better understand without inserting our experience.

Defining family constructs

Consider the changing definition of family that is occurring throughout the U.S. currently. The social construction of "family" is key to what we do as systemic thinkers (Mills & Sprenkle, 1995). If we traveled back in time to the 1950s in the U.S., everything about how we define family would look different. Family social constructions consisted of a male (husband/father), who was the head of the home in decision-making, financial contribution, and setting the rules and expectations. Aside from this role, there was a female figure who tended household and childcare duties. Children were to mind parents. There were constructions about communication, behavior and appearance (i.e., what was labeled as a "normal" family was White and middle class). Fast-forward to today, family can take on many different social constructions. Larger social systems (including laws) have recognized differences in family and family therapy has followed suit. We can no longer assess family dynamics based on this 1950s construction. In addition, because of the varied definitions of family, we can no longer assume that we understand from our own perspective of family. The social construction of family is at the root of what we as MFTs do on a daily basis.

Postmodern therapy constructs and applications

This section will identify some of the concepts and interventions that are used by postmodern family therapy models. The core of postmodern therapy is a belief, a true understanding, that social construction is what generates reality. Interventions are part of some of the postmodern models and will be addressed here as well; however, it is important to state that the "interventions" are merely a result of the social constructionist's mindset. Throughout the next few chapters in this book, you will consider different postmodern models. This chapter will specifically tie in the constructs of postmodernism and social constructions as they provide underlying assumptions as to how change happens in postmodern models. Interventions will be brought in to describe the connection between the assumptions of how change happens and what this looks like in interventions. Visit the chapters on Solution-Focused, Narrative and Collaborative for more detailed explanations on the models themselves.

Second-order cybernetics

The systemic concept of second-order cybernetics plays an important role in the understanding of postmodernist models (Mills & Sprenkle, 1995). In the mid-1900s, systemic theorists explored the idea of cybernetics to explain family systems (Hanson, 1995). Cybernetics is the way a family adapts to maintain their comfort level (their homeostasis). If a family seems to live in constant chaos, each family member seems to have a role in this chaos. One member may "cause trouble", another may come in to "save the day" and another may over-react and pull in other members of the family; this is cybernetics. Cybernetics is the way the system "stays on course" or maintains its direction. If the family starts to move in a different direction, the family members will jump back into their roles to keep this chaos in their lives because it is what is comfortable to them.

Early modernist theorists (most notably those in MRI brief, Milan, Intergenerational and Structural) identified the role of the therapist as an "objective observer" to the family's cybernetic process (Mills & Sprenkle, 1995). They noted that our role as family therapists was to help the family identify and change the process that was not working for them. As postmodernists began to look at family process and, more specifically, cybernetics, there was a realization that once the therapist was working with the family, they were part of the system, playing a role in the family cybernetic process. This is what is known as second-order cybernetics.

Consider what you know about social construction and how you think second-order cybernetics fits with the recognition that we each have a different social construction. As therapists, who are part of the family system, postmodernist ideas help us see how we are influencing the family social construction. It is a reminder about recognizing our own social constructions and working to maintain that recognition while understanding the clients' reality. Second-order cybernetics has led to a focus on the importance of "self-of-the-therapist" work because of the likelihood of our experiences and understandings playing a major role in the family system.

Deconstruction

Freedman and Combs (1996) introduce the ideas of deconstructive listening and deconstructive questioning. In deconstructive listening, the therapist listens to the client in a way that makes no assumptions about the meaning behind what they are sharing. Postmodernist therapists ask questions to follow up and make sure we are understanding their meaning. The process of asking questions in essence generates new social constructions because the questions lead the client to explore their meaning in a new way.

Deconstruction can also be a more active and mindful process for individuals, families and society as a whole (Freedman & Combs, 1996). Consider a man comes in and shares he feels weak and does not "feel like a man". The postmodernist therapist might ask questions that allow that client to deconstruct his meaning about masculinity. For example, maybe the man mentioned that he cries a lot and this makes him feel weak. The postmodern therapist will ask: "Where did you learn that crying was a weakness?", "Have you seen men in your life crying?", "What message did you get as a child around crying?" or "does your sister cry? How has your family reacted to her when she cries?" By thinking through these questions, the client might begin to question his own previous social constructions and adopt a new social construction by looking at where and how this social construction developed.

We can also consider the deconstruction of social messages that may integrate power and/ or biases in a way that is harmful. For example, let us assume there is an African American man in therapy who shares some challenges with depression and anxiety. He mentions that he fears governmental officers and social settings. It would make sense, from a postmodern perspective, to deconstruct the role of racism in his life and the influences of his experiences with racism on the presenting problem. The postmodern therapist might dive into this context as a way to tap into the connection between social injustices and mental health. Some examples of deconstructing questions could include: "Tell me more about how you personally have experienced microaggressions in your life" or "Do you have moments where you feel a sense of safety in your world, what do these look like?"

Collaboration

Postmodernists seek to explore the collaborative components of the therapeutic relationship (Hoffman, 1992). Prior to postmodernism coming into scope, therapy took on an "expert" approach and the therapist held the role of power in the relationship.

Postmodernists challenge this thinking and push to create a more level relationship between client and therapist. To create this collaborative dynamic, therapists must be aware of their power, their own social constructions and their identity. Therapists should not dictate changes, rather learn from their client and suggest and "check-in" with their client about possible challenges. Postmodern therapy embraces the idea that the therapist works "with" the client, taking in the client's goals, direction and understanding as a way to move the client toward change. Rather than the therapist jumping in and stating "if you did X, you would see a resolution in your symptoms", the postmodern therapist would open up the dialogue around what "X" would look like. For example, the postmodern therapist might ask "Was there a time that your symptoms were not there, what was that like?" or "If you had a resolution in your symptoms, what do you imagine that would look like?"

Not-knowing

One way to conceptualize how postmodern therapies work is through what is called "not-knowing" (Anderson & Goolishian, 1992). The theory behind this idea of not-knowing comes from the recognition of how language is communicated. For someone to share "I feel sad about my loneliness" brings with it constructs that may mean something different for the person saying it and the person hearing it. By taking a not-knowing stance, the therapist assumes they do not know or understand these constructs; they might say, "Tell me what sad feels like to you" or "When you feel lonely, what does that look like?" Each one of us comes from a place of understanding from our own social constructions and we cannot project that to the clients. If a client states "I am an awful mother", this evokes many images to the therapist. Rather than assuming these images exist for the client, the postmodern therapist would ask "What does a good mother look like?" or "What about your experience led you to think you were an awful mother?" Using this not-knowing approach allows us to better understand the social constructs of these words for the client. Anderson and

Goolishian (1992) state that the not-knowing stance is not a technique, rather it is a mindset through which the client approaches therapy. This stance allows the therapist to truly honor where the client is coming from. Not-knowing is asking questions that we, as therapists, do not have a pre-set understanding or even expectation about what the answer might be (Freedman & Combs, 1996). Anderson (1997; Anderson, 2005) states that "not-knowing means humility about what one knows. In effect, a therapist is more interested in learning what a client has to say that in pursuing, telling, validation, or promoting his or her know-ledge or preoccupations" (p. 136). One important characteristic of not-knowing is that this does not mean the therapist is without thoughts or opinions, it is more the recognition that the client's may differ.

Client as expert

Postmodernist approaches identify the client as the expert of their lives (Anderson, 1997). In contrast to modernist models where the therapist enters the room, engages in a series of questions, and provides an assessment and a direction for therapy, postmodernist therapists approach each session to learn more about what the client wants from the therapeutic relationship and their personal goals. Being aware of our own social constructions and working to put these aside to truly listen to the client's social constructions is a major part of the postmodern models. Social construction and postmodernism identify that the clients know themselves better than anyone else. There is a focus on collaboration and better understanding the client's goals (rather than the therapist's goals). Consider this example. a family comes in for therapy and there is a parent, stepparent and two children. One child is clingy to the biological parent at all times. If you look back at a modernist model, like the Structural or Bowen models (see Chapters 9 and 12), the therapist immediately develops a clear therapeutic direction. The Bowen therapist might state as a goal "we need to define clear differentiation between child and parent". The structural therapist might say "the family has developed an unhealthy hierarchy and clear parental subsystems need to be established". In contrast, the postmodern therapist would not make these directional assumptions and might ask the family members, "What would you want your family to look like?" Therapeutic goals would be developed collaboratively based on what the client feels is best for them.

Mapping the influence of the problem

One technique that is used by narrative therapists that builds in the idea of social construc-tion is mapping the influence of the problem (White & Epston, 1990). As the postmodern therapist is taking into consideration the client's story, mapping the influence of the problem explores many of the elements around the family that could be influencing the presenting problem. When I think about this technique, I think about really getting as many details about the problem as possible from the clients' social constructions. This could include asking about how the problem influences each person individually, how the problem is seen by larger social venues (culture, community, school, friends, extended family, etc.), how the problem influences emotions, functioning, daily life or any number of possible influences. The goal of mapping the problem is to deeply explore this problem story and identify the family's constructions around the problem. By asking questions, the socially constructed "space" that exists within the conversation leads to new social constructions. Postmodern models often pull in strengths as they map the influence of the problem as well. This allows the client to start socially constructing what "works well" in their lives already and apply this to creating change.

Consider an example of this process, there is a family of five (two parents and three children under 10) that come into therapy. The family shares that the middle child is constantly picking fights with the other two children and is not listening to the parents. The postmodern therapist begins to ask all the members of the system about their experience with the problem. Often questions are more strength-based in format. For example, they might ask one sibling "When is (middle sibling) less likely to pick on you?" Or, the therapist might ask one of the parents "When do you see the three siblings getting along?" If there is a response, the therapist will continue to build on this mapping process. For example, maybe the parent shares that the three siblings get along well when they go to the park. The therapist will check-in with the others in the family, "What do you think is different about being at the park?" Maybe the middle child says: "I enjoy playing in the tire swing with my brother because he makes me laugh a lot." The therapist can ask, "When are other times when the family can laugh a lot?" Mapping the influence of the problem helps the family look at exceptions to the problem, it helps the therapist (and the family) better understand contextual factors around what is happening, it allows for collaboration between therapist and client, and it generates a new social construction around looking at the dynamics.

Conversation

Conversation is the main "tool" for postmodern therapists. Considering postmodernists approach therapy from the social constructionist lens, defining this as meaning created between individuals, conversation is crucial to the process of therapy (Anderson & Goolishian, 1992). The development of a conversation about what the client brings into the room both defines the story or situation from the client's perspective, while also contributing thought and dialogue about possible changes to the story in that "space between". Therapy is conversing and the definition of therapy is that change occurs as a result of the therapeutic connection and resulting dialogue. Conversation is simply asking about the stories around the "problem". It is asking about what the family wants in life, what they have tried and what they have not tried.

Dominant narratives

The idea of "dominant narrative" can be explored individually or through a social lens. Individually, when we think of a dominant narrative, this is the narrative the client brings into therapy. This dominant narrative is the "story" that has challenged the client and becomes a major force in their presenting problem. I think of this as being "stuck" in the story. For example, assume a family comes in and a parent and teen are at odds. The family is constantly sharing how awful the relationship between the two are and consistently discuss how difficult it has been in the home because of the bickering. This has become the dominant narrative of the family. Dominant narratives can be social constructions in themselves (almost like self-fulfilling prophecies). The family constructs that this "problem" (the dominant narrative) is the way things are. By exploring other ways of looking at this narrative, change happens. Creating space for a new narrative to evolve allows the family to get out of the social construction that this is the way things are.

One aspect of stories that is addressed by the postmodernist lens is the dominant narratives of one's social environment (Freedman & Combs, 1996). Dominant narratives can be defined as the social constructions in our environment that are more generated by those in power, those in the majority. Consider an example of the 1950s U.S. and the social construction of family at the time. This was a dominant narrative because if one's family did not fit into the idea of a heterosexual, White, middle class, 2.5 kids and white picket fence construction, that family was thought of as on the fringe, even abhorrent. Social construction around difference (or non-majority communities) tend to negate or problematize those populations. Social construction processes indicate that minority communities can internalize some of the negative social constructions that exist to describe their uniquenesses. Consider a couple that may share they are struggling with intimacy. They are a same-sex couple. The therapist starts to unpack their experience and one individual shares they struggle with religious messages from their past and also some of the opinions of their family. This is leading to a dominant narrative that they are internalizing the dominant narrative from their environment that same-sex relationships are not appropriate. Through asking questions about this dominant narrative of homophobia, the client starts to recognize that this narrative has contributed to their challenges with intimacy with their partner.

Externalization

Externalizing is a construct that developed out of the narrative model (Freedman & Combs, 1996). The idea behind externalization is the construct of a different reality behind the presenting problem or "story" the client brings to therapy. To externalize is to put the problem outside of the person. Oftentimes, social constructions equate the person in the problem. Consider the difference between saying "he is anxious" and "he has anxiety". From a social constructionist perspective, the second example allows the system around the family (and the identified client) to explore this construction a bit differently. A narrative therapist might ask the question, "Tell me how anxiety influenced you today?" as a way to externalize the problem and allow the story to develop out of this externalization. Michael White and David Epston (1990) state that this kind of externalization allows families to "open up possibilities for them to describe themselves, each other, and their relationships from a new, nonproblem-saturated perspective" (p. 39). Externalization changes the social construction.

Locating strengths

Collaborative, Narrative and Solution-Focused models all address strengths differently; however, each of these models value the importance of highlighting strengths to become part of the client's social construction. As the therapist highlights the strengths within the client's conversation, the client is able to better see these strengths and utilize them as they move toward change. Narrative therapists have identified looking for "unique outcomes" in therapy sessions (White & Epston, 1990). With unique outcomes, the therapist observes and shares moments within the client's story where the problem was not as prevalent as times when the client's strengths helped them through the problem. In the Narrative model, this unique outcome directly becomes part of the "new" story.

The overall goal of the Solution-Focused model is to locate strengths ("solutions") to incorporate change through these solutions. The Solution-Focused model has many techniques that hone in on how to explore client's strengths; I will only mention a couple here. The miracle question is a way to better understand the client's reality and expectation. The miracle question, quite simply, is asking the client "if a miracle were to happen tomorrow and things were exactly the way you would want them to be, what would that look like?" (Strong & Pyle, 2009). In the Solution-Focused model, the idea is that this conversation will lead to social constructions about the future and the client's goals and ask questions about strengths and resources that the family has to get to this solution. Another technique, called scaling questions, asks clients to rate (i.e., on a scale of 1–10) where they feel they are related to the problem each week. This allows the conversation to open up and better understand the strengths (and solutions) involved in helping the situation become "better" some weeks. Locating strengths through conversation can generate new social constructions around the problem. These techniques are often utilized by modernists and postmodernists as a way to identify strengths.

As you can see, there are many ideas and techniques that make up postmodernist models. These embrace the role of the therapist as collaborative and open to the client's constructions. Postmodern models highlight the role of conversation and constructions as they move toward change.

Addressing social justice

Aside from constructs and technique, one area that also utilizes postmodern perspectives is related to social justice. Postmodernism embraces external experiences and constructions, for many postmodernist thinkers, this ideology also incorporates the experiences of those that experience inequalities in our communities (Elliott, 1998).

Through the deconstruction of power in our social spheres, many postmodernist therapists explore the role of dominance, discrimination and prejudices in the clients' lives. We, as therapists, might recognize the inequities that we have developed from our own social constructions and use these to explore this with the client in front of us. A White male therapist seeing an African American female, for example, might share, "In my own life, I have seen a lot of racism and sexism from White men toward African American women. Are there ways that racism and sexism influence you?" Language and the predominate ways that language is presented in respect to groups or "categories" of people influence how these individuals are treated in society (Burr, 1995). Buying into ideas of social construction, many postmodern thinkers feel that we have a responsibility, as therapists, to address some of these inequities and use language as a way to de-construct and develop new constructions that embrace and celebrate uniquenesses.

Postmodern models in MFT

Several notable postmodern models have developed from the ideas of postmodernism and social construction. These have been mentioned before in talking about constructs. I will touch on a couple of these briefly and how social construction and postmodernism influenced the origins of these models.

Solution-Focused Brief Therapy

Solution-Focused Therapy is based in the understanding that an individual can get completely wrapped up in a dominant "problem"-focused meaning (Sutherland, Dienhart & Turner, 2013). The problem and the social constructions around the problem work in a recursive way, keeping the client from embracing other meaningful elements that exist in their lives. Therapists, in the Solution-Focused model, attempt to explore solutions that exist within the client's perspective to move the client into a different social construction, while utilizing their strengths and noted solutions.

Narrative Family Therapy

The way that Narrative Therapy embraces postmodernism is through the language of one's story (Lax, 1992). The idea is that we understand our "presenting problems" are based on a construction of a story around our lived experience. Change in Narrative Therapy is related to the de-construction of this story and identifies the newly constructed story, which is the direction the client wants their life to go in. The therapists' role in Narrative Therapy is to collaborate with the client to make suggestions or highlight elements of the client's self-stated story as a way to construct a new story around a more positive direction.

Collaborative Language Systems

Harlene Anderson (1997) developed the Collaborative approach directly from the understanding of the role of language in the therapeutic relationship. When I think about this approach, I think about a book-club meeting. All the members in the book-club read the same book, yet, when they meet together and discuss elements of that book, they arrive at different (collaborative) ideas that result from the discussion. Anderson's approach begins by engaging with the client and learning about their language and constructions. She identifies that change can occur through the use of sharing. That "space between" the therapist and the client constructs a better understanding of direction for the client. With this, the therapist asks questions and encourages the presentations around the constructions related to the "problem" the family system has introduced into therapy. During this constructing process of therapy, the collaborative therapist might challenge elements of the story, reorganizing meaning to some constructs, opening up options or bringing awareness to other elements of the discourse. This "conversation" provides different ways of looking at the "problem" that are consistent with what the client brings to the room.

The role of research and science

The goal of postmodern therapy is to tap into the client's reality in order to gain a clearer picture of what clients bring and where they want to go in life. Postmodernism is the rejection that there is "one" way or idea. Think about science and medical practice. Consider a disease like cancer. Science can describe, define, medicate, etc. for cancer. That being said, there tends to be more complex issues that science sometimes cannot explain. Why cancer in one person can progress quickly and be completely cured in another leaves the reality of that scientific explanation missing something that is a different reality. When it comes to practice, specifically systemic therapies, postmodernism is about looking at multiple ideas and perspectives. It is about looking at the individual and the family within the context of their social constructions.

The idea is that there is a reinventing or re-constructing going on all the time. This is the focus of change (Gergen & McNamee, 1992).

A consideration when it comes to science and postmodernist family therapies is related to diagnosing (Iversen, Gergen & Fairbanks, 2005). Given the insurance and medical social constructions that are often involved in our therapeutic work, understanding diagnosing and assessing from a postmodernist perspective can be essential. Even modernist systemic therapists assess clients (i.e., there is a lack of differentiation/Bowen, the family hierarchy does not support the parents/Minuchin). Genograms are commonly used to highlight relationship patterns and identify them as problematic. Social constructionist ideas find assessments to only embrace the constructions around the assessment, and may not embrace the constructions of the client. Iversen et al. (2005) argue that it is important that social constructionists add to the dialogue about the usefulness of evaluations and assessment. They stress that the dialogue within the field is essential to the new constructions of the way mental health and family dynamics are viewed. Being that the use of these is common and expected, viewing these as "new options or possibilities" (Iversen et al., 2005, p. 11) is one way postmodernist therapists can build in these expectations. Presenting ideas to clients and "checking-in" with them about their experiences and emotions around the assessment, I have found that sometimes a diagnosis or a concept that defines a way of looking at family dynamics leads clients to a different story that they embrace. It can be empowering to put language and meaning behind an experience.

Consider evidence-based practice and the connection to postmodernism or social construction. Evidence-based practice is research that explores different theories, presenting problems, techniques and other therapeutic encounters to indicate the "best" direction for the therapist to go in therapy. If you are postmodern, would you ignore the research because you know that people do things differently? If you were a modernist, would you do exactly what the research said because you believe it to be truth? Many modernists and postmodernists have debated certain elements or results of evidence-based practice. Some research (typically qualitative) explores certain situations rather than apply the research to large groups. Other research identifies itself as generalizable to larger populations because it is "founded" in scientific methodology. Ramey and Grubb (2009) highlight the importance of looking at both of these philosophies and valuing what both bring to research and practice. Modernism can highlight "common" trends and postmodernism can build in specifics that may not fit with the trends. Currently, research that highlights a mixed-method approach builds in these strengths that explore both modernism and postmodernism.

Tilsen and McNamee (2015) shared the challenges that some postmodern and social constructionist therapists highlight in evidence-based practice research.

Research is summative and highlights a meaning or direction. Less frequently, research identifies variants or multiple perspectives. Also, it is important to note, the process of therapy isn't part of the "outcome" identified in much quantitative research. Clients may not respond the same to data-supported measures of therapeutic success. These researchers highlight rethinking research and Feedback Informed Therapy (FIT). Rather than the therapists' knowledge of the "evidence" gathered on a particular presenting problem or technique, the therapists may introduce some researched directions to the therapy room, while allowing the feedback from the client to guide the process. FIT involves a deliberate checking-in process.

Summary

We have discussed the foundational philosophies of postmodernism and social construction. These play a major role in understanding the narrative model, which is built on the understanding that language can shift reality. Keep in mind that postmodernism and social construction – just like their meanings – can vary slightly depending on the user. There is no one reality, there is no one definition of postmodernism (Anderson, 1997). In my own experience with students and early clinicians who are exploring models, defining themselves as a postmodern therapist or adopting one of the postmodern models is about really embracing the constructs of social construction and postmodernism first. It is about fully believing in the idea that our worlds are socially constructed through language and that therapy is a way of tapping into that meaning and helping explore new meanings.

References

Anderson, H. (1997). *Conversation, language, and possibilities: a postmodern approach to therapy*. New York, NY: Basic Books.

Anderson, H. (2005). Myths about "not-knowing." *Family Process, 44*(4), 497–504.

Anderson, H. & Goolishian, H. (1992). The client is the expert. In S. McNamee & K. J. Gergen, *Therapy as a social construction* (pp. 25–39). Thousand Oaks, CA: Sage Publications.

Burr, V. (1995). *Social constructionism*. New York, NY: Routledge.

Elliott, H. (1998). Postmodernism, feminism, and narrative therapy. In S. Madigan & I. Law (Eds.), *Praxis: situating discourse, feminism, and politics in narrative therapies* (pp. 35–59). Vancouver, BC: The Cardigan Press.

Freedman, J. & Combs, G. (1996). *Narrative therapy: the social construction of preferred realities*. New York, NY: WW Norton.

Gergen, K. J. & McNamee, S. (1992). *Therapy as Social Construction*. Thousand Oaks: CA: Sage, 1–240.

Hanson, B. G. (1995). *General systemic theory beginning with wholes*. Washington, DC: Taylor & Francis.

Hoffman, L. (1992). A reflexive stance for family therapy. In S. McNamee & K. J. Gergen, *Therapy as a social construction* (pp. 7–24). Thousand Oaks, CA: Sage Publications.

Iversen, R. R., Gergen, K. J. & Fairbanks, I. P. (2005). Assessment and social construction: conflict or co-creation? *British Journal of Social Work, 35*(5), 689.

Lax, W. D. (1992). Postmodern thinking in a clinical practice. In S. McNamee & K. J. Gergen, *Therapy as a social construction* (pp. 69–85). Thousand Oaks, CA: Sage Publications.

Mills, S. D. & Sprenkle, D. H. (1995). Family therapy in the postmodern era. *Family Relations, 44*, 368–376.

Ramey, H. L. & Grubb, S. (2009). Modernism, postmodernism and (evidence-based) practice. *Contemporary Family Therapy, 31*, 75–86.

Strong, T. & Pyle, N. R. (2009). Constructing a conversational "miracle": examining the "miracle question" as it is used in therapeutic dialogue. *Journal of Constructivist Psychology, 22*(4), 328–353.

Sutherland, O., Dienhart, A. & Turner, J. (2013). Responsive persistence part II: practices of postmodern therapists. *Journal of Marital and Family Therapy, 39*(4), 488–501.

Tilsen, J. & McNamee, S. (2015). Feedback informed treatment: evidence-based practice meets social construction. *Family Process, 54*(1), 124. doi:10.1111/famp.12111

White, M. & Epston, D. (1990). *Narrative means to a therapeutic ends*. New York, NY: W.W. Norton.

19 Solution-Focused Brief Therapy

Vanieca Kraus

Introduction

In the early 1980s, the developers of more traditional models of marriage and family therapy (MFT), such as strategic therapists at the Mental Research Institute (MRI) in Palo Alto, California (Connie, 2013; de Shazer et al., 2012), were focusing on defining the problem and observing the interactions of the family to develop a hypothesis of what was happening in the family/couple system. Their goal was to determine what was going awry in the system so that they could create an intervention to solve the couple/family's problem (Watzlawick, Weakland & Fisch, 1974). Having been trained by this original group, Steve de Shazer, Insoo Kim Berg and colleagues at the Brief Family Therapy Center in Milwaukee were attempting to get more detailed information about the problem so that they could more quickly solve client problems. They started asking clients to go home and observe the problem and come back to the next session with more details. What they noticed is that clients returned reporting, not only about the problem, but also about what they were doing to solve it and what was going well that they wanted to increase. Through this experiment, the observation of hundreds of sessions and being influenced my Milton Erikson, this team learned that it is not necessary to focus on the problem in order to solve it. Rather, they became convinced that clients are resourceful and have solutions within to resolve their problems (de Shazer et al., 2012; Walter & Peller, 1992; Weiner-Davis & Durrant, 2014). Walter and Peller (1992) explained, "We realized that only solution or goal talk was necessary, that solution construction was independent of problem processes" (p. 8). Thus, Solution-Focused Brief Therapy (SFBT) was born.

Philosophical underpinnings

As they developed the SFBT model, Berg, de Shazer and their team were significantly influenced by **social constructionism** and **postmodernism**. At the core of these philosophies are the ideas that reality is relative and socially constructed. That means that there is no one right answer, no one right way that families must be or behave. Rather, reality or meaning is developed through interaction with others, largely through conversation (Gergen, 1985; de Jong & Berg, 2012). In fact, SFBT therapists believe that change occurs when clients change how they talk about a problem because this changes how they experience the problem and the meaning of the problem. Thus, through language, Socratic questioning and conversations, therapists help clients identify their path and determine what they want out of therapy. Rather than bringing a pre-determined set of beliefs of how clients should

DOI: 10.4324/9781003382621-23

function to be healthy, SFBT therapists work with clients to co-construct their goals. This shifts the focus of the therapy session away from problem-oriented language to solution-focused language (de Jong & Berg, 2012). With this understanding, we will look at the core tenets and the systemic foundation of SFBT.

Main concepts

Social constructionism and postmodernism at the core, the focus of therapy becomes positive, strengths-based and future-focused. With that in mind, de Shazer et al. (2012) identified **eight key tenets** of SFBT. These core beliefs are the foundation for everything therapists do in sessions with clients.

If it's not broken, don't fix it. Clients come into therapy stressed and experiencing significant problems. As therapists, it is tempting to focus on these problems; in fact, this is exactly what therapists from other approaches do. As they focus on clients' problems, these therapists will also look for other areas of the clients' lives that are problematic.

However, solution-focused therapists believe that clients are resilient and able to resolve many problems themselves; and thus, they do not address issues that clients do not identify as being a problem (Connie, 2013; de Shazer et al., 2012).

Do more of what's working. Solution-focused therapists understand that clients are capable of solving their own problems and that there are areas of the clients' lives in which they are experiencing success. Through collaborative conversations, SFBT therapists encourage clients to identify areas of success and do more of what is working. Therapists collaborate with clients to discover what is working well and help them use it to accomplish change. Furthermore, SFBT therapists do not offer judgment about these solutions and believe that those successes may very well be solutions for the current problem (Connie, 2013; de Shazer et al., 2012).

Change it up. SFBT therapists are flexible with interventions. Thus, if therapists have been working with clients around a particular intervention that is not working, they will change strategies. Therefore, instead of trying to fit clients into a certain intervention, they will change the intervention to fit the clients. Additionally, when solution-focused therapists hear clients talk about things they are doing that are not helpful, they encourage them to stop doing them and shift the focus to what is working (Connie, 2013; de Shazer et al., 2012).

Even a small change matters. As systemic therapists, SFBT therapists believe that even a small change in the system will affect the whole system; thus, they take a minimalist approach and focus on small manageable changes (Connie, 2013; de Shazer et al., 2012). De Shazer et al. (2012) explained, "…small steps toward making things better help the client move gradually and gracefully forward to accomplish desired changes in their daily life and to subsequently be able to describe things as 'better enough' for therapy to end" (p. 2).

The solution does not need to fit the problem. Remember that the group at the Brief Therapy Center in Milwaukie (see introduction to this chapter) found that it was not necessary to focus on the problem to find a solution. Thus, unlike previous more traditional models, SFBT therapists do not spend a long time gathering historical information and analyzing the problem to determine the "perfect" solution. Rather, they ask about exceptions right away, "Tell me about a time when the problem is or was not happening?", and build on those exceptions. Therapists may use an intervention, such as the miracle question (see below for a more complete explanation), to help clients describe what their lives would look like without the problem. Once they have described a full picture of their lives without the problem, therapists help clients identify their strengths and solutions, which are often not even directly related to the problem (Connie, 2013; de Shazer et al., 2012).

Solution versus problem language. Earlier theorists who were problem-focused spent a lot of time looking at the history of the problem and the family through exploring generational patterns and family legacies (Backhaus, 2011). In contrast, examining solutions rather than problems allows solution-focused therapists to use positive language that focuses on the future. Rather than spending hours talking about the problem and the negative things that go along with it, SFBT therapists help clients talk about positive aspects of their lives and a future that is hopeful. SFBT therapists call this solution talk (Connie, 2013; de Shazer et al., 2012).

No problem is always present; there are always exceptions. Regardless of the amount of time the problem has persisted or the perceived severity of the problem, solution-focused therapists remember that there are always exceptions or times when the problem is not happening. Through collaborative conversations, SFBT therapists seek to identify these exceptions and to develop goals, even very minimalist goals, to increase these times (de Shazer et al., 2012).

The future is created and negotiable. This tenet relates to what we discussed earlier about social constructionism. Rather than seeing clients as being locked into their problems and unable to change, therapists view clients as resourceful and resilient.

Regardless of what the problem is, therapists approach clients believing that they can co-construct a future without the problem (de Shazer et al., 2012).

Keeping all of these tenets in mind, and the philosophical foundations of postmodernism and social constructionism, we will next look at the unique way that SFBT therapists integrate systems theory into their work with clients.

Systemic foundation

Whether seeing one person, a couple or a family, as marriage and family therapists, we work from a systemic perspective. This means that we conceptualize problems within the client's context and recognize that the entire system contributes to problems, through creating, maintaining or solving them (von Bertalanffy, 1968). Given their positive, future, solution-focused philosophy, SFBT therapists believe that all members of the family play a part in identifying, developing and maintaining solutions. What follows is a review of key systems theory ideas and how SFBT therapists integrate these in their work with clients without compromising their assumptions founded in postmodernism and social constructionism.

Homeostasis. Homeostasis is the systems tendency to remain the same (Watzlawick, Bavelas & Jackson, 1967; Whitchurch & Constantine, 1993). This is not a conscious process that clients are aware of; rather, the family will automatically adjust to maintain the status quo. SFBT therapists use interventions to both maintain and disrupt homeostasis, whichever will lead to solution-focused change. One way to do this is to consider how interventions can facilitate either positive or negative feedback.

Positive and negative feedback. When you hear the words positive and negative feedback, you might think, "That's what I get from my professor each week. Feedback that I either did or did not do well on my assignment". However, this is not what these systemic terms refer to. Rather than thinking of positive as good and negative as bad, think about positive meaning change and negative meaning no change. A simple example of this is a woman taking a pregnancy test. If the test is negative, it means she is not pregnant, there was no change (negative feedback), and positive means she is pregnant, there is change (positive feedback) (Watzlawick et al., 1967; Whitchurch & Constantine, 1993).

Solution-focused therapists seek to help clients identify areas of their lives that they should not change. For example, they may use a coping question or a formula first session task (see section on intervention for further explanation of these interventions) to highlight what clients are already doing well and do not want to change. This is negative feedback because clients do not change their thoughts, feelings or behavior as a result of the intervention.

Example: negative feedback

Imagine that you are seeing a couple who is struggling with feeling connected to each other. To elicit negative feedback, you might ask, "What do you want to make sure you do not change as a result of therapy?"

However, when SFBT therapists help clients make changes, it is positive feedback. Two common techniques that can be used to elicit positive feedback are the miracle question and identifying exceptions.

While there are many versions of the miracle question, they all seek to get the client thinking about what life would be like without the problem. The miracle question often goes something like this, "Imagine that you were to wake up tomorrow morning and this problem was solved, what would be different?" When clients answer this question, the therapist will ask more questions to help them provide enough detail that they envision and experience what things will be like without the problem; and thus think, feel and/or do something different (de Jong & Berg, 2012). Because the goal is for clients to change, this is positive feedback.

Another way solution-focused therapists elicit positive feedback is to ask exception questions. These questions help clients view themselves in a different way and thus act differently (de Jong & Berg, 2012).

Example: positive feedback

In the same example above, to elicit positive feedback, you may ask, "Tell me about a time this week when you felt connected to your partner." This helps clients to experience feeling connected in session and recognize activities or communication that helps them feel closer to their partner. The therapist would then follow with other questions to help clients see how they can do more of that in the week to come, which brings about change.

First-order versus second-order change. First-order change is a simple straightforward solution to a problem (Watzlawick et al., 1974). As a solution-focused therapist, you may elicit first-order change by using scaling questions.

Example: first-order change

With the couple above who are working on connecting more, you may ask, "How would you rate your connection on a scale of 1 to 10?" Let's say they answer is 4. You would then ask questions to learn about what they are doing that makes it a 5 and not a 4. Then you could ask, "How can you do just a little bit more of what you are already doing to move from a 5 to a 5½ this week?" The reason this is a first-order change is that it helps them change their behavior, but it doesn't necessarily change their system (Watzlawick et al., 1974).

Whereas first-order change allows the system to keep functioning in the same manner, second-order change requires the system to change (Watzlawick et al., 1974). To elicit second-order change as an SFBT therapist, you would help clients change how they talk about the problem. Through conversation and focusing on positives, you would help them shift from problem-focused to solution-focused language. Shifting their beliefs about the problem leads to a new perspective or view. As clients move from feeling hopeless and overwhelmed that the problem is always happening to hope and belief that change is possible, they will shift in how they talk about the problem, which is second-order change.

Interdependence of subsystems. Changes in one part of the system lead to changes in other parts of the system (Whitchurch & Constantine, 1993). You will see this important systems concept in SFBT therapists' belief that small changes lead to bigger changes (de Shazer et al., 2012). Thus, SFBT therapists look for and encourage small steps or changes clients can make with the belief that this creates positive feedback, leading to bigger changes not just with the individual, but the whole system.

Role of the client and therapist

As you may recall from our earlier discussion, SFBT was developed within the context of postmodernism and social constructionism and, thus, therapists acknowledge that clients develop meaning within relationships, both within their family and within their larger communities (de Jong & Berg, 2012). These philosophical underpinnings have a direct effect on therapists' stance in the therapy room. Rather than taking an expert stance in therapy, SFBT therapists believe that clients are the experts and they join clients in a collaborative relationship to cultivate meaning and help them accomplish their goals. Furthermore, therapists assume that clients have the insights, strength and abilities to solve their own problems (de Jong & Berg, 2012). As a therapist, you will be trained in MFT theory, communication and development. However, you do not have detailed knowledge of clients' thoughts, perceptions, definitions of reality and experiences; thus, the client is the expert regarding him/herself. With this in mind, solution-focused therapists respectfully take a not-knowing stance. This means that they do not claim to know what clients need to do to solve a problem (de Jong & Berg, 2012). As Anderson and Goolishian (1992) as sited in de Jong & Berg, 2012) explained:

> The not-knowing position entails a general attitude or stance in which the therapist's actions communicate an abundant, genuine curiosity. That is, the therapist's actions and attitudes express a need to know more about what has been said, rather than

convey preconceived opinions and expectations about the client, the problem, or what must be changed. The therapist, therefore, positions himself or herself in such a way as to always be in a state of "being informed" by the client. (p. 29)

This non-knowing position is shared with the Collaborative Language Systems Therapy model, which you will read about later in this book. Solution-focused therapists sometimes refer to this as leading from behind because, while you are learning from the client, you are still leading in what you choose to highlight/comment on and the questions you ask. Given the view of the clients' expertise, clients are the ones to set goals for themselves and decide when these goals have been accomplished (de Jong & Berg, 2012).

Last, acknowledging client expertise means that we need to let go of the idea that clients are resistant. While other theorists consider clients, who are not making certain changes, or who question the therapist, to be resistant, de Shazer and colleagues (2012) questioned this notion. De Jong and Berg (2012) explained:

Once we accept the notion of client competence, we are left with a humbling and challenging conclusion: What we once thought of as client resistance is more accurately regarded as practitioner resistance. Impasses and apparent failures in our work do not result from clients' resistance to our best professional efforts to make them well. Rather, they result from our failure to listen to clients and take seriously what they tell us. (p. 79)

The fact that SFBT therapists view clients as the expert, co-collaborators in meaning making, and being ready and capable of making needed changes, affects the way that therapists view change in therapy.

How change happens

Solution-focused therapists assume that clients come into therapy ready and willing to change and that change is constant. In fact, SFBT therapists assume that the client has already started changing just by making the decision to come to therapy.

Furthermore, the client, not the therapist, defines change. During therapy, change happens through solution talk – positive solution-focused conversations. Through this dialogue, therapists work to create hope and an expectation of change. Interventions are not imposed on clients; rather, therapists work collaboratively with clients to set goals. From there, they will facilitate conversations to highlight strengths, resiliency, and identify and expand upon exceptions. As mentioned previously, SFBT therapists believe that even **a very small change can bring about a big change**. This is why they assume that any therapy session could be the last session, i.e. brief therapy (Connie, 2013; de Jong & Berg, 2012; de Shazer et al., 2012). As we move to a discussion of assessment and core interventions, look for the beliefs articulated above related to how clients change and the fact that SFBT therapists assume they will.

Assessment

It will likely not be a surprise to you to learn that assessment looks different in SFBT. SFBT therapists are "not bound by traditional assessment and diagnostic categories, nor does it limit itself to preferred interventions for particular diagnosed problems. Instead, it follows each client from one step behind as the client develops an individualized solution" (de Jong & Berg, 2012, p. 258). Rather than assessing for the scope of the problem, SFBT therapists assess for change, coping strategies and strengths.

Therapists begin this assessment in their first interaction by looking for pre-session change. For example, the therapist may ask, "What changes have you noticed that have happened or started to happen since you called to make the appointment for this session?" (de Shazer et al., 2012, p. 5). De Shazer et al. (2012) identified three possible outcomes of this question. If the client states that there has been no change, the therapist will ask how he/she can be helpful and begin therapy. If the client identifies change, the therapist will start asking questions to elicit detail about the change, i.e., solution talk and help the client continue moving toward this change.

Last, if the client states that things have stayed about the same, the therapist might ask, "How have you managed to keep things from getting worse?" (de Shazer et al., 2012, p. 5). Throughout this conversation, the therapist highlights change, solution and client strengths.

Assessment, identifying client strengths and successes, is a part of every conversation, from the first session to the last, and is seen in every intervention.

Interventions

Compared to their predecessors, interventions in SFBT happen more organically. Remember that strategic therapists were trying to figure out what the problem was so that they could develop a hypothesis about what was happening in the family system and create an intervention to interrupt the homeostasis (Watzlawick et al., 1974). In contrast, solution-focused therapists accept that they become part of the system and, thus, are not able to "observe" what is going on and develop an intervention to "change" people. Rather, as we discussed in the previous sections, solution-focused therapists see clients as resilient, capable and ready to change. Through collaborative conversations with clients, they seek to highlight strengths and resiliency and build upon solutions that are already occurring or open up possibilities for clients. So, the question becomes, what do these collaborative conversations look like?

Collaborative conversations. Our first goal in therapy, as solution-focused therapists, is to have collaborative conversations with clients. Thus, solution-focused therapists often start by asking, "How can we be useful to you?" (de Jong & Berg, 2012, p. 17).

Notice that this question is not focused on the problem and thus it sets the therapist up as a collaborator/partner in helping the client. Because SFBT therapists are not expected to focus on the problem and they believe that anything can become a solution, therapists engage in these conversations with curiosity and openness. As therapists, we are looking for direction from the client about what they want to do differently and what they want their life to look like. However, being a solution-focused therapist is not all about listening; rather, you initiate this process through asking Socratic questions (de Jong & Berg, 2012).

Miracle question. As mentioned above, one of the first things we want to know is how we can be useful to clients, what their goals are for therapy. To discover these goals, solution-focused therapists ask the miracle question, designed by Insoo Kim Berg to help clients paint a picture of what they want their life to look like. This question can take different forms, but is often phrased like this: "Now I want to ask you a strange question. Suppose that while you are sleeping tonight and the entire house is quiet, a miracle happens. The miracle is that the problem that brought you here is solved. However, because you are sleeping you don't know that the miracle has happened. So, when you wake up tomorrow morning, what will be different that will tell you that a miracle has happened and the problem that brought you here is solved?" (de Shazer, 1988,p. 5, as cited in de Jong & Berg, 2012)

This question is helpful because it helps clients think of new possibilities for their future. It takes their focus away from the problem and helps them imagine their preferred future. When using the miracle question with clients, it is important to take your time and ask follow-up questions to help you get quite a bit of detail. Example of follow-up questions might be, "What's the first thing you'd notice about the miracle? What else did you notice? What would your partner notice? How did that happen?" Notice that you are asking questions about the how, when, why and what of the miracle (or solution), and not the problem. The more detailed you help clients be, the more they will be able to picture their life without the problem and identify small manageable goals/solutions that can lead them more toward that preferred future (de Jong & Berg, 2012).

Formula first session task. Because SFBT therapists believe that clients are resilient and resourceful, they enter therapy believing that there are things that clients are already doing successfully. To help bring these successes out in session, de Shazer (1985) developed the formula first session task. That is, at the end of the first session, the therapist asks something like, "What do you want to make sure you do not change as a result of therapy?" This helps clients to talk about what they are already doing successfully.

Exceptions. While listening to clients talk about their preferred future, through asking the miracle question, and the formula first session task, therapists identify and highlight exceptions. "Exceptions are those occasions in clients' lives when their problem could have occurred but did not – or at least were less severe" (de Jong & Berg, 2012, p. 11). An example of a question to help you identify exceptions is, "Tell me about a time when you noticed this miracle, even just a little bit?" or "Tell me about a time when the issue you are struggling with did not exist?" Then, you will ask follow-up questions to gather as much detail as possible about this exception. Pay close attention because in this detail you will learn how the client wants to change (de Jong & Berg, 2012).

Scaling questions. To help clients identify progress toward goals and what behaviors are needed for further progress, solution-focused therapists use scaling questions (de Jong & Berg, 2012; de Shazer et al., 2012). For example, therapists might ask, "On a scale of 1–10, 1 being not at all and 10 being all the time, how often do you and your partner [whatever the exception and/or solution that was identified]?" Additionally, scaling questions may also be used to identify and build on past solutions. For example, the client might note that the problem is a 6 whereas it used to be a 5. The therapist would then ask, "What happened that made it a 6 and not a 5?" The therapist and client would examine the change together and identify what and who helped the client move from a 5 to a 6. Then they would talk about how the client could do more of that solution, even just to move a small amount, such as from a 6 to a 6.5 (de Jong & Berg, 2012).

Presuppositional questions. Therapists ask questions with the presupposition that what they are asking for is possible or already exists. For example, if you want to look for exceptions, you would not ask, "Is there a time that you don't experience this problem?" Rather, you would say, "Tell me about a time when you didn't experience this problem this week." You can then follow up with comments and questions to help clients talk about the solution they experienced and help them to know what they need to do to build on those.

Complimenting. All clients have strengths, things they have done or qualities they possess that help them to resolve their problems. Solution-focused therapists look for evidence of these strengths and identify them through complimenting clients (de Jong & Berg, 2012). Imagine you are working with a couple that is looking for a way to work together to do housework instead of arguing. As you are talking to them, you hear about a time that they went to a food pantry to volunteer. You might say, "You seem to be a couple who care very much for others, working together to help others have food to eat." After giving the compliment, you can ask a follow-up question to learn about other times they used this strength (de Jong & Berg, 2012), "When else have you worked together to help others?" De Jong and Berg (2012) identified two types of compliments, direct and indirect. The examples given are both direct compliments. An indirect compliment is when you phrase a question in a way that it presupposes a strength, "How did you manage to work together so calmly?"

Solution talk. Because we want clients to envision their life without the problem, therapists will work hard to help clients talk as if the problem does not exist, to focus on the solutions or use solution talk. This is easier for some clients than others; thus, as the therapist, you will need to continue to redirect the client back to the solution. Furthermore, you will work to amplify the solution through the questions you ask. For example, working with the same couple, you could ask them, "What would you be doing differently when this problem is solved?" As they are answering the question, stay with that topic and ask follow-up questions to get more and more detail. The idea is that you want clients to be talking in detail about when the problem does not exist. So, in the case of this couple, one partner might say, "We'll be spending more time together." The therapist might follow up with, "What will you be doing together? How often?" Speaking in detail about how their lives will be different gives clients a sense of power and hope that they did not have when they entered therapy (de Jong & Berg, 2012).

Termination of therapy

Solution-focused therapy is considered a brief therapy. This does not mean that it needs to be ten sessions or less; rather, therapists enter therapy believing that any session could be the client's last session. In other words, we do not put limitations on how long therapy should last. SFBT therapists believe that change can happen quickly and that not every problem needs to be resolved for therapy to end. If a client says that they are happy with their life and their problem is resolved, then we end therapy. When and if clients feel they could use more support, they are welcomed back at any time, but there is no expectation that they will be back (de Jong & Berg, 2012).

Ethical considerations

Having learned that SFBT therapists, being strongly influenced by postmodernism and social constructionism, view clients as capable, resourceful and experts in their lives, when is it then, if ever, appropriate for the therapist to take the expert role? Is it truly best for clients to be able to make these decisions in therapy? What if you have clients that are breaking a law or they are engaging in self-harm or harming someone else? What if the therapist can see how the clients can be "healthier" but the clients are just not seeing it? Let's consider this unique position of SFBT therapists, seeing the client as the expert, while examining two provisions of the American Association for Marriage and Family Therapy (AAMFT, 2015) Code of Ethics.

Informed consent

The AAMFT Code of Ethics (2015) requires therapists to obtain informed consent from clients. This means therapists clearly explain the scope of treatment along with risks and benefits, which clients must independently agree to. At the beginning of treatment, we obtain informed consent just like therapists of other models. However, understanding that clients are the experts and have the innate ability to know what they need and how much information to share helps us respect and not move past the consent given. For example, therapists of other models may probe and ask clients poignant questions about their past or problematic experiences, while SFBT therapists respect that clients may not want to talk about the intimate details of their situation/relationships, past or present. SFBT therapists trust clients to know what they need to share and do not push to find out more about these sensitive topics. This means clients truly have the ability to give consent in deciding what information they share and do not share (de Jong & Berg, 2012).

As mentioned above, an aspect of informed consent is to discuss the risks and benefits of treatment. Inherent in this is the idea that therapists should not promise clients unrealistic outcomes, i.e., raise false hopes. Because clients are the experts, they are responsible for identifying what they want changed in a session, not the therapist. The risk here is when clients have unrealistic expectations; for example, when they identify miracles they want to see in their lives that are clearly not attainable. This is when therapists need to step into an expert role and guide the client to a more realistic expectation; however, they do this through asking questions and leading from behind, continuing to respect the client's expertise. De Jong and Berg (2015) explained that therapists ask "clients, as experts about their situations, to clarify what parts of their miracle picture can and cannot happen and, in this way, encourages clients to think about and explain what is realistic in their contexts" (p. 258).

Client autonomy

The AAMFT Code of Ethics (AAMFT, 2015) requires marriage and family therapists to give clients autonomy in their decision-making. In SFBT, therapists accept the clients' view of their problems without judgment. De Jong and Berg (2012) explained, "All aspects must be accepted... strengths, limitations, positive and negative attitudes, seemingly unhealthy and healthy behaviors, and attractive and unattractive qualities and habits" (p. 256). This approach certainly encourages autonomy. However, what about times when clients are clearly making decisions that are not good for them? As therapists, we want what is best for our clients and it can be tempting to tell them how to do that. However, the AAMFT Code of Ethics explains that part of giving clients autonomy is to allow them to make their own decisions, good or bad, "respect the rights of clients to make decisions and help them to understand the consequences of these decisions" (2015, no. 1.8). This is where the therapists' expertise comes in. When we are concerned about the decisions clients are making, we can ask clarifying questions to help clients explore their strengths and recognize other potential more beneficial solutions. When these decisions are potentially life threatening, for the clients or someone else, we must make a decision to make an issue the focus of the session or break their confidentiality (AAMFT, 2015).

Non-discrimination

To maintain a position of non-discrimination, SFBT therapists should engage in practices that align with cultural competence and cultural humility. Because of its postmodern stance, SFBT integrates cultural humility values of awareness of therapist influence on the therapy process and is curious and respectful of client values. Some have criticized the model for not being more overt in addressing how social justice issues of discrimination or marginalization contribute to problem formulation (Dermer, Hemesath & Russell, 1998). Therefore, it's recommended that SFBT therapists integrate this into the existing model.

Research support

SFBT was developed through inductive research. As we discussed previously, Steve de Shazer, Insoo Kim Berg and colleagues observed countless hours of therapy at the Brief Family Therapy Center in Milwaukee (de Jong & Berg, 2012; de Shazer et al., 2012; Walter & Peller, 1992; Weiner-Davis & Durrant, 2014). Out of these observations came the core assumptions of SFBT. Since its inception, SFBT has been a well-researched therapy model that has been used with culturally diverse populations, children, adults, individuals, couples and groups to resolve a variety of client problems.

After reviewing randomized controlled trials or quasi-experimental designs on SFBT with Latinos in the U.S., Suitt, Franklin and Kim (2016) suggested that SFBT is applicable among Latino populations. Moosa, Koorankot and Nigesh (2017) studied solution-focused art therapy among 30 refugee children in India. These children, who all had a variety of emotional disturbances, showed significant improvement in depression, anxiety and stress. Additional populations where SFBT has been used include siblings and families of children with Autism (Jordan & Turns, 2016; Turns, Eddy & Jordan, 2016, and foster children (Koob & Love, 2010). Furthermore, SFBT has been used in behavioral health, counseling clinics, school counseling and mental health services, organizational consulting, management, child protective services and coaching (Kim & Franklin, 2015).

In addition to being used with diverse groups of people and across multiple settings, SFBT has been shown to be effective with specific client issues. In a review of 43 outcome studies, Gingerich and Peterson (2013) concluded that SFBT consistently yields positive results for a variety of client issues, such as childhood behavioral and academic problems (e.g., Cepukiene & Pakrosnis, 2011; Fearrington, McCallum & Skinner, 2011), adult mental health issues (e.g. Smock et al., 2008), and marriage and family related concerns (e.g., Kenney, 2010). Additional researched problems include substance abuse (e.g., Kim, Brook & Akin, 2018), domestic violence (e.g., Bolton, Lehmann, Jordan, Frank & Moore, 2016) and parent training (e.g., Carr, Hartnett, Brosnan & Sharry, 2017).

Summary

SFBT is a strengths-based positive systemic therapy that can be used with diverse individuals, couples and families across a number of settings, such as clinics, schools and organizations. Furthermore, there is growing evidence that SFBT may be shorter and more cost effective than other approaches (Gingerich & Peterson, 2012). All of which make it an excellent choice! Keep in mind, SFBT is not an "easy" therapy. SFBT therapists are focused in every session with clients looking for ways to support the client by identifying strengths, exceptions and solutions to help them create their preferred future.

References

American Association for Marriage and Family Therapy. (2015). AAMFT code of ethics. Retrieved from www.aamft.org/Legal_Ethics/Code_of_Ethics.aspx

Anderson, H. & Goolishian, H. (1992). The client is the expert: a not-knowing approach to therapy. In S. McNamee & K. J. Gergen (Eds.), *Therapy as social construction* (pp. 25–39) Sage Publications, Inc.

Backhaus, K. (2011). Solution-focused brief therapy with families. In L. Metcalf (Ed.), *Marriage and Family Therapy: a practice-oriented approach* (pp. 287–312). New York, NY: Springer Publishing Company. https://doi.org/10.1891/9780826106827.0012

Carr, A., Hartnett, D., Brosnan, E. & Sharry, J. (2017). Parents plus systemic, solution- focused parent training programs: description, review of the evidence base, and meta-analysis. *Family Process, 56*(3), 652–668. doi:10.1111/famp.12225

Cepukiene, V. & Pakrosnis, R. (2011). The outcome of solution- focused brief therapy among foster care adolescents: the changes of behavior and perceived somatic and cognitive difficulties. *Children and Youth Services Review, 33*, 791–797. doi:10.1016/j.childyouth.2010.11.027

Connie, E. (2013). *Solution building in couples therapy*. New York, NY: Springer.

de Jong, P. & Berg, I. K. (2012). *Interviewing for solutions* (3rd ed.). Belmont, CA: Brooks/Cole.

de Shazer, S. (1985). *Keys to solution in brief therapy*. New York, NY: W. W. Norton & Company, Inc.

de Shazer, S., Dolan, Y., Korman, H., Trepper, T., McCollum, E. & Berg, I. K. (2012). *More than miracles: the state of the art of solution-focused brief therapy*. New York, NY: Routledge.

Dermer, S. B., Hemesath, C. W. & Russell, C. S. (1998). A feminist critique of solution-focused therapy. *American Journal of Family Therapy, 26*(3), 239–250.

Fearrington, J. Y., McCallum, R. S. & Skinner, C. H. (2011). Increasing math assignment completion using solution-focused brief counseling. *Education and Treatment of Children, 34*, 61–80.

Gergen, K. J. (1985). The social constructionist movement in modern psychology. *American Psychologist, 40*(3), 266.

Gingerich, W. J. & Peterson, L. T. (2012). Effectiveness of solution focused brief therapy: a systematic qualitative review of controlled outcome studies. *Research on Social Work Practice, 23*(3), 266–283. doi:10.1177/1049731512470859

Gingerich, W. J. & Peterson, L. T. (2013). Effectiveness of solution-focused brief therapy: a systematic qualitative review of controlled outcome studies. *Research on Social Work Practice, 23*(3), 266–283.

Jordan, S. S. & Turns, B. (2016). Utilizing solution-focused brief therapy with families living with autism spectrum disorder, *Journal of Family Psychotherapy, 27*(3), 155–170. doi: 10.1080/08975353.2016.1199766

Kenney, J. (2010). *Solution focused brief intervention for caregivers of children with autism spectrum disorder: a single subject design*. Minneapolis, MN: Walden University.

Kim, J. S., Brook, J. & Akin, B. A. (2018). Solution-focused brief therapy with substance using individuals: a randomized controlled trial study. *Research on Social Work Practice, 28*(4), 452–462. doi:10.1177/1049731516650517

Kim, J. S. & Franklin, C. (2015). Understanding emotional change in solution-focused brief therapy: facilitating positive emotions. *Best Practice in Mental Health, 11*(1), 25–41.

Koob, J. J. & Love, S. M. (2010). The implementation of solution-focused therapy to increase foster care placement stability. *Children and Youth Services Review, 32*, 1346–1350. doi:10.1016/j.childyouth.2010.06.001

Moosa, A., Koorankot, J. & Nigesh, K. (2017). Solution focused art therapy among refugee children. *Indian Journal of Health and Well-being, 8*(8), 811–816.

Smock, S. A., Trepper, T. S., Wetchler, J. L., McCollum, E. E., Ray, R. & Pierce, K. (2008). Solution-focused group therapy for level 1 substance abusers. *Journal of Marital & Family Therapy, 34*, 107–120.

Suitt, K. G., Franklin, C. & Kim, J. (2016). Solution-focused brief therapy with Latinos: a systematic review. *Journal of Ethnic & Cultural Diversity in Social Work, 25*(1), 50–67. doi:10.1080/15313204.2015.1131651

Turns, B., Eddy, B. P. & Jordan, S. S. (2016). Working with siblings of children with autism: a solution-focused approach. *Australian & New Zealand Journal of Family Therapy, 37,* 558–571. Doi:10.1002/anzf.1183

von Bertalanffy, L. (1968). *General systems theory; foundations, development, applications.* New York, NY: George Braziller.

Walter, J. L. & Peller, J. E. (1992). *Becoming solution focused in brief therapy.* New York, NY: Brunner/Mazel.

Watzlawick, P., Bavelas, J. B. & Jackson, D. D. (1967). *Pragmatics of human communication: a study of interactional patterns, pathologies, and paradoxes.* New York, NY: Norton.

Watzlawick, P., Weakland, J. H. & Fisch, R. (1974). *Change: principles of problem formation and problem resolution.* New York, NY: W. W. Norton & Company, Inc.

Weiner-Davis, M. & Durrant, M. (2014). *Seve de Shazer and Insoo Kim Berg: storried reflections about genuine pioneers.* Keynote presentation at the American Association for Marriage and Family Therapy Annual Conference, Milwaukie, WI.

Whitchurch, G. & Constantine, L. L. (1993). Systems theory. In P. G. Boss, W. J. Doherty, R. LaRossa, W. R. Schumm & S. K. Steinmetz's (Eds.), *Sourcebook of family theories and methods: a contextual approach* (pp. 325–355). New York, NY: Plenum Press.

20 Narrative Family Therapy

Valerie Q. Glass

Introduction

This chapter will highlight some important elements of the Narrative Therapy model. Narrative Therapy embraces postmodernist and social constructionist ideologies and is particularly concerned with the role of social interaction (specifically between the therapist and client) in creating change. The following will highlight the history of the narrative model, the philosophies of social constructionism and postmodernism, the assumptions of the narrative model, the techniques of the model, a discussion on evidence-based research and cultural competency related to the narrative model.

History of the model

The Narrative model evolved during the 1980s from early modernist models, such as strategic, Ericksonian and feminism (Freedman & Combs, 1996), while integrating social constructionist and postmodernist thinking. The Narrative model interjects that individuals and families generate stories around the problem in their lives and gives it meaning to the point that the story is actually the problem (White & Epston, 1990).

Some therapists were drawn to the idea that clients were active participants in the creative solutions that might guide their directions. Family systems thinkers and clinicians started to put themselves in a more "co-creator" role where they would connect to the clients' stories and, rather than being directive, there was a focus on collaboration between therapist and client.

Philosophical underpinnings

Foucault was a 20th-century philosopher and many of his ideas influenced the origins of the narrative model (White & Epston, 1990). One of his fundamental ideas was that larger social experiences and understandings of social experiences left out or marginalized those voices and experiences that were part of the majority culture or did not have power in their community context. Foucault's ideas are easily seen in the concept of social construction, which identifies that our identity and reality is constructed by our social environment.

Social construction further informed Narrative and other postmodern models. Social construction is the idea that our understanding of who we are, what we do, what things mean is based on the social connections that we have with those around us (Freedman & Combs, 1996). As we move through our communities, laws are created, expectations

DOI: 10.4324/9781003382621-24

evolve, and ideas expand based on these connections and conversations that we have with one another. Consider *beauty* as a social construction. People view beauty in so many different ways. In one area of the word, beauty might be about a longer neck, another might view beauty as a slight slant in the eye, another might focus on the shape of a person's feet, another might view dark curly hair as a beauty standard, while another sees straight light hair as representing beauty. Even beauty constructions shift overtime. What was seen as attractive in the 1950s may not have the same appeal in the 2020s. Consider what things attract your eye and where you might have developed these thoughts on what is attractive. Often stories are what leads us to view attraction in certain ways. In Western cultures, for example, many children watch princess movies and develop an expectation of beauty based on these characters. Through this social construction of beauty, people can develop personal narratives around their own view of beauty and/or how they fit into this construction of beauty. You might hear someone say "my feet are too big" or "my legs look too bony" or "my hair is too thin". They are interacting with this socially constructed view of beauty and creating narratives around how this plays a role in their own experiences. Taking this even further, these narratives around beauty and how one describes themselves filter back into society. A person sharing with a friend "my feet are too big" leads to the friend considering their own feet and paying more attention to the feet around them and how they fit this construction. This dominant narrative that "feet should be small" becomes a key social construction of beauty in their world. This can lead to an over-representation in advertising and media of "small feet" that contributes to how people view themselves and others.

Freedman and Combs (1996) go so far to say that people's stories "create culture" (p. 17). Social constructionism is the key philosophical understanding behind the narrative model because of how shifts happen in therapy. There is an understanding that, through social constructions, the therapists learn to understand the client's reality, join with them in that reality and contribute to their story to "shift" or move them to another place, creating change.

Postmodernism is a philosophy that highlights the fact that realities are socially constructed. This is the understanding that social "groups" or environments generate ways of understanding experience. Consider if you were to ask 100 college students about their experiences in college. They might each share slightly different realities (i.e., "it is so hard", "my classes are boring", "it is really challenging me", "it is fun," etc.) With all these stated experiences there is an understanding of what college is and what is expected. This can change or "adapt" with the college student's experience in their environment. Maybe professors, peers and even family/friends are adding to this reality. A postmodernist therapist identifies that they understand their context may not fit with the clients' context. My understanding of being a woman, a student, etc., will be different to the person sitting in front of me. I am not there to make their reality into mine, but to accept and understand their context. Some major points identified in postmodernism are: "Realities are constituted through language, realities are organized and maintained through narrative, and there are no essential truths" (as cited by Freedman & Combs, 1996, p. 22).

Another philosophy that provides a foundation for the Narrative model is that of family systems. The Narrative model developed from the early systemic thinkers within the marriage and family therapy (MFT) field. White and Epston (1990) shared that the concept of cybernetics played a role in considering the way the Narrative model creates change. Cybernetics is a concept that describes how a system will function and reorganize to maintain its course. One way to visualize this in a family context is to consider how a family might maintain homeostasis by restructuring constantly to stay in a place that is comfortable or fits their sense of "normal". Narrative therapists were increasingly interested in the concept of second-order cybernetics (also known as "cybernetics of cybernetics") where they consider the therapist's role within this family system as it relates to keeping the system on course. Considering the role of social construction, the therapist's "person" may contribute to changing the understanding of the story or the direction of the course. When the narrative therapist points out elements of client's stories or contributes some other ideas or curiosities to the story, the client's narrative shifts because of the new social constructions that come into play.

Founders

Michael White is considered one of the major founders of the narrative model.

Michael White was curious about Foucault's philosophies and how they related to some of the systemic ideas of cybernetics and cybernetics of cybernetics (White & Epston, 1990; Freedman & Combs, 1996). His ideas came together to consider the role of the therapist in both listening to the client's story, understanding their story and identifying elements in their story that might lead to the creation of a story that would work better for them. **David Epston** contributed to the flow of the model and how questions were asked to help clients build on their story during therapy (White & Epston, 1990). Jill Freedman and Jill Combs (1996) contributed to the philosophy of the Narrative model through their perspectives on social justice, the importance of one's context as a contribution to the story, and the role of power and privilege in individuals' lives.

Main concepts and assumptions

One major assumption of the Narrative model is the idea that the therapist is a co-creator of the "new" story (Freedman & Combs, 1996). To examine this assumption a bit more, let us use an example. Consider the stories that you often hear at funerals. Often, we will share with the grieving "they are in a better place", "they aren't suffering anymore" or "good thing you have such a strong family to help you through this". These are strength-based elements of the families' story. This is one way to describe the process of co-creating a more positive/strength-based story. Being supportive relatives or friends, we are not likely to reiterate that the family is sad, which is really likely the dominant narrative in their life at the moment; rather, we look for the good things in the event and help them recognize the direction according to our observations of their strengths. Narrative works in a similar way by locating what is working (and maybe what is not working) that has become a primary story in the life of the family.

Dominant narratives or **internalized discourses** are somewhat similar terms to describe the rut that people get into by viewing the story through a problem-saturated lens (Freedman & Combs, 1996; Muntigl, 2004). Families have spent a great deal of energy constructing the story around the "problem", which has highlighted it and given it meaning to the deficit of the strengths that would positively contribute to a new story or new direction. The language involved in constructing the family's story around the problem is negatively influencing where the family wants to be (Muntigl, 2004). The therapist connects to aspects of the clients' stories that are elaborated on through questioning skills. This evolves into a new narrative that better suits the family.

Techniques and interventions

Listening

It may sound intuitive to consider that listening is an intervention. In the Narrative model, listening is an active process. A major tool in the building of a therapeutic alliance in the narrative model is the openness to hearing another person's story.

Listening, in the Narrative model, requires being aware and present. It requires us to attempt to forego what we think we know about the other person's experience and really try to listen from their perspective (Freedman & Combs, 1996). Narrative therapists ask questions to fully hear the story and the details. Freedman and Combs (1996) suggest a style of deconstructive listening where the therapist finds elements of the story that are unclear and explores those gaps. This exploration is done through asking questions about the meaning behind pieces of the story that may not make sense or seem left out. For example, if a child says "everyone is always angry at each other", the therapist dives into this by listening and asking questions. The therapist might ask, "What does angry look like?", "Who is less likely to be angry with you?" or "When people are angry, what happens?" The narrative therapist is mindful, aware and in-tune with the voices and words that are presented in therapy.

Mapping the influence of the problem

Mapping the influence of the problem is a technique to aid in the discussion of the dominant story (White & Epston, 1990). In this technique, the narrative therapist is exploring many facets of the problem and the story around the problem. They may ask each member about their relationship with the problem. Through these questions the therapist can understand the connections and struggles that the family perceives as part of this story. In the above example of the family who shares "everyone is always angry at each other", the therapist carefully asks each member about the role of anger, when anger is and is not present, and each person's relationship with this anger and how it influences them. Mapping the influence of the problem can build on itself. As the family starts to answer one question, it can lead to starting the process over again. For example, maybe a parent shares something like "we are not really angry, we just talk loudly". The therapist can start to dive into this narrative and ask the rest of the family about being loud or how they distinguish between "loud" and "anger".

Witnessing structure

Similar to mapping the influence of the problem, witnessing is a technique where family members are questioned during another family member's discussion of a "story" (Freedman, 2014). The idea is that the therapist is aware of the way the family all views the story. It provides much richer context for understanding the meanings surrounding the problem-saturated story as well as identifying more strengths within the story. This can be done simply by asking other family members about their perspectives of the story. This is similar to mapping the influence, but the focus is more on really getting each family member to engage in the discussion around the story, the dominant narrative and the exceptions to the dominant narrative. For example, if a parent shares they are not angry, they are just "loud", the therapist may turn to a child and ask them "tell me about when things are not so loud in your home".

Not-knowing

The not-knowing technique is crucial to listening. At times, in conversation, we may ask a question seeking a particular answer. Not-knowing assumes that you are not looking for a particular direction. It is about exploring. It is putting our own assumptions to the side or at least being aware of them and working to put ourselves into the client's reality. An example might be when a client shares, "you know being a parent is hard". I can look into my reality and simply nod. A narrative therapist would put on a **"not-knowing" stance** and ask more about the client's reality of parenting. They might ask, "What is most difficult about parenting?" The not-knowing approach is critical to understanding a client's experience and their social constructions. If a child says "Dad is so mean", from a not-knowing perspective the therapist might ask, "What does mean look like?" The child's answer reflects their constructions around the word mean and allows the therapist to consider this context.

Recognizing cultural influence

From the postmodern lens, one of the techniques used is to listen to the parts of the clients' stories that seem to be rooted in their culture or community messages (Suddeath, Kerwin & Dugger, 2017). This goal of recognizing the influence of these cultural messages is not to change client's views, but to offer up alternative ways of considering these dominating ideas. For a parent to share, "I am not a good parent", for example, the narrative therapist would help the client explore where the messages of what a "good parent" is has come from. The client may share their history, their experiences with their own family of origin, their religious and cultural background, and how all these things help them to understand what being a good parent looks like. The narrative therapist would listen and appreciate this cultural experience. The therapist might also open up dialogue (in a respectful and embracing way) that would offer alternative views on parenting.

Externalization

Externalization is where you separate the person from the problem (Freedman & Combs, 1996; White & Epston, 1990). This is also known as deconstruction questions. Rather than stating, "you have an anger problem", the narrative therapist would ask, "What is your relationship with anger?" The narrative therapist would view the problem as external to the person and help them see that they are not "the problem", rather they are a person with a problem. By viewing the problem as external to the person, a whole different vision of the story can take place because the family can work to visualize themselves on "one side" and the "problem" on another. It can bring families together to look at how to conquer the "problem" as a team. Another positive benefit of externalization is that it separates the story and allows a family or individual to see their story when the problem is not present. Perhaps just as important, the therapist is able to join the family "on their side" against the problem, aiding in the building of a therapeutic alliance (O'Hanlon, 1994).

Unique outcomes

Unique outcomes (also known as "sparkling moments") are when the therapist searches through listening for moments when the problem either did not exist or was not as bad (Freedman & Combs, 1996; White & Epston, 1990). If a family comes in and shares that they are arguing "all the time", the therapist will look for times within the story where the family is getting along and bring these out through deeper questions or curious observations. For example, the therapist would ask: "Are there moments when people are not arguing? What is happening in these moments?" Or "Why do you suppose Gia and Lamar do not argue?" Narrative therapists look for moments that the problem is not happening and ask about these. For example, maybe a family returns after a week and it comes out that they have not argued in the last couple of days. The therapist would ask, "What has been different that led to you all not arguing?" Unique outcomes can also explore hopes and dreams for the future, where the therapist is seeking out parts of the story that the family presents that indicate how they might "beat" the problem in the future or even what the future might look like without the problem present.

Letters

White introduced the idea of letter writing as a tool for Narrative Therapy (White & Epston, 1990). He incorporated letters for several reasons: as a way to build comfort when he sensed clients were resistant or uncomfortable with the idea of therapy, to highlight elements of the client's story, to further explore unique outcomes and to build in growth or change that he observed. Writing clients letters is a way to validate the story, while suggesting alternatives. After a difficult session, the therapist might send a client a letter: "You mentioned at the end of session that the emotion was very difficult. I wanted to follow up with you and share how much I appreciate your openness and your willingness to share with me." The therapist will reiterate strengths, "the way that you stood up for yourself was really admirable and I can see how your persistence and determination will get you through difficult moments in your future". Writing letters is a way to reinforce the new narrative while validating the client.

Reflecting teams

Reflecting teams are a tool utilized with some narrative therapists, particularly those with access to training facilities (Freedman & Combs, 1996). Reflecting teams were introduced in early MFT training programs. The narrative model utilizes social constructions and strength-based language differently to modernist predecessors. Essentially, to conduct a reflecting team, a family is observed by a group of therapists during their therapy session.

The team behind the mirror is also listening to the family discourse with the understanding that their voices will contribute to the social construction of a new story. The therapists are seeking to identify strengths within the story. At some point within the session, the family observes the team discussing their case. The team may share observations and curiosities in a supportive and affirming manner. They particularly might explore ideas that do not fit within the family's dominant problem-saturated story. After the reflecting teams' response and discussion, the therapist and family meet to process their understanding of the team's reflections. For example, with the family that is "arguing all the time", the therapists behind the mirror may notice things like: how well one parent really listens to the children, how the younger child tries to have conversation around issues rather than argue, how the family really seems to love one another, how humor is a big part of the family dynamic and how willing it seems everyone was to come to therapy and that this is a step in change. The team will bring these strengths and positive directions up in a discussion that the family listens to. The idea is that the family starts to integrate these more strength-based social constructions into their life and into their preferred narrative.

Research support

The effectiveness of narrative therapies and research supporting narrative work with many types of presenting problems and populations is expansive, only a portion of the current research in this area is mentioned here. The medical field and the mental health fields have adopted some of the narrative techniques or language to help bring families into the discussion of health (Williams-Reade, Freitas & Lawson, 2014).

Mental health services have benefited from integrating systemic and narrative perspectives. Adolescent residential programs (Merritts, 2016) and wilderness programs (DeMille & Montgomery, 2016) have found that narrative is a helpful model for bridging family work. Research has explored the effectiveness of narrative techniques in connecting spirituality to therapy through the use of spiritual narratives and meanings (Olson et al., 2016).

Some of the re-storying techniques in the Narrative model have been useful for stepfamilies and blended families who are adjusting to a new narrative (Shalay & Brownlee, 2007). In addition, families that are experiencing adoption have found that narrative allows them to explore messages and expectations of expanding families and identify their own personal story of family creation (Stokes & Poulsen, 2014).

Narrative allows LGBTQ individuals to look at their gender or minority status, explore how this does not fit with dominant cultural narratives and then re-write a new narrative. Transgender clients have benefited from exploring gender narratives in their lives and re-storying future narratives (Piper & Mannino, 2008). In addition, same-sex couples have benefited from Narrative Therapy because of the focus on cultural expectations and how, at times, these expectations have been internalized (Cohn, 2014).

Narrative model techniques and underlying philosophies have been found to be effective with many different cultures and communities. Bell-Tolliver, Burgess and Brock (2009) noted that the postmodern models were better for African American families because of the strength-based focused approach that does not pathologize or assume. In addition, the Narrative model can bridge kinship networks and spirituality that is common for some African American families (Bell-Tolliver & Wilkerson, 2011). Some research has explored using Narrative with Hispanic families. One method included using the strengths offered in some spiritual elements of Hispanic families for building the "new story" (Bermudez & Bermudez, 2002). Another study explored the social construction around machismo and how to build this into the therapeutic environment (Falicov, 2010).

Chen (2012) identifies the benefits of utilizing narrative techniques with Chinese population. She explored narrative with Chinese children born under the "one-child-only" law in China. She noted that these children have developed a specific story based on their scenario and narrative aids in better understanding this perspective. She noted that the style of narrative (including respectful curiosity) are beneficial to many Chinese cultures.

The Narrative model and the technique have been explored in many other cultures, communities and populations. The previous three listed here are only a sampling of the research done with a narrative, which focuses on specific cultural or other differences. Some of the narrative techniques, such as storytelling, respectful questioning, listening and externalizing have been found to be useful for populations globally (Roberts et al., 2014). The openness to understanding context really opens up the model to reach many different populations.

Cultural humility and Narrative Therapy

One of the core components of the narrative model is the focus on context, which nicely opens up the process to understanding difference. The model arose out of a perspective that, at times, voices were marginalized based on larger, dominant discourses (Freedman & Combs, 1996). The very essence of the narrative model is to understand cultural context. O'Hanlon (1994) stated that models in the postmodern era draw:

> ...attention to far larger systems, such as the daunting cultural sea we swim in – the messages from television advertisements, schools, newspaper 'experts,' bosses, grandmothers and friends – tell us how to think and who to be.
>
> (p. 23)

One way to understand cultural humility within this model is to look more at social construction and context of the therapist (Richert, 2003). The therapist should be aware of the inherent power and privilege that comes with their professional position as therapist. Therapists can be insightful about their own background and experiences and how these directly influence the questions and expectations within the therapeutic relationship. Being that one of the primary goals of the narrative therapeutic relationship is a collaborative re-building of a story, the therapist must be acutely aware of their presence within that story and weed out what is more representative of their own life and understanding.

Some theorists have even expounded on the ideas within the narrative models to posit challenges to dominant cultural expectations and discourses (Elliott, 1998). The idea is that the therapist assists clients in seeing the (perhaps controlling or limiting) discourses in their own lives. For example, consider a woman enters therapy feeling overwhelmed with expectations and demands on her. The therapist might ask about her sense of the cultural ideal in her own community (i.e., "Where did you learn these messages about women?") to help the client get a better picture of social expectations. In addition, race, gender and other identities could be part of the exploring process (i.e., "How do you think being a woman has played a role in this part of your story?"). The thought is that this could lead to questioning these expectations and empowering clients.

Summary

The Narrative model explores, in detail, the story that the family presents. The Narrative model is a way of looking at families and their presenting problems. It is a "way of being". Narrative therapists embrace the understanding that reality is understood through our social interactions with others and that therapy is one way to interact. Therapy works to help clients identify the strengths in their story. It is through conversation that the story shifts and the clients are exposed to a new way of visualizing the problem they once presented.

References

Bell-Tolliver, L., Burgess, R. & Brock, L. J. (2009). African American therapists working with African American families: an exploration of the strengths perspective in treatment. *Journal of Marital and Family Therapy, 35*(3), 293–307. doi:10.1111/j.1752-0606.2009.00117.x

Bell-Tolliver, L. & Wilkerson, P. (2011). The use of spirituality and kinship as contributors to successful therapy outcomes with African American families. *Journal of Religion & Spirituality in Social Work, 30*(1), 48–70. doi:10.1080/15426432.2011.542723

Bermúdez, J. M. & Bermúdez, S. (2002). Altar-making with Latino families: a narrative therapy perspective. *Journal of Family Psychotherapy, 13*(3–4), 329–347. doi:10.1300/J085v13n03_06

Chen, R. (2012). Narrative therapy for Chinese adults raised as an only child. *Contemporary Family Therapy: An International Journal, 34*(1), 104–111. doi:10.1007/s10591-012-9177-7

Cohn, A. S. (2014). Romeo and Julius: a narrative therapy intervention for sexual-minority couples. *Journal of Family Psychotherapy, 25*(1), 73–77. doi:10.1080/08975353.2014.881696

DeMille, S. M. & Montgomery, M. (2016). Integrating narrative family therapy in an outdoor behavioral healthcare program: a case study. *Contemporary Family Therapy: An International Journal, 38*(1), 3–13. doi:10.1007/s10591-015-9362-6

Elliott, H. (1998). Postmodernism, feminism, and narrative therapy. In S. Madigan & I. Law (Eds.). *Praxis: Situating Discourse, Feminism, and Politics In Narrative Therapies* (pp. 35–59). Vancouver, BC: The Cardigan Press.

Falicov, C. (2010). Changing constructions of machismo for Latino men in therapy: 'the devil never sleeps'. *Family Process, 49*(3), 309–329. doi:10.1111/j.1545-5300.2010.01325.x

Freedman, J. (2014). Witnessing and positioning: structuring narrative therapy with families and couples. *Australian & New Zealand Journal of Family Therapy, 35*(1), 20–30. doi:10.1002/anzf.104

Freedman, J. & Combs, G. (1996). *Narrative therapy: the social construction of preferred realities.* New York, NY: W. W. Norton Company, Inc.

Merritts, A. (2016). A review of family therapy in residential settings. *Contemporary Family Therapy: An International Journal, 38*(1), 75–85. doi:10.1007/s10591-016-9378-6

Muntigl, P. (2004). Ontogensis in narrative therapy: a linguistic-semiotic examination of client change. *Family Process, 43*, 109–131.

O'Hanlon, B. (1994). The promise of narrative: the third wave. *Family Therapy Networker, 18*, 18–29.

Olson, T., Tisdale, T. C., Davis, E. B., Park, E. A., Nam, J., Moriarty, G. L. & … Hays, L. W. (2016). God image narrative therapy: a mixed-methods investigation of a controlled group-based spiritual intervention. *Spirituality in Clinical Practice, 3*(2), 77–91. doi:10.1037/scp0000096

Piper, J. & Mannino, M. (2008). Identity formation for transsexual individuals in transition: a narrative family therapy model. *Journal of GLBT Family Studies, 4*(1), 75–93. doi:10.1080/15504280802084472

Richert, A. J. (2003). Living stories, telling stories, changing stories: experiential use of the relationship in narrative therapy. *Journal or Psychotherapy Integration, 13*, 188–210.

Roberts, J., Abu-Baker, K., Diez Fernández, C., Chong Garcia, N., Fredman, G., Kamya, H. & … Zevallos Vega, R. (2014). Up close: family therapy challenges and innovations around the world. *Family Process, 53*(3), 544–576. doi:10.1111/famp.12093

Shalay, N. & Brownlee, K. (2007). Narrative family therapy with blended families. *Journal of Family Psychotherapy, 18*(2), 17–30. doi:10.1300/J085v18n02_02

Stokes, L. D. & Poulsen, S. S. (2014). Narrative therapy for adoption issues in families, couples, and individuals: rationale and approach. *Journal of Family Psychotherapy, 25*(4), 330–347. doi:10.1080/08975353.2014.977681

Suddeath, E. G., Kerwin, A. K. & Dugger, S. M. (2017). Narrative family therapy: practical techniques for more effective work with couples and families. *Journal of Mental Health Counseling, 39*(2), 116–131. doi:10.17744/mehc.39.2.03

White, M. & Epston, D. (1990). *Narrative means to therapeutic ends.* New York, NY: W. W. Norton Company, Inc.

Williams-Reade, J., Freitas, C. & Lawson, L. (2014). Narrative-informed medical family therapy: using narrative therapy practices in brief medical encounters. *Families, Systems, & Health, 32*(4), 416–425. doi:10.1037/fsh0000082

21 Collaborative Language Systems Therapy

Siva Perera

Introduction

Collaborative language systems (CLS), also referred to as collaborative therapy, is a post-modern approach to therapy built on language and communication. It can be described as "a language system and a linguistic event in which people are engaged in a collaborative relationship and conversation – a mutual endeavor toward possibility" (Anderson, 1997, p. 2). The theory and therapeutic approach to CLS was a joint venture between Harlene Anderson and Harry Goolishian developed in the 1980s. However, the foundational roots of this model can be traced all the way back to the ideas of David Jackson, Gregory Bateson and Kenneth Gergen, and later to that of the Mental Research Institute (MRI) team (Anderson & Gehart, 2012).

This model is based on **social constructionist** theory and **hermeneutics**. Collaborative therapists believe that our experiences of reality are constructed via the ways in which we interact with other people, a central idea behind social constructionism. Hermeneutics on the other hand deals with the methodology of interpretation. Combined together, CLS therapists rely on assessing the language clients' use in therapy to help navigate the process of finding solutions to their clinical problems.

As the name implies, this approach relies on a nonhierarchical, collaborative relationship between the client and therapist that is built on mutual understanding and respect for each other. Because collaborative therapists believe that knowledge and language are constantly interacting and evolving, they also believe that clients are capable of coming up with solutions to their problems via a shift in language. In other words, problems can be dissolved through dialogueue between the therapist and client.

Founders

Harlene Anderson and the late Harry Goolishian developed the CLS approach, an approach to therapy that originally evolved from the early works of family therapy. Sometime in the 1970s, Goolishian led an interdisciplinary team at the University of Texas Medical Branch in Galveston. They employed an approach called Multiple Impact Therapy (MIT) and worked intensively with adolescents with psychiatric problems. This was a short-term family-centered approach and they included the adolescents, their families and other professionals as well in their treatment and care.

Around the same time, members of this group became interested in the work of the MRI team based out of Palo Alto, California. The MRI team recommended that therapists

DOI: 10.4324/9781003382621-25

use and speak the clients' language in therapy rather than teach the client to speak the therapist's language. This way of thinking caused the team at Galveston to move away from cybernetics and general systems theories and they now began to focus on the clients' language as being central to therapy. Anderson and Goolishian (1988) then assumed that human beings are language systems, language-meaning-making system. This gave way to the possibility of exploring therapy as a conversational dialogue and hence the beginning of therapy based on a CLS approach.

Main concepts of CLS

CLS therapy is a **postmodern approach** that revolves around dialogueic conversations between therapist and client. This relationship leads to the potential of finding new possibilities within these therapeutic conversations.

Anderson and Goolishian (1988) believed that the client is the author of their stories and only they have the power to change the outcome of their story. They also stress that problems are maintained by language or dialogueue. Hence, a collaborative therapist helps the client to deconstruct their story thereby allowing the possibility for new stories to emerge. Through conversation, new possibilities can arise and this is what leads to the idea of transformation in collaborative therapy.

Duration of therapy can vary drastically when working with clients from a CLS approach as there is no set number of therapy sessions that need to be fulfilled. Some might benefit from a single, one-time session, while others may continue to seek therapy for years, most likely off and on. Since each session is considered unique, the therapist and client will decide if therapy needs to continue and when. Termination is collaboratively decided and mutually ended.

Philosophical underpinnings and conceptualization of issues

Anderson and Goolishian (1988) present CLS as a philosophical stance rather than a therapy model. They believe that meaning is created via language, which also means that problems are maintained by language. Hence potential solutions can be constructed via a change in language. This way of thinking places the therapist and client as partners in a mutual inquiry. Together, they create or co-create new meaning using language and hence develop a new way of finding solutions.

Because collaborative therapists take on a stance of truly not knowing a client's experience, they refrain from labeling, diagnosing and giving instructions. So, for instance, collaborative therapists do not take any particular stance regarding medication. If it plays a role in the client's life and will influence the process of therapy, then it will be addressed when necessary. If not, then collaborative therapists will apply this same attitude of not knowing toward each therapy session, which is viewed as a unique meeting with no preconceived goals or notions. They will continue to work with what the clients bring in in order to dissolve problems and discover new meaning.

How change occurs

Language and conversation are the key players in the CLS approach to therapy. Drawing from social construction theory and hermeneutics, Anderson and Goolishian (1988) propose that, for change to occur from a collaborative therapy approach, a two-way dialogue needs to occur, allowing for new meaning to evolve.

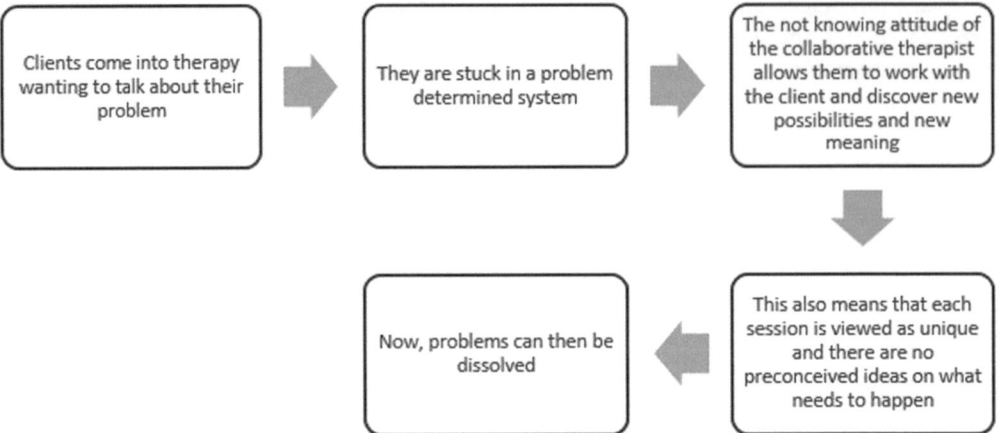

Figure 21.1 Change Process in Collaborative Language Systems.

Here is another way of looking at it from a clinical standpoint:

Role of the client and role of the therapist

In CLS, the client is considered to be **a teacher** and the therapist a learner. There is the absence of hierarchy and the presence of a mutual, collaborative relationship between the therapist and client. The therapist offers a space in which clients can come up with new meaning to their situation. The therapist is not considered to be an expert but rather a participant in this therapeutic relationship, while the client is recognized as the expert with the most useful knowledge on his or her experience. So, in short, to be consistent with other systemic models, therapists practicing from a CLS perspective should:

- avoid a judgmental position
- ask relevant questions
- listen deeply
- ensure that they have understood the situation clearly
- provide a safe space to facilitate the therapeutic process

Interventions

Collaborative therapists do not follow a series of steps or design interventions as part of their therapeutic approach. Instead, they maintain a collaborative attitude based on a number of concepts that determine how they approach their clients as well as their sessions. These concepts include the following:

a. conversational partners
b. therapy as research
c. client as an expert
d. not-knowing
e. uncertainty

f. being public
g. everyday ordinary life

- **Conversational partners.** Anderson (2006) notes that the therapist and clients are "conversational partners who engage in collaborative relationships and in dialogueical conversations with each other" (p. 45). The therapist will focus on what the client is saying and constantly listen and try to understand the situation from the clients' perspective and in their own language. The therapist will continue to demonstrate that they are paying close attention to what the clients are saying and also check in with them about their satisfaction regarding the direction of the conversation.

- **Therapy as research.** Collaborative therapists often play the role of a researcher and probe clients to tell their stories in detail. The therapist will remain curious and show deep interest in what the clients share about their experience and situation. During this process, they will ask for clarification and ensure that they are on the same page as their clients. Therapists will ask questions about the clients' perspective on the problem and, through conversation, they will explore their situation and discuss what the future might hold.

- **Client as an expert.** Keeping in line with other postmodern therapies, collaborative therapists also consider clients to be the expert in their own lives. The client is the expert on the presenting problem and the solution. They know what resources will work best and what will not. On the other hand, the therapist is the expert on providing an environment that makes inviting and maintaining a collaborative relationship possible (Anderson, 2006).

- **Not-knowing.** Collaborative therapists encourage clients to come up with their own goals for therapy because they truly believe that the clients themselves know best how they should live their lives. The therapist will present a humble attitude and create a sense of truly not knowing privileged information about their clients. Simply put, the therapist avoids assuming anything about the client or their circumstance.

- **Uncertainty.** This is somewhat connected to not knowing in the sense that both the therapist and client does not know where a therapeutic conversation will lead them to. When a therapist and client engage in conversation, it gives way to the development of ideas and possibilities that neither party could have generated on their own. It is the spontaneous development of ideas and possibilities that lead to transformation in a client's story.

- **Being public.** Collaborative therapists maintain an open stance with their clients and often share their internal thoughts, opinions and ideas rather than keeping them hidden. The therapist will make public private thoughts so that there is openness and honesty in the therapeutic relationship. On another note, narrative therapists refer to this as transparency. The distinction between transparency and being public is that we cannot see through someone, but we can be public with our own experiences as per Anderson (2001).

- **Everyday ordinary life.** Just like life, therapy too is a social event for collaborative therapists. The conversation that occurs during a collaborative therapy session, and questions asked, often resembles everyday conversations. Therapists avoid jargon and do not use technical language, but rather an informal one.

Case example

A therapist asks her clients (husband and wife) why they are coming to therapy, and the husband states they are there because of "money trouble" and the wife's lack of responsibility. The therapist takes on a **not-knowing stance** and asks the client to help her understand "money trouble". The therapist then goes on to display a sense of *uncertainty* and inquires what responsibility will look like within the context of this couple's relationship.

The conversation revolves around the different perspectives on money and responsibility based on the couple's individual backgrounds. The therapist picks up on some key words that the clients repeat during the conversation, such as money, cheap and responsibility, and repeats these words in her dialogueue showing the clients that she is paying close attention to what they are saying. This is an example of the clinician being a *conversational partner*. The therapist then asks each client to delve deeper into what these words, money, cheap and responsibility, mean for them based on their backgrounds and upbringing. The therapist is playing the role of a researcher to draw out detailed definitions for these terms and is thereby practicing *therapy as research*.

Use with diverse clients

Collaborative Language Systems-based therapists always maintain a not-knowing stance and this, coupled with their therapeutic dialogueical conversations, lend them the unique ability to appreciate differences that arise as a result of culture, class, gender and sexuality. Therefore, such topics will be included in therapy only if there is a need or if the participants (therapist or clients) find it to be necessary and relevant. This does not mean that a collaborative therapist negates the presence of these issues, but they would rather see the client for who they are and not as a representation of a larger group or label.

The therapeutic relationship is based on language and the therapist is focused on local knowledge and how to best fix the problem. To elaborate, the therapist works closely with the client and any others involved by attending to local discourses on determining the nature of the problem and how to resolve it. Each client is unique and every problem is different, but the therapist's position regarding the client always remains the same. Language connects the therapist and client, thereby enabling intercultural communication. Therefore, this approach is a good fit for therapists working with clients that come from different cultures, backgrounds and have varying social beliefs.

Research support

Collaborative therapists rely on giving new meaning to problems and work with clients to generate solutions through the use of language. They take on a not-knowing stance, regard the client as the expert and decentralize power. Due to these ideas, collaborative therapy has been noted as beneficial for several populations. However, Chenail, deVincentis, Kiviat & Somers (2012) noted that research available exists in the form of case studies, literature review and client-therapist feedback from sessions, and that research based on CLST is much more limited than its other postmodern counterparts. At the same time, Anderson (1997) has explored the usefulness of collaborative therapy with people from various countries and found that the effectiveness of this approach can be understood by examining articles that include narratives of the clients' experiences.

There are many pieces of work that support the effectiveness of collaborative work with diverse populations. Among several, Levin (2006) looked into the application of this approach with battered women. Feinsilver, Murphy and Anderson, (2006) examined its use with homeless women and Fernandez, Cortez and Tarragona, (2006) with eating disorders. Anderson (2003) found collaborative therapy to be useful when working with challenging populations such as court-mandated clients, women in shelters, patients experiencing chronic psychiatric conditions, etc. Anderson, Carleton and Swimm (1999) and Sesma (2011) explored the effectiveness of this model from a couples perspective.

A 20-year study conducted in Finland reported impressive results when the collaborative approach was employed with psychosis patients returning to work after two years in treatment (Haarakangas, Seikkula, Alakare & Aaltonen, 2007). Boyd-Franklin (2013) noted that postmodern approaches including collaborative therapy were useful when working with African American clients. The same is true for immigrant families (Taylor, Gambourg, Rivera & Laureano, 2006). Paynter and Estrada (2009) found that, because collaborative therapists regard the client as the expert, it was an effective approach when working with immigrants from Mexico.

CLS practice has also been employed in educational settings to engage with students and to aid in the learning process (Anderson, 1997; Gehart, 2007; London & Rodriguez-Jazcilevish, 2007; McNamee, 2007). Gehart, Tarragon and Bava (2007) also found that qualitative interviews based on a collaborative approach as employed in therapy were useful in obtaining rich, quality data from participants.

Strengths and limitations

Anderson (2016) noted that the strengths of this model are in "the relationships and conversations that are created between the client and a therapist and in the inherent possibilities" (p. 190). There are few limitations with the main one being that "limits are considered therapist-created: a therapist for instance slips out of a collaborative way" (Anderson, 2016, p. 190).

References

Anderson, H. (1997). *Conversation, language, and possibilities: a postmodern approach to therapy.* New York, NY: Basic Books.

Anderson, H. (2001). Postmodern collaborative and person-centered therapies: what would Carl Rogers say? *Journal of Family Therapy, 23,* 339–360. doi:10.1111/1467-6427.00189

Anderson, H. (2003). Postmodern social construction therapies. In G. Weeks, T. L. Sexton & M. Robbins (Eds.), *Handbook of family therapy* (pp. 125–146). New York, NY: Brunner- Routledge.

Anderson, H. (2006). The heart and spirit of collaborative therapy: the philosophical stance – "A way of being" in relationships and conversations. In H. Anderson & D. Gehart (Eds.), *Collaborative therapy: relationships and conversations that make a difference* (pp. 43–59). New York, NY: Routledge.

Anderson, H. (2016). Postmodern-poststructural-social construction therapies: collaborative, narrative and solution-focused. In T. Sexton & J. Lebow (Eds.), *Handbook of family therapy.* New York, NY: Routledge.

Anderson, H., Carleton, D. & Swim, S. (1999). A postmodern perspective on relational intimacy: a collaborative conversation and relationship with a couple. In, J. Carlson & L. Sperry (Eds.), *The intimate couple* (pp. 208–226). New York, NY: Brunner/Mazel.

Anderson, H. & Gehart, D. (Eds.). (2012). *Collaborative therapy: relationships and conversations that make a difference*. New York, NY: Routledge.

Anderson, H. & Goolishian, H. A. (1988), Human systems as linguistic systems: preliminary and evolving ideas about the implications for clinical theory. *Family Process*, 27(4), 371–393. doi:10.1111/j.1545-5300.1988.00371.x

Boyd-Franklin, N. (2013). *Black families in therapy: understanding the African American experience*. New York, NY: Guilford.

Chenail, R. J., DeVincentis, M., Kiviat, H. E. & Somers, C. (2012). A systematic narrative review of discursive therapies research: considering the value of circumstantial evidence. In A. Lock & T. Strong (Eds.), *Discursive perspectives in therapeutic practices* (pp. 224–244). Oxford, UK: Oxford University Press.

Feinsilver, D., Murphy, E. & Anderson, H. (2006), Women at a turning point: a transformational feast. In H. Anderson & D. Gehart (Eds.), *Collaborative therapy: relationships and conversations that make a difference* (pp. 269–290). New York, NY: Routledge.

Fernandez, E., Cortes, A. & Tarragona, M. (2006). Las conversaciones reflexivas en el trabajo clinic, el eltrenaniento y la supervision. In H. Selicof, I. Y. Pakentin & G. Licea (Eds.), *Voces, voces y mas voces: El equipo reflexive en Mexico*. Mexico: D. F. Alinde.

Gehart, D. (2007). Process-as-content: teaching postmodern therapy in a university context. *Journal of Systemic Therapies*, 18, 39–56.

Gehart, D., Tarragona, M. & Bava, S. (2007). A collaborative approach to inquiry. In H. Anderson & D. Gehart (Eds.), *Collaborative therapy: relationships and conversations that make a difference* (pp. 367–390). New York, NY: Brunner/Routledge.

Haarakangas, K., Seikkula, J., Alakare, B. & Aaltonen, J. (2007). Open dialogue: an approach to psychotherapeutic treatment of psychosis in northern Finland. In H. Anderson & D. Gehart (Eds.), *Collaborative therapy: relationships and conversations that make a difference* (pp. 221–233). New York, NY: Routledge.

Levin, S. B. (2006). Hearing the unheard: advice to professionals from women who have been battered. In H. Anderson & D. Gehart (Eds.), *Collaborative therapy: relationships and conversations that make a difference* (pp. 109–128). New York, NY: Brunner/Routledge.

London, S. & Rodriguez-Jazcilevich, I (2007). The development of a collaborative learning and therapy community in an educational setting: from alienation to invitation. In H. Anderson & D. Gehart (Eds.), *Collaborative therapy: relationships and conversations that make a difference* (pp. 235–250). New York, NY: Brunner/Routledge.

McNamee, S. (2007). Relational practices in education: teaching as conversation. In H. Anderson & D. Gehart (Eds.), *Collaborative therapy: relationships and conversations that make a difference* (pp. 313–336). New York, NY: Brunner/Routledge.

Paynter, C. K. & Estrada, D. (2009). Multicultural training applied in clinical practice: reflections from a Euro-American female counselor-in-training working with Mexican immigrants. *Family Journal*, 17(3), 213–219.

Sesma, M. (2011). Pathways to dialogueue: the work of collaborative therapists with couples. *International Journal of Collaborative Practices*, 2(1), 48–66.

Taylor, B. A., Gambourg, M. B., Rivera, M. & Laureano, D. (2006). Constructing cultural competence: perspectives of family therapists working with Latino families. *American Journal of Family Therapy*, 34(5), 429–445. doi:10.1080/01926180600553779

Glossary

Causality in systemic thinking implies that one person is not the "cause" of the problem; rather, there is a systemic response to specific challenges (Flaskas, 2010).

Circular causality is related to the circular or reciprocal causation patterns (Rasheed, Rasheed & Marley, 2011). Rather than the A leads to B example of linear thinking, circular causality is more recursive, A leads to B, which leads back to A and so on. In addition, in a systemic scenario there might be more than just "A" and "B", but, for simplification purposes, reflect on an example of this recursive process with just two people in a system.

Closed system is a system that is not interacting or engaging with external systems. The functioning of a closed family system is not influenced by external systems. An example of a closed system is a family that has deep secrets and challenges and these are only known within the family.

Complementary system of communication is one that communicates differently; they "mirror" each other. For example, one person is the authoritarian and the other is submissive; or, one person is the substance abuser, the other person is the enabler.

Conjoint Family Drawing in this technique from Experiential Family Therapy, family members are asked to draw a picture of their family. The family does this together and the pictures they create can highlight differences in viewpoints between family members and help them to acknowledge roles or emotions in the family that they had not previously considered.

Context is what is around the family system or even the individual, the extended systems that are part of the family's experience (Cox & Paley, 1997). Bateson (1979) called context "a piece of the world of ideas limited and isolated by closing the door" (p. 14), meaning each system's context is "isolated" and "different" to another system's context. The system understands and develops related to how it perceives the meaning of the context around them.

Continuous change is taking things step by step (Smith-Acuna, 2011). The idea is that change occurs progressively over time in smaller minor changes.

Cybernetics is a field of study focused on "the mechanism of feedback by which a system corrects itself, like the steering of a ship" (Weiner, 1948 as cited in Becvar and Becvar, 2012, p 16). Cybernetics looks at the behavior of all sorts of things that are capable of adjusting their behavior based on information from the environment.

Cybernetics is the way that any system will keep correcting itself as a way to maintain "normality" (Keeney, 1983). A major element of cybernetics is feedback and how feedback causes the family system to recalibrate to maintain their equilibrium – how the family roles adjust to the feedback to maintain homeostasis (Keeney & Thomas, 1986).

Differentiation   is a multifaceted Bowen concept that deals with a person's ability to manage their need for both intimate connection with others and personal autonomy.

Discontinuous change   is a sudden, more pronounced change. An example might be a family's first baby; there is a sudden need to adapt to this change. In a homeostatic system, discontinuous change can add an interesting dynamic because the change is inevitable and homeostasis typically restructures to some degree after the system gets over the shock.

Double bind   is an intense message that has contradictory content (Hanson, 1995). It is a difficult situation within a family systems context where there is a request or statement that has two meanings and there is not a way the person receiving the meaning can get out of the situation.

Emotional Cutoff   In response to a difficult family emotional process, some people employ Emotional Cutoff as a mechanism to survive. This is sometimes done geographically when the child moves far away and stops communicating with the rest of the family. However, one can also live right next door to one's parents and be emotionally cutoff. Emotional Cutoff is about the person's relationship to the family emotional process (Bowen, 1978; Friedman 1991; Kerr & Bowen, 1988). The person who is emotionally cutoff has been unable to resolve their emotional attachments in their family of origin.

Epistemology   is the way one understands what is in front of them, and the root with which decisions are made.

Equifinality   describes how many possible variables could lead to one specific result (Smith-Acuna, 2011).

Externalization   is where you separate the person from the problem (Freedman & Combs, 1996; White & Epston, 1990). This is also known as Deconstruction Questions. Rather than stating "you have an anger problem", the narrative therapist would state "what is your relationship with anger?" The narrative therapist would view the problem as external to the person and help them see that they are not "the problem", rather they are a person with a problem. By viewing the problem as external to the person, a whole different vision of the story can take place because the family can work to visualize themselves on "one side" and the "problem" on another.

Family Projection Process   this Bowen concept is the idea that parents project onto their children their own anxieties and lack of differentiation.

This social feedback goes into the family as input and the family adjusts by teaching the child the expectations and putting a different punishment and reward expectation in place.

Family Sculpting   in this intervention, popularized by Virginia Satir, family members are asked to pretend as though their other family members are clay and arrange them (both in tableau and in action). This serves as a visual portrayal of each person's take on the family system and their place within it (Nicholas & Schwartz, 2006). It can also be used as a way of re-enacting important moments from the past.

Feedback   is when the system takes in information to "feed into" the whole and adjusts as needed to that feedback (Hanson, 1995). A family example might be a family that is in the public eye and has an expected public image. One of the children misbehaves in public. The media sends the message that the family is not what it wants to present.

First-order change   is a small change or immediate change that is typically temporary and does not make major changes to the larger system and how it works (Smith-Acuna, 2011).

Homeostasis is a system's natural restructuring to maintain the intended function (Messer, 1971).

Joining the intervention of joining is seminal to the work of family therapists. Through joining, family therapists are able to become a part of the family system and ultimately help to realign the system. There are several key aspects of joining, which includes accommodating to the system and their ways for interacting, matching the language of the client and displaying empathy (Gehart & Tuttle, 2003; Minuchin, 1974).

Linear Causality is when one aspect causes another aspect (Flaskas, 2010). Simply put, it is when "A" causes "B". For example, a rock in your path "causes" you to trip or exposure to a virus "causes" you to get sick.

The Mental Research Institute (MRI) it was "originally conceived of as an institute dedicated to the relationship of family members to each other and how those relationships evolved into the health and illness of its members" (Satir, 1982 as cited in Becvar & Becvar, 2000, p. 33). MRI's lasting impact on family therapy would be in the form of two very important contributions: one is the creation of strategic therapy and the other is the formation of the field's first academic journal, *Family Process* (originally edited by Don Jackson and Nathan Ackerman), which exists to this day.

Modernism was a dominant epistemology and paradigm during the turn of the 1900s, during the time of the industrial period and the evolution of science. Modernism highlights that science is an accurate and complete explanation for knowledge and understanding why things are the way they are.

Multifinality is when there are multiple possible "endings" from one action (Hanson, 1995).

Multigenerational Transmission Process this Bowen concept transmits the idea that the family emotional process is passed down from one generation to the next.

Naïve realism implies that people generally only see part of the whole (Keeney, 1983).

Negative feedback is when whatever happens does not lead to any change in the system (Hanson, 1995).

Nonsummativity is the idea that the whole of the system is more than each piece of the system individually.

Not-knowing one way to conceptualize how postmodern therapies work is through what is called "not-knowing" (Anderson & Goolishian, 1992). The theory behind this idea of not-knowing comes from the recognition of how language is communicated. For someone to share "I feel sad about my loneliness" brings with it constructs that may mean something different for the person saying it and the person hearing it. By taking a not-knowing stance, the therapist assumes they do not know or understand these constructs, they might say "tell me what sad feels like to you" or "when you feel lonely, what does that look like?" Using this not-knowing approach allows us to better understand the social constructs of these words for the client.

Nuclear Family Emotional Process it's a Bowen concept that includes how the family (as individuals and a unit) thinks, feels, behaves and responds to one another.

Open system an open system is a system that is not completely independent (Becvar and Becvar, 2012). An open system interacts with systems around it and is influenced by systems around it.

Ordeal is an intervention in which the therapist assigns a task that would be more of a problem to engage in than the presenting problem. Every time the symptom occurs, clients are assigned to also follow through with an ordeal. Assigning an ordeal can also be useful, in which the therapist makes it more difficult for the clients to carry out the problem than the solution. The ordeal not only has the purpose of making it more difficult to engage in the symptom, but it also creates a second-order shift in a system, as it requires a change in the usual sequence of interactions.

Positive feedback   leads to some kind of change (Hanson, 1995).

Postmodernism   a philosophy that rejects the existence of an objective reality or "truth" and questions the necessity for a search for one truth, but rather encourages the embracing of multiple perspectives. There are several postmodern assumptions; the most important of which is that reality is constructed by our experiences and the interactions in which we engage.

Reciprocal systems   are more balanced (Smith-Acuna, 2011). Think of reciprocal systems as families that encourage healthy competition, where relationships are on equal playing fields, and there is a sense of both connection and independence within the system.

Reframing   is a technique that helps to expand the manner in which clients understand their problems. Specific to structural family therapy, problems are reframed to be understood within the context of the larger family system. For example, an African American father and mother enter therapy with their 16-year-old son, citing complaints that his parents are too strict when it comes to curfew and hanging out with his friends. After conversations in which the parents share their concern for the son's safety due to fear of being stopped by the police, a structural family therapist might reframe the parents' actions as a loving attempt to protect the son, rather than an attempt to be overly restrictive.

Second-order cybernetics   the therapist starts to become part of the family's cybernetic processes. An example of cybernetics in the therapy room is when the therapist may feel anger toward the reactions of a father and, despite her personal work on this outside the therapy room, this puts the therapist on a side against the father, unintentionally. As a result, the family dynamics (the family homeostasis) shift because of the therapist's reactions and responses.

Sibling position   this concept is based on the work of Toman (1993), who examined the impact of sibling position of child development. Bowen theory suggests that, based on one's sibling position, the experience of the family emotional process may differ.

Social constructionism   this is a specific theory of knowledge that was an important part of the postmodern movement. Social constructionism, as a theory, suggests that what we consider to be true and real is largely shaped by the complex interactions of social groups. At its most basic level, social constructionism states that our understanding of our world and everything in it is based on the collective, subjective truths of our society. Language is not a representation of reality, but rather shapes how we see the world. When we attach words to the world around us, we are actively attributing meaning to the world. It is through social processes, particularly our use of language, that things take on meaning.

Societal Emotional Process   the final concept in Bowen theory may seem less applicable to specific therapy sessions, but it is in fact a vital component of the theory and its application. Since Bowen theory seeks to explain all human relationship interactions, it is easily extended beyond the nuclear family system. In fact, the theory virtually demands that we consider larger societal contexts since all human relationships face the same systemic patterns. Likewise, larger social systems – schools, churches, hospitals, political groups, social movements – all have an ongoing impact on the nuclear family system since each of these is also a relational system.

Subsystem   is a smaller "part" of a larger system (Smith-Acuna, 2011). If you examine an extended family system, grandparents might be one subsystem, parents another and siblings another.

Symmetrical system is a sense of similarity, almost a competition of sameness (Smith-Acuna, 2011). Bateson (1979) explains that a symmetrical system occurs when one part of a system does things one way, another part of the system will follow suit and do the same thing. A way to think of symmetrical system is that two or more members are competing for control.

System a group where the members of the group are affected by and affect each other.

Triangles Bowen theory says that all families make use of triangles in their relationships as a means of keeping stability in the family.

Unique outcomes (also known as "sparkling moments") are when the therapist searches through listening for moments when the problem either didn't exist or wasn't as bad (Freedman & Combs, 1996; White & Epston, 1990). If a family comes in and shares that they are arguing "all the time", the therapist will look for times within the story where the family is getting along and bring these out through deeper questions or curious observations.

Validation this is an intervention originally proposed in Experiential Family Therapy. When the therapist validates a client's experience or emotional response, they are giving the message that that experience is valid and that it is not wrong to feel a particular way. Like with reflection, this intervention helps create emotional safety and strengthen the therapeutic alliance. It is especially important to help clients gain comfort with emotions that they have not previously been aware of or expressed (Freedman & Combs, 1996).

"The whole is greater than the sum of its' parts" means that an individual cannot be understood unless the individual's system is considered and analyzed (Watzlawicz, Beavelas & Jackson, 1967),

Bibliography

Anderson, H., & Goolishian, H. (1992). The client is the expert: a not-knowing approach to therapy. In S. McNamee & K. J. Gergen (Eds.), *Therapy as social construction*. (pp. 25-39). Sage Publications, Inc.

Bateson, G. (1979). *Mind and nature: a necessary unity*. New York: E. P. Dutton.

Becvar, D., & Becvar, R. (2012). *Family therapy: a systemic integration*. Pearson.

Bowen, M. (1975). *Family therapy in clinical practice*. Lanham, MD: Rowman & Littlefield.

Cox, M. J., & Paley, B. (1997). Families as systems. *Annual Review of Psychology*, 48, 243-267.

Flaskas, C. (2010). Frameworks for practice in the Systemic Field: part 1 – Continuities and transitions in family therapy knowledge. *The Australian and New Zealand Journal of Family Therapy*, 31(3), 232-247.

Friedman, S. D. (1991). Sibling relationships and intergenerational succession in family firms. *Family Business Review*, 4(1), 3-20.

Friedman, J., & Combs, G. (1996). *Narrative therapy: the social constructions of preferred realities*. New York: W. W. Norton & Co.

Gehart, D. R., Tuttle, A. R. (2003). *Theory-based treatment planning for marriage and family therapists*. Cengage.

Hanson, B. G. (1995). *General systems theory*. New York: Taylor & Francis.

Kerr, M. E., & Bowen, M. (1988). *Family evaluation: an approach based on Bowen theory*. New York: W. W. Norton & Company.

Keeney, B. (1983). *Aesthetics of change*. New York: Guilford.

Messer, A. A., (1971). Mechanisms of family homeostasis. *Comprehensive Psychiatry*, 12(4), 380-388.

Minuchin, S. (1974). *Families and family therapy*. Boston, MA: Harvard Press.

Nichols, M. P., & Schwartz, R. C. (2006). *Family therapy: concepts and Methods*. Boston, MA: Pearson/ Allyn & Bacon.

Rasheed, J. M., Rasheed, M. N., & Marley, J. A. (2010). *Family therapy: models and techniques*. Thousand Oaks, CA: Sage, Inc.

Smith-Acuna, S. (2011). *Systems theory in action: applications to individual, couples, and family therapy*. Hoboken, NJ: John Wiley & Sons, Inc.

Toman, W. (1993). *Family therapy & sibling position*. Lanham, MD: Jason Aronson.

Watzlawick, P., Beavin Bavelas, J., & Jackson, D. D. (1967). *Pragmatics of human communication*. New York: W. W. Norton.

White, M., & Epston, D. (1990). *Narrative means to therapeutic ends*. New York: Norton Professional Books.

Index

Note: Page locators in **bold** and *italics* represents tables and figures, respectively.

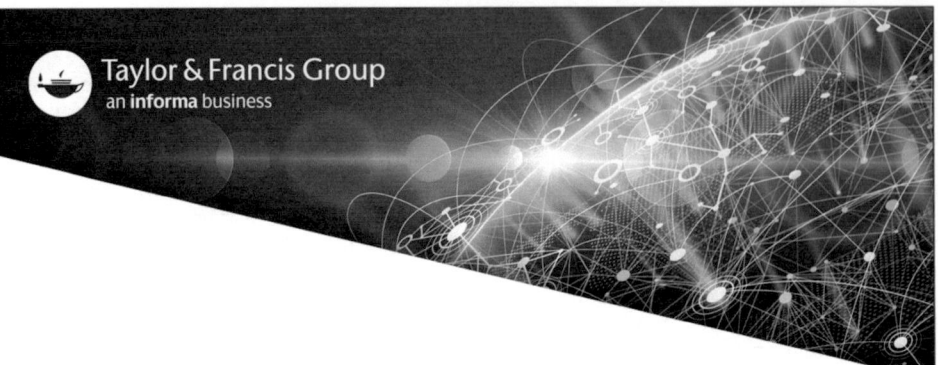
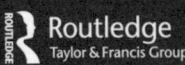
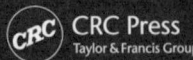